Illustrated Pediatric Dentistry

(Part I)

Edited by

Satyawan Damle

Former Professor of Pediatric Dentistry,
Dean Nair Hospital Dental College,
Mumbai, India

Former Vice Chancellor,
Department of Pediatric Dentistry,
Maharishi Markandeshwar University,
Mullana, Ambala, India

Ritesh Kalaskar

Department of Pedodontic and Preventive Dentistry,
Government Dental College & Hospital, Nagpur,
India

Dhanashree Sakhare

Founder, Lavanika Dental Academy
Melbourne
Australia

&

Abdulkadeer Jetpurwala

Department of Pediatric Dentistry
Nair Hospital Dental College, Mumbai,
Maharashtra
India

Illustrated Pediatric Dentistry (Part I)

Editors: Satyawan Damle, Ritesh Kalaskar, Dhanashree Sakhare & Abdulkadeer Jetpurwala

ISBN (Online): 978-981-5051-48-3

ISBN (Print): 978-981-5051-49-0

ISBN (Paperback): 978-981-5051-50-6

First published in 2022.

need for a court order if at any point you breach any terms of this License Agreement. In no event will any delay or failure by Bentham Science Publishers in enforcing your compliance with this License Agreement constitute a waiver of any of its rights.

3. You acknowledge that you have read this License Agreement, and agree to be bound by its terms and conditions. To the extent that any other terms and conditions presented on any website of Bentham Science Publishers conflict with, or are inconsistent with, the terms and conditions set out in this License Agreement, you acknowledge that the terms and conditions set out in this License Agreement shall prevail.

Bentham Science Publishers Pte. Ltd.
80 Robinson Road #02-00
Singapore 068898
Singapore
Email: subscriptions@benthamscience.net

BENTHAM SCIENCE

CONTENTS

FOREWORD 1

It is my great pleasure to pen down a foreword for this tremendous book on Pediatric Dentistry for a legend and doyen of the subject, a mentor and guide to the brightest of minds in the field of dentistry.

Rising from the fundamentals, comprehensive in-built, contemporary and authoritative in construct and approach, and hands-on to the core, ***Illustrated Pediatric Dentistry*** is a wonderful work engineered by some of the best-known academics in this noble realm. The chief author, ***Professor Satyawan Damle***, is a colossus among giants, having been a celebrated teacher, distinguished leader, and dynamic policymaker at several dental institutions and universities, including the most prized, the University of Mumbai.

Prof. Satyawan Damle is the rare blend of a gifted clinician and a carved-out academic guru whose intellect has emerged with decades of practice. It is no secret that the degree of acquisition of knowledge by students is one of the measures of the effectiveness of a medical curriculum; and with Pediatric Dentistry being one of the crucial epicentres of growth, it has the potential to make momentous advancements in the evolutionary trajectory of oral and general health.

His co-editors ***Ritesh Kalaskar, Abdulkadeer Jetpurwala***, and ***Dhanashree Sakhare*** are examples excellence in their arena. The work reflects their collective understanding of where pediatric dentistry stands today, what have been the treasures and well-kept secrets of the past, and where this tree of knowledge finds fruition today pawing way for the future.

Embedding best care practices of all times, ***Illustrated Pediatric Dentistry*** is a comprehensive yet concise work, which fulfils the essentials of the pediatric dentistry curriculum both for graduates and postgraduates across all universities.

Walking you through the nitty-gritties of preventive, curative and restorative childhood dentistry, be it the behavioral challenges, cariology, endodontics, traumatology, para-surgical themes such as the use of conscious sedation and general anaesthesia at that age, and the management of medically compromised children, the work is a tree of knowledge, nurtured with experiential learning, and carries wonderful blossoms of practical wisdom.

Let us savour and celebrate the chef-d'oeuvre. Indeed, Illustrated Pediatric Dentistry is a must-read and must-assimilate work for each one of us. Students, practitioners and teachers of Pediatric dentistry will cherish it as a treasured possession on their shelves. I congratulate Prof. Damle and Bentham Science, Singapore, for publishing this irreplaceable tome.

Prof. (Dr.) Mahesh Verma
Vice Chancellor
Guru Gobind Singh
Indraprastha University,
New Delhi,
India

FOREWORD 2

I am delighted to write this foreword for a Book of Illustrated Pediatric Dentistry authored by Professor Satyawan Damle and other academicians. Prof. Satyawan Damle is a well-known researcher and academician with over 44 years of clinical and teaching experience in Dentistry. Besides the several posts and hats he wore in the various roles he played for the profession, he is also a recipient of several awards and recognitions, including the Lifetime Achievement Awards, Outstanding Public Servant Awards, and Research Awards and Fellowships. He is an active member of the Indian Council of Medical Research. Despite his extraordinary achievements as a Pediatric dentist, researcher, and academician, Prof Satyawan Damle will always be known as the longest-serving chief editor of Indexed journals. For almost 35 years. He dedicated himself to overseeing the publication of the highest-quality peer-reviewed studies and opinion pieces on child dental health.

Prof. Damle is actively involved in writing several books on Pediatric Dentistry and Dentistry, which is the testimony of his in-depth knowledge of the subject. The Book of Illustrated Pediatric Dentistry is their new venture initiated by him. I am confident that this book will be accepted by students and faculty involved in teaching Pediatric Dentistry. His work as a teacher, researcher, innovator, visionary and extraordinary academician made him a legend. His role as a mentor and friend made him a role model to those of us who know him and worked with him. His legacy persists not only in academics but also as an able administrator, as he proved his mettle as the Dean of a dental school, Director of Medical Education, Joint Municipal.

Commissioner of Mumbai and, ultimately, the Vice Chancellor of a University. Prof. Damle has worked conscientiously and untiringly to present an unmatched educational endeavour. The topics in this book display a clear and succinct clinical expertise and the capability of imparting updated education and information to Oral Health Professionals. The entire volume of this book deals with ultramodern and current state-of-the-art techniques. I take this opportunity to congratulate Prof. Satyawan Damle and his team of contributors - Ritesh Kalaskar, Abdulkadeer Jetpurwala and Dhanashree Sakhare for having published this Textbook for Bentham Sciences.

Dr Ashok Dhoble. Hon. Secretary
General, Indian Dental Association H.O.
India

PREFACE

It is imperative to have an established approach to handling Children's oral diseases. **'Illustrated Pediatric Dentistry,'** is an unpretentious endeavour to integrate the latest developments and up-to-date reviews in the field of Pediatric dentistry by distinguished writers. The book intends to allow students to understand the conceptions of Pediatric dentistry and create a spur to discover the subject by advance reading. Several illustrations, descriptions and graphic drawings have been included to attract the students and make the subject simple to comprehend. A healthy mouth is a gateway to a healthy body and the best time to inculcate healthy habits is through childhood. Prevention of the initiation of oral diseases and training appropriate oral hygiene methods are commenced best throughout the formative years of the child. With a substantial percentage of the worldwide population being in the Pediatric age group, it is imperious to have a scientific approach in the behaviour management, prevention and treatment modalities in the dental office, as Pediatric dentistry is a fast-growing division of dental disciplines that lays the basis for the impending dental health of the populace.

The book has been divided into several sections. The sections on child psychology and the emotional development of children are important to learn the basics of various behaviour management strategies. The section on dental caries sensitizes the reader towards the most common dental disorder that is seen in children, and preventive procedures aimed towards lessening dental caries are the necessity of the hour. While an endeavour has been made to include the growth and development of the facial structures and dentition and along with their disturbances and the interceptive and preventive procedures to monitor the erupting teeth.

Pediatric Operative techniques, including endodontics and management of teeth with immature apices affected due to Dental caries and traumatic injuries have been given prominence. Innovations in the field of Pediatric dentistry are transpiring amazingly fast, and it is crucial to stay up to date with the latest materials, equipment and techniques to deliver the highest quality of care to our little patients.

The New Book cannot be successfully compiled without the collective contribution regarding meticulous reviews of the manuscript to keep pace with the latest innovative novelties. The credit for introducing a New Textbook goes to the contributors for their engrossment, devotion and dedication in presenting a manuscript after applying prudent and well-adjudged scrutiny and analytical approach and have excelled in exploring the things to the ultimate.

Accumulation of information and its cogent management would not have been conceivable without the efforts of the contributors who have painstakingly submitted their manuscripts to shape this gargantuan task and to introduce this book in the service of Pediatric dentistry.

Satyawan Damle
Former Vice-Chancellor,
Maharishi Markandeshwar University,
Mullana (Ambala), India

Ritesh Kalaskar
Department of Pedodontic and Preventive Dentistry
Government Dental College & Hospital, Nagpur
India

Dhanashree Sakhare
Founder,
Lavanika Dental Academy,
Melbourne
Australia

&

Abdulkadeer Jetpurwala
Department of Pediatric Dentistry
Nair Hospital Dental College, Mumbai
Maharashtra
India

ACKNOWLEDGEMENTS

We do not find such appropriate words to praise the unique nature of Dr. Mahesh Verma, Vice Chancellor of Guru Gobind Singh Indraprastha University, New Delhi, who himself being a great resolute and connoisseur of dentistry occupying an illustrious position with an eminent background in dentistry, has spared his valuable time from his busy schedule to inscribe the foreword for the Textbook of" Illustrated Pediatric Dentistry." We take it as inventiveness and encouragement rather than a morale-boosting for us to uphold and keep up our determination to satisfy our hunger for academics for the advantage of budding dental professionals.

We also do not find such befitting words to laud the unique nature of Dr. Ashok Dhoble Hon, General Secretary Indian, Dental Association Head Office, who himself being a great advocate and connoisseur of dentistry occupying a distinguished position with an illustrious background in dentistry has spared his precious time from his busy schedule to write the foreword for the Textbook of Illustrated Pediatric Dentistry. I take it as an inspiration and encouragement rather than a morale-boosting for us to uphold and keep up our determination to satisfy our hunger for academics for the advantage of budding dental professionals.

We are also indebted and beholden to the contributors for their altruistic and substantial contribution to make this Textbook of Illustrated Pediatric Dentistry, a great academic endeavour. The contributors are highly competent and knowledgeable clinicians known for their aptitude and capability, which have successfully recognized the most complex and convoluted details of each topic, duly integrating and blending the latest advancements and innovations in Pediatric Dentistry. They are a terrific hard worker and legendary luminaries known for their admirable accomplishments and remarkable involvement in dental education. They have made lots of efforts to lead things to excellence. Credit goes to these patrons and benefactors for the benevolent bequest of their vast knowledge and experience for the betterment of dental education.

We would also like to thank Dr. Priyanka Bhaje, Dr. Parag Kasar, Dr. Sharath Chandra, Dr. Prachi Goyal and Dr. Vidya Iyer for their painstaking efforts and intransigent toil during the editing of this book. They displayed exceptional patients, forbearance, and commitment during the preparation of the book Our dream has come true due to the support of our past and present students. Credit also goes to our family members for their tolerance, Love, and affection.

We would like to appreciate the efforts of Mrs. Humaira Hashmi of Bentham Science and the publishers Bentham Sciences for giving us an opportunity to pen down our ideas and academic work to reality. We also convey our kind and sincere appreciation to Pascali Pascalis.

Representative of Porter Instrument Business Unit of Parker Hannifin Matrx by Parker and Parker-Porter Product for permitting us to use the company products in our book.

Lastly, we would like to state that fortune favours those who defy complexities and overcome them on their own. We also passionately believe that Man is the architect of his own destiny, and God is on the side of those who toil and perspire to make their providence.

We place our sincerest admiration and gratitude to all those who have delightfully contributed to this cause and for their wishes and devotions made for understanding our dream.

Satyawan Damle
Ritesh Kalaskar
Dhanashree Sakhare
Abdulkadeer Jetpurwala

List of Contributors

Aditi Pashine Associate Dentist, MyDentist, Aberystwyth, UK

Aman Chowdhry Professor, Faculty of Dentistry, Jamia Milia Islamia (A Central University), New Delhi, India

Armelia Sari Widyarman Department of Oral Biology, Faculty of Dentistry, Universitas Trisakti, Jakarta, Indonesia
Departmental Head of Microbiology, Faculty of Dentistry, Universitas Trisakti, Jakarta, Indonesia

Arun M Xavier Department of Pediatric and Preventive Dentistry, Amrita School of Dentistry, Cochin, Kerala, India

Bhavna Dave Department of Pediatric and Preventive Dentistry, K. M. Shah Dental College, and Hospital, Sumandeep Vidyapeeth Deemed to be University, Vadodara, Gujarat, India

Bhavna Gupta Saraf Department of Pedodontics and Preventive Dentistry, Sudha Rustagi College of Dental Sciences and Research, Faridabad, Haryana, India

Deepika Bablani Popli Department of Oral Pathology and Microbiology, Faculty of Dentistry, Jamia Millia Islamia, New Delhi, India

Dhanashree Sakhare Founder Lavanika Dental Academy, Melbourne, Australia

Eko Fibryanto Department of Conservative Dentistry, Faculty of Dentistry, Universitas Trisakti, Jakarta, Indonesia

Enrita Dian R. Department of Pedodontic, Faculty of Dentistry, Universitas Trisakti, Jakarta, Indonesia

H. Sharath Chandra SJM Dental College and Hospital, Chitradurga, Karnataka, India

Jay Gopal Ray Professor and Head, Burdwan Dental College and Hospital, West Bengal, India

M. Vijay Department of Orthodontics, CSI College of Dental Sciences and Research, Madurai, Tamil Nadu, India

M.H. Raghunath Reddy Professor and Head, SJM Dental College and Hospital, Chitradurga, Karnataka, India

Monika Rathore Department of Pedodontics and Preventive Dentistry, BBD College of Dental Sciences, BBD University, Lucknow, U.P, India

Neerja Singh Department of Pedodontics and Preventive Dentistry, BBD College of Dental Sciences, BBD University, Lucknow, U.P, India

Parag Kasar Chief Pediatric Dentist at Deep Dental Clinic, Nerul, Navi Mumbai, India

Prachi Goyal Maharishi Markandeshwar College of Dental Sciences and Research, Ambala, India

Pratik Kariya Department of Pediatric and Preventive Dentistry, K. M. Shah Dental College, and Hospital, Sumandeep Vidyapeeth Deemed to be University, Vadodara, Gujarat, India

Priyanka Bhaje Rungata College of Dental Sciences and Research Center, Bhilai, Chhattisgarh, India

Raghavendra M. Shetty	Department of Clinical Sciences, College of Dentistry, Center of Medical and Bio-allied Health Sciences Research, Ajman University, Ajman, UAE
Satyawan Damle	Former Professor of Pediatric Dentistry, Dean Nair Hospital Dental College, Mumbai, India Former Vice Chancellor, Department of Pediatric Dentistry, Maharishi Markandeshwar University, Mullana, Ambala, India
Shailaja Chatterjee	Department of Oral Pathology, Yamuna College of Dental Sciences and Research, Yamuna Nagar, Haryana, India
Shruti Balasubramanian	Department of Pediatric and Preventive Dentistry, Government Dental College and Hospital, Nagpur, India
Tri Erri Astoeti	Department of Dental Public Health and Preventive Dentistry, Faculty of Dentistry, Universitas Trisakti, Jakarta, Indonesia
Trisha Gadekar	Department of Pediatric Dentistry, Mamata Dental College, Khammam, Telangana, India
Vidya Iyer	Department of Orthodontics, CSI College of Dental Sciences and Research, Madurai, Tamil Nadu, India

CHAPTER 1

Introduction to Pediatric Dentistry

Satyawan Damle[1,2,*]

[1] *Former Professor of Pediatric Dentistry, Dean Nair Hospital Dental College, Mumbai, India*

[2] *Former Vice Chancellor, Department of Pediatric Dentistry, Maharishi Markandeshwar University, Mullana, Ambala, India*

Abstract: Pediatric dentistry is the only speciality that has an abundance of knowledge for the management and treatment of the oral health care needs of infants and children. Pediatric dentistry concentrates on the integration of appropriate tactics and knowledge of various specialities into a framework of quality oral health care for children. It is necessary to implement procedures that are safe, comprehensive, accessible, affordable, high quality, and respectful for children. The role of a Paediatric dentist is to promote the dental health of children as well as serve as a resource person to the parents.

Keywords: Pediatric Dentistry, Infants, Children, Parent, Management.

INTRODUCTION

Various authors have rightly equated children with flowers. A few of them quoted: *Let them bloom by giving them our warm smiles, our soft gentle words falling on them like rain and our art of confidence. Water them with love, nourish them with praise, and compliment them every day. Be their sun when all you see is rain. Protect them from storms and shelter their pain. Children are like flowers that blossom every day* (Fig. **1**).

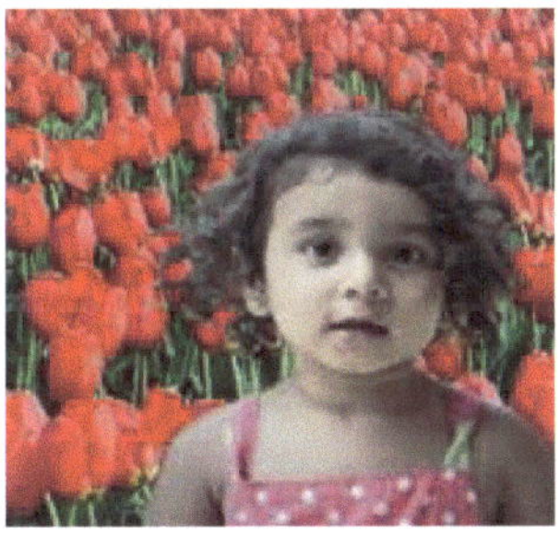

Fig. (1). Children are as lovely as flowers.

* **Corresponding author Satyawan Damle:** Former Professor of Pediatric Dentistry, Dean Nair Hospital Dental College, Mumbai, India & Former Vice Chancellor, Department of Pediatric Dentistry, Maharishi Markandeshwar University, Mullana, Ambala, India; Tel: +91 9729062515; E-mail: sgdamle@gmail.com

Satyawan Damle, Ritesh Kalaskar, Dhanashree Sakhare & Abdulkadeer Jetpurwala (Eds.)

To put it into a nutshell, children are the flowers of life! They bring joy and happiness to our world. Let us be kind to them, let us make them happy and let us help them to save that child inside them for the rest of their lives!

Pediatric dentistry a branch of Dentistry deals with these delightful children.

Definition

It is an age-specified speciality that provides both primary and comprehensive preventive and therapeutic oral health care for infants and children through adolescence, including those with special health care needs (Fig. **2**). Pediatric dentistry is a speciality that adjusts techniques and procedures from general dentistry and other specialities to provide primary and comprehensive preventive and therapeutic oral health care for children [1, 2].

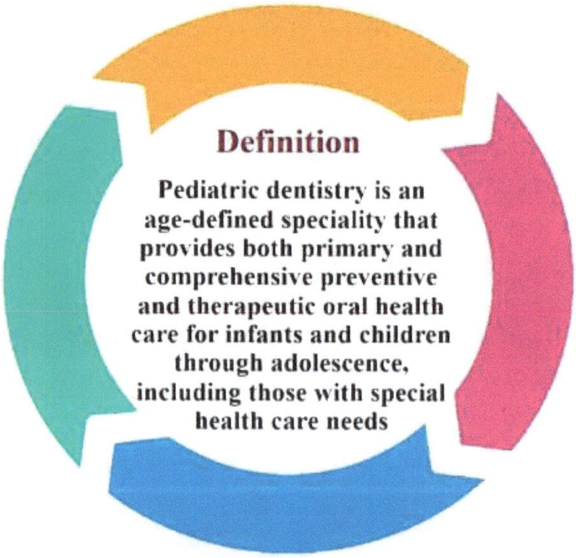

Fig. (2). Definition of Pediatric Dentistry (AAPD 2020).

Pediatric dentistry encompasses a variety of disciplines, techniques, procedures, and skills that reveal a common basis with other specialities however these practices are modified and adapted to the unique requirements of infants, children, adolescents, and those with special health care needs (Fig. **3**). Being an age-specific speciality, pediatric dentistry encompasses disciplines such as behaviour guidance, care of medically and developmentally compromised and disabled patients, supervision of orofacial growth and development, caries prevention, sedation, pharmacological management, and hospital dentistry, as well as other traditional fields of dentistry. These skills are applied to the needs of children during their ever-changing stages of development and to treating conditions and diseases unique to growing individuals [3].

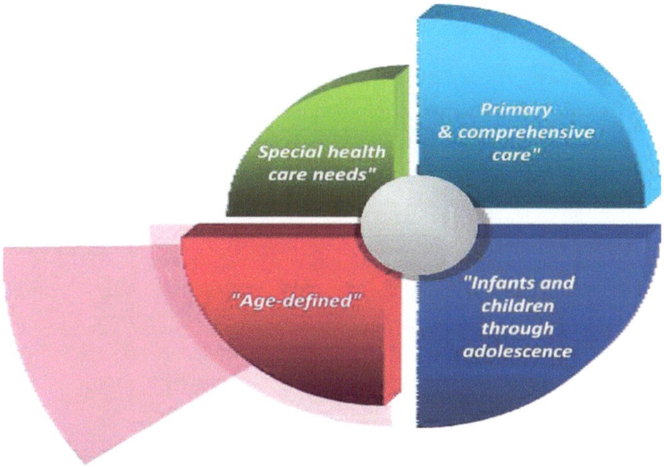

Fig. (3). Pediatric Dentistry Encompasses Different Aspects.

DENTISTRY ENCOMPASSES DIFFERENT ASPECTS

An Important Aspect of Children Being Treated in a Separate Speciality.

What is the most appealing about children?

Is it their cute faces?

Their playfulness?

Their smile? Of course, yes, however!

Beyond all these aspects, children are beautiful because they possess something unique, that we as adults have lost and that is innocence as well as purity (Fig. **4A**).

Pediatric dentists encourage the oral and dental health of children as well as provide educational resources for parents. It is advised that a dental visit should occur: within six months after the presence of the first tooth or at least by a child's first birthday. It is important to create a comprehensive and accessible ongoing association between the dentist and patient, so the healthy and beautiful smile and natural teeth always remain beautiful (Fig. **4B**).

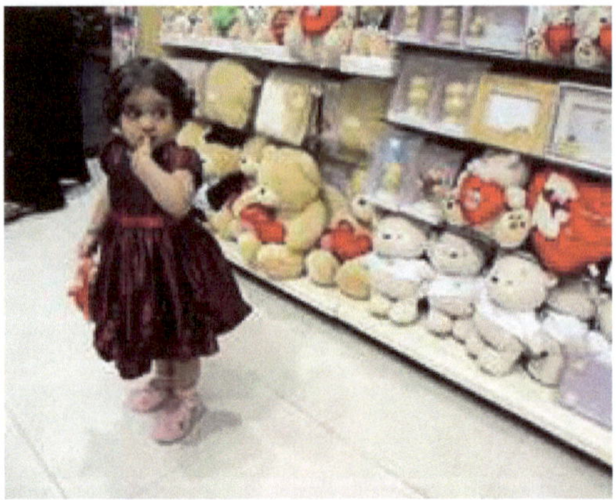

Fig. (4A). A Child: A Picture of Innocence.

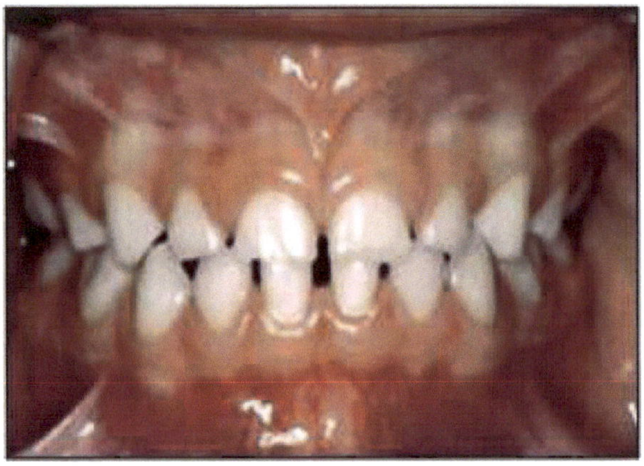

Fig. (4B). Healthy Primary Dentition.

The Key Role of a Pediatric Dentist is

1. To identify the treatment, need and devise a suitable treatment plan keeping in mind the child's age.
2. Discuss the treatment to be delivered to the child must be acceptable to the child and the parent.
3. Therefore, the dentist must possess child management skills to be able to do the needful (Fig. **5**).

However, it is also true that all Pediatric dentists, even today, do not practice dentistry exclusively for children. Though, a few do believe that they have the necessary knowledge, skill, and love for the subject they had been taught. It is also true that many general dentists are willing to practice dentistry for children but encounter difficulties due to a lack of practical training on key areas in child behaviour management in dentistry.

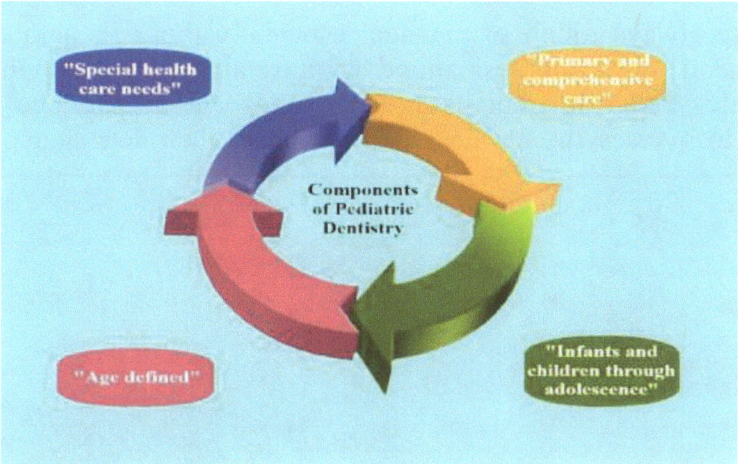

Fig. (5). Components of Pediatric Dentistry.

Responsibilities of a Pediatric Dentist Include

- Diagnose and manage oral diseases (preventive and restorative) and pathology pertains to the oral cavity.
- Interpret x-rays and other diagnostic tests.
- Devise treatment plans to restore the oral health of children, including those with special health care needs.
- Monitor growth and development of the jaws and teeth.
- Correct malocclusion through interceptive orthodontic treatment.
- Perform surgical procedures on teeth, bone, and soft tissues of the oral cavity,
- Provide emergency care (dental infection, pain, and dental trauma)
- Treat patients under various stages of sedation (minimal, moderate, or deep), general anaesthesia (Fig. **6**).

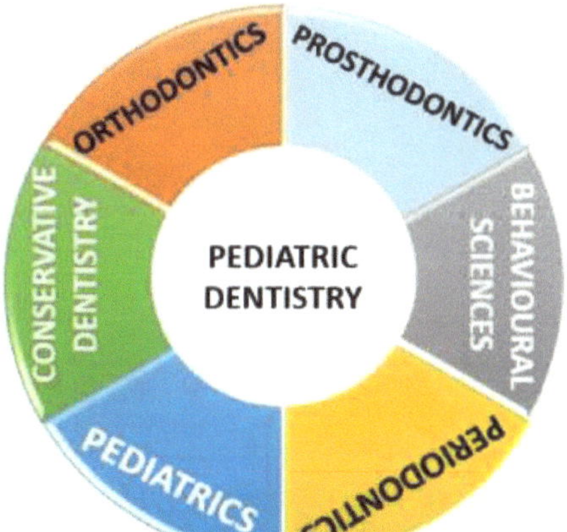

Fig. (6). Pediatric dentistry – Multispecialty in itself.

Children are always tough to manage, especially those in pain due to oral or dental ailments. They possess mood swings, and their behaviour is entirely unpredictable. Pediatric dentists need to show great patience and effective techniques to oversee the children and eliminate their fear and pain (Fig. **7**).

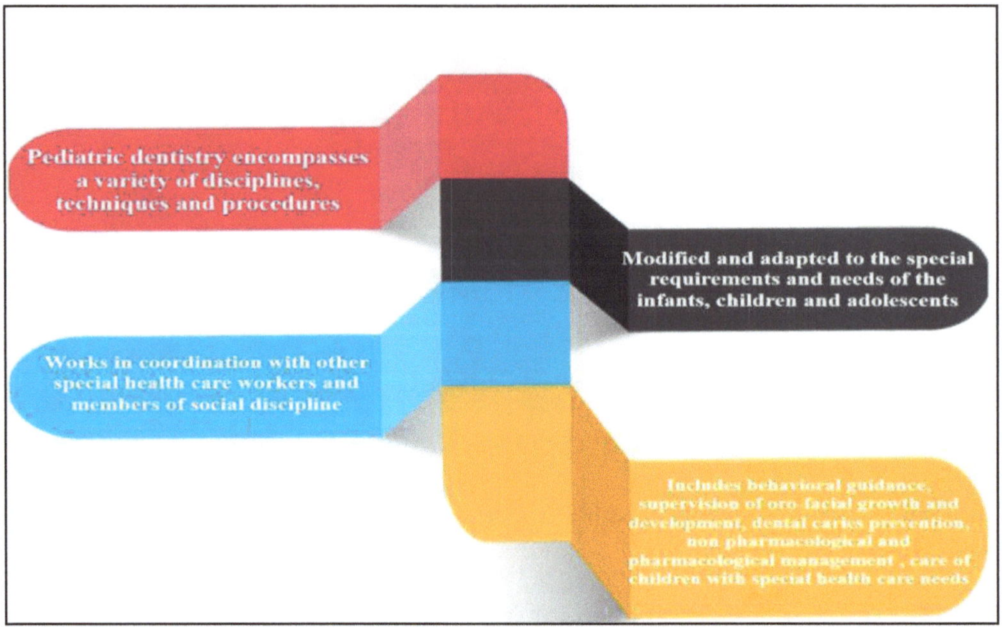

Fig. (7). "Pediatric Dentistry: Why?"

Aims and Objectives of Pediatric Dentistry

The health of the child specifically concerned with oral health.

Early diagnosis and prompt treatment timings for better outcomes (Fig. **8**).

- Restoring good oral health
- Relief of pain
- Increasing knowledge of dental care
- Instituting positive behaviour
- Restoring lost tooth structure
- Management of patients with specific needs.

Dentists and patients(parents/children) should have a strong relationship. Pediatric dentists should effectively and efficiently need to perform the treatment of children. They should have a clear, constructive, and positive attitude.

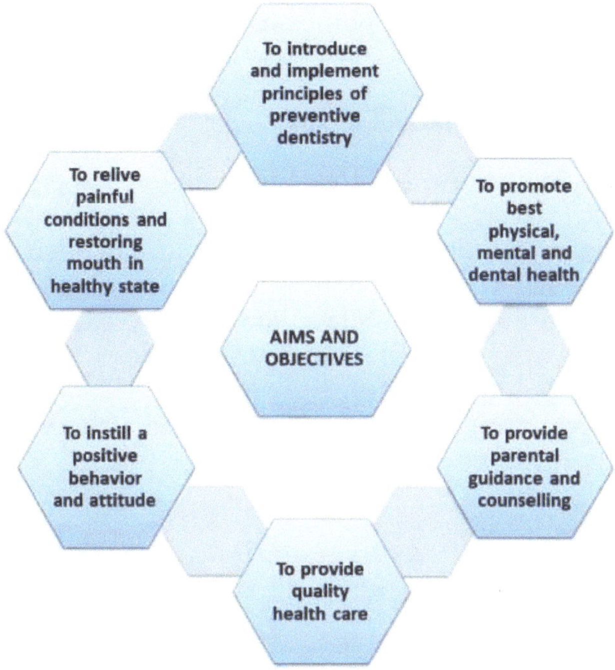

Fig. (8). Aims and Objectives of Pediatric dentistry.

Establishing and maintaining communication with the child who is cooperative or uncooperative will result in the successful completion of dental procedures.

Interaction, Communication as well as the consultation will also lead the child to develop a positive attitude towards dentistry.

Every hour, in a dental office, a pediatric dental patient enters the treatment room. Immediately there is increased commotion, quivering knees and lips, tears rolling down cheeks. Unfortunately, this scenario can apply to both the patient and the treating dental team.

For a variety of reasons, there are dental practitioners and staff that have an aversion to treating pediatric patients, especially infants and toddlers. This is unfortunate for both the patients and the dentist.

By the institution of early oral health education and the application of preventive dentistry procedures, the pediatric dental patient can be insured for a lifetime of Excellent Dental health.

For the dental practice, ignoring or rejecting the infant and toddler population results in a missed opportunity to contribute to improved oral health for the overall population, establish dental homes early, and attract new patients to the practice.

HISTORY OF PEDIATRIC DENTISTRY

- In 1909, Minnie Evangeline Jordon created the first dental practice in the United States dedicated exclusively to pediatric patients.
- In 1925, she published the first textbook on pediatric dentistry, titled Operative Dentistry for Children.
- The first dental care brought to public school was by Alfred C. Fones in 1914, which was 6 decades after the first woman, Lucy Hobbs Taylor, who received a DDS.
- Plenty of things have changed and improved in pediatric dentistry since it was first revolutionized in 1900's (Figs. **9** & **10**).

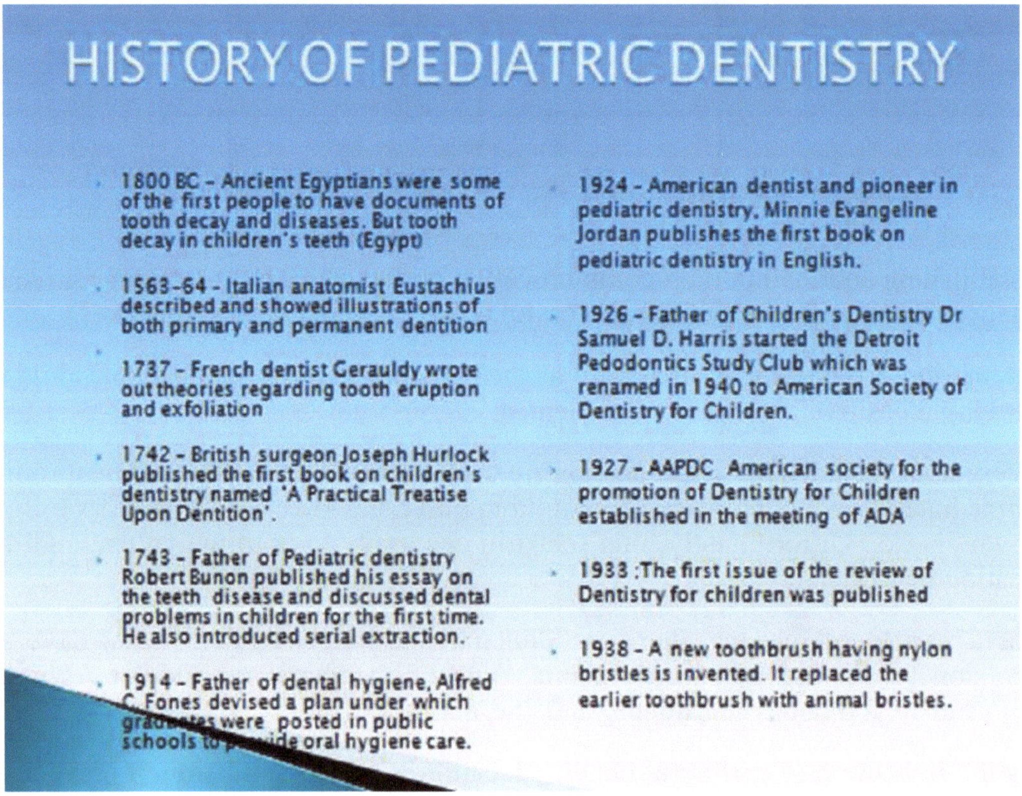

Fig. (9). History of Pediatric Dentistry.

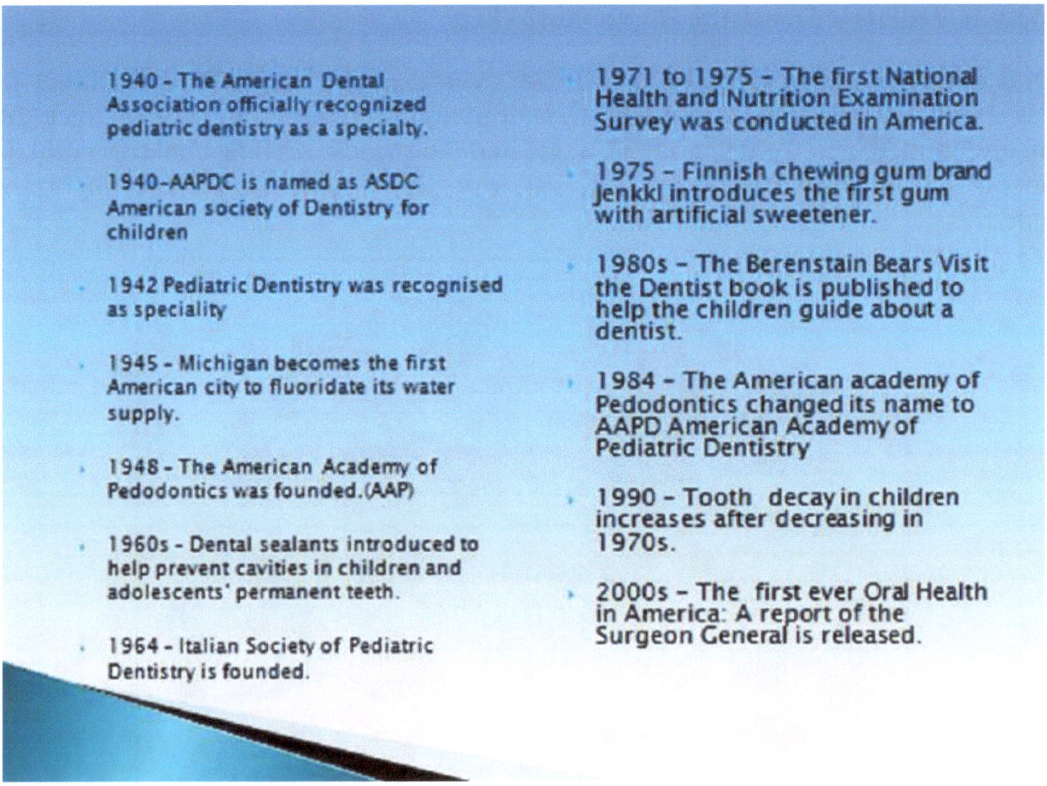
1940 - The American Dental Association officially recognized pediatric dentistry as a specialty.
1940-AAPDC is named as ASDC American society of Dentistry for children
1942 Pediatric Dentistry was recognised as speciality
1945 - Michigan becomes the first American city to fluoridate its water supply.
1948 - The American Academy of Pedodontics was founded.(AAP)
1960s - Dental sealants introduced to help prevent cavities in children and adolescents' permanent teeth.
1964 - Italian Society of Pediatric Dentistry is founded.
1971 to 1975 - The first National Health and Nutrition Examination Survey was conducted in America.
1975 - Finnish chewing gum brand Jenkki introduces the first gum with artificial sweetener.
1980s - The Berenstain Bears Visit the Dentist book is published to help the children guide about a dentist.
1984 - The American academy of Pedodontics changed its name to AAPD American Academy of Pediatric Dentistry
1990 - Tooth decay in children increases after decreasing in 1970s.
2000s - The first ever Oral Health in America: A report of the Surgeon General is released.

Fig. (10). History of Pediatric Dentistry.

PEDIATRIC DENTISTRY PROCEDURES

A. It is important to make it easy for the child to be comfortable. The dentist / pediatric dentist must decide whether the parents should be present in the operatory during the dental procedure or not.

B. The dentists should also practice non-verbal communication if needed during the procedure. It may be necessary if he cannot talk and guide the patient by facial expressions.

C. It is also important to distract the child's attention to decrease the pain intensity; for example, the child can be given a mirror to hold or sunglasses to wear to avoid light exposure.

D. The dentist should be fully aware of the child's history and prescribe suitable pediatric dentistry procedures for him.

Why Is Pediatric Dentistry Important? (Fig. 11)

Oral hygiene is a vital component of the overall health of a person. Without it, human beings' health is incomplete. It is of paramount importance to convince the parent/child that if oral health is neglected, the body suffers and the child is unable to eat and drink anything, and the body gets insufficient important nutrients.

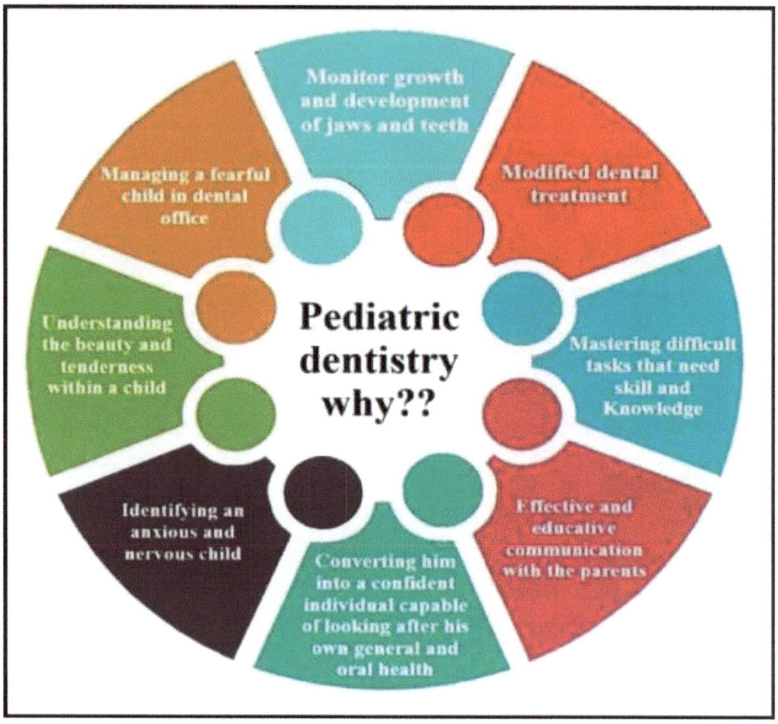

Fig. (11). Importance of pediatric dentistry.

Pediatric Dentistry takes into Consideration

1. The advent of social medicine in pediatric health care.

2. Expanding knowledge about pediatric oral health risk and disease management.

3. Trends in oral health and dental care disparities and forces that propel them.

4. Perceived needs for dental care services and other barriers that propel the need for dental home utilization.

5. Dentistry as an independent profession.

6. Dental capacity system for all children, including children with special dental care needs.

The First Dental Visit

- Parents are always excited about different milestones in their child's life.
- The first syllable convey, crawling, standing, and walking, and the parents celebrate the eruption of the first tooth.
- There is a need to create a similar desire and preparation of the parent for the child's first dental visit. Dentists should urge patients to give importance to pediatric dentistry as soon as their child gets their first tooth (Fig. **12**).
- It is suggested that a child should have his first visit to the dentist when he turns one year old. Early engraining of oral hygiene habits will develop strong teeth and gums in the child throughout life. A Paediatric dentist can be the child's best friend and protect him from long term problems and lifelong complications.
- The first visit often sets the tone for the future dental behaviours of an individual. When a child comes to the dental operatory in a non-threatening environment for a check-up, which often goes uneventful after a thorough oral and dental examination of the teeth [4], hence first visit makes the child look forwards to future visits.
- On the other hand, if the first visit of the child is overdue until the child shows signs of tooth decay or the presence of a dental emergency, it is conducted in a stressful situation for the child and prepares the child's mind to look forward to an unpleasant experience that would involve some form of dental treatment.
- Delay in the first dental visit may also lead to irreversible progression and an increase in the severity of dental caries.
- Conditions involving improper feeding habits can be detected, and counselling of the involved caregivers can be done to prevent early childhood caries. Certain developmental disturbances like cleft lip and palate and natal and neonatal teeth also require prompt diagnosis and intervention. Hence the American Academy of Pediatric Dentistry have recommended it to conduct the first dental visit within six months of the eruption of the first tooth but not later than twelve months of age.
- At the first dental visit, the dentist should take a thorough medical history and review the pre-natal and post-natal history with an emphasis on any medications taken by the mother, access to fluoride supplements during pregnancy, and the presence of any maternal conditions that may affect the child's oro-dental development.
- The examination of the child should be done in a comfortable environment keeping the child as the focus of attention of both parent and the dental surgeon.
- The dentist may choose to seat the child in a child-friendly low chair or examine in the knee-to-knee position commonly used for small children. The parent's

presence in the operatory is encouraged as they may help to relieve the anxiety and participate in keeping the child relaxed [2 - 4].

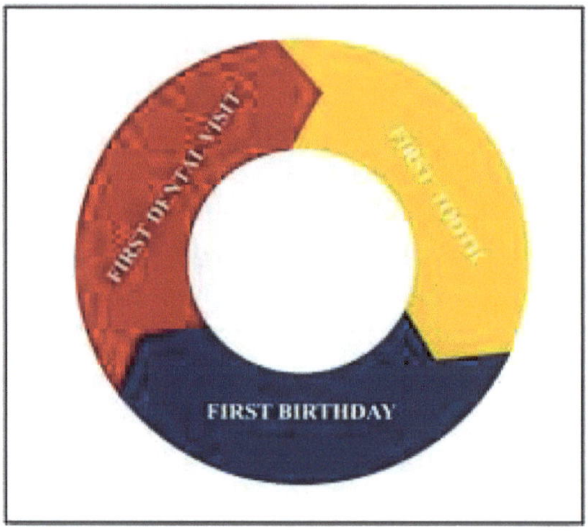

Fig. (12). First visit of a child to Pediatric Dentist.

Outcomes of a First Dental Visit

- Counselling of parents towards age-appropriate oral hygiene methods
- Counselling of parents for diet and nutrition
- Evaluation of the fluoride programme and supplementing fluoride wherever necessary
- Advice on breastfeeding and discuss methods and the right time for weaning
- Inform the parent about cariogenic habits like the use of honey-dipped or sweetened pacifiers
- Thorough oral examination of the teeth and supporting structures if present
- Examination of gum pads
- Identify any development disorders of hard and soft tissues
- Inform parents about the different preventive methods

Anticipatory Guidance

- One of the important aspects of the first dental visit is anticipatory guidance. It involves identifying present problems and informing the parents about future anticipated problems due to the present condition.
- When a child with improper feeding or highly cariogenic habits is discovered, the parents should be informed about the future effects and sequelae of dental caries.
- Similarly, if developmental disturbances like ankyloglossia are noticed the parents should be informed about the anticipated speech problem later [5, 6].

- As compared to general dentists, pediatric dentists have specific skills and expertise to treat oral diseases in infants, children, and teens.
- Having a single pediatric dentist from the beginning will help the child in finding the right treatment for a child. They do not have to find a different dentist each time. The dentist will know the child's history and treat him accordingly instead of adopting a new procedure every other time.
- The child will also be saved from the additional pain, and he will become familiar with the Pediatric dentist, and their bond will get stronger, resulting in a better understanding. This will be helpful in the successful treatment of the child and creates no worries for parents.

Considerations of Child Management in Dentistry

1. To desire, decide and learn the practice of dentistry for children is a great step in terms of patient care in dentistry.

2. The dentist willing to practice dentistry for children should possess good skills in general dentistry, including restorative procedures, extractions, endodontic treatment and above all, diagnosis and treatment planning (Fig. **13**).

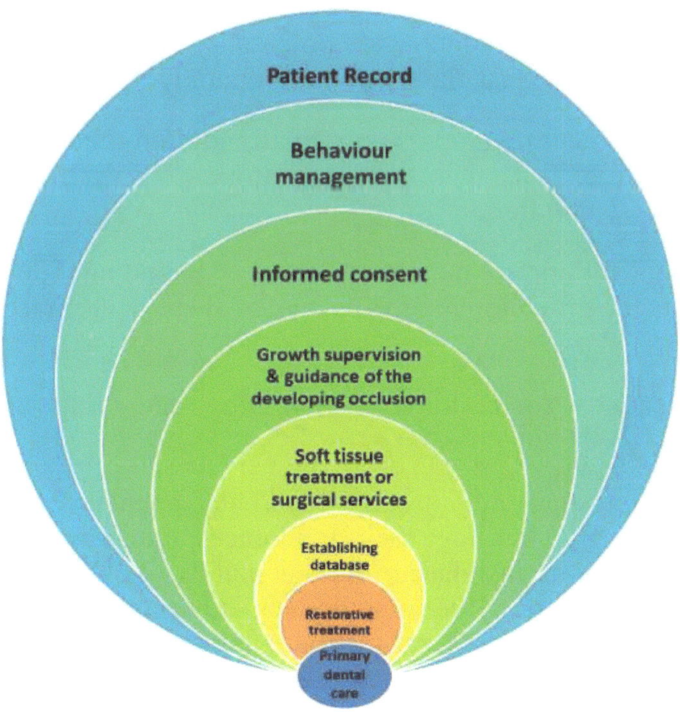

Fig. (13). Comprehensive Pediatric Dental Care.

3. They must have dealt with children to an extent during their graduation or during their initial years of association with senior practitioners to understand what difficulties can be encountered while dealing with children.

4. To learn the art and science of child management in dentistry, they must either observe the work of a pediatric dentist or a dentist with reasonable skills in practicing dentistry for children.

5. The most difficult hurdle to overcome while beginning to practice dentistry for children is 'to believe' that child management principles work! Those who do, accept that, like most sciences, despite limitations,

'child management' can be practised with a certain predictability.

6. The dental surgeon must develop a team that he/she heads for practising dentistry for children. The team must continuously acquire knowledge and learn from experience while dealing with children. It is also important to decide policies in practice about specific child management techniques or aspects (for example: whether parent/s should be present in the operatory during the dental treatment of a child; whether a restraining technique is to be used.

7. Most children beyond a certain age are potentially cooperative for most dental procedures. They cannot be just classified as 'cooperative' or 'uncooperative'.

8. The 'child management methods' apply to all children- cooperative as well as initially uncooperative. It is therefore mandatory to learn for the successful management of most children.

9. Children account for approximately one-third of the population; thus the onus of practising dentistry for children remains on dental surgeons practising dentistry with children.

10. Practicing dentistry for children is rewarding, satisfying and challenging profession.

11. Children are not small adults (Fig. **14**). They behave and relate to their surroundings differently. They have their preferences, likes and dislikes. A dentist for children has to have an insight into their demands.12. There are certain rules for successful dental practice; for example, achieving adequate anaesthesia is a rule before tooth extraction; a correct instrumentation technique, working length determination, and use of proper irrigation are the basics of endodontic success. The success story of practising dentistry for children begins with good child management. It is important to have patience and sustained interest for success in the practice of dentistry for children.

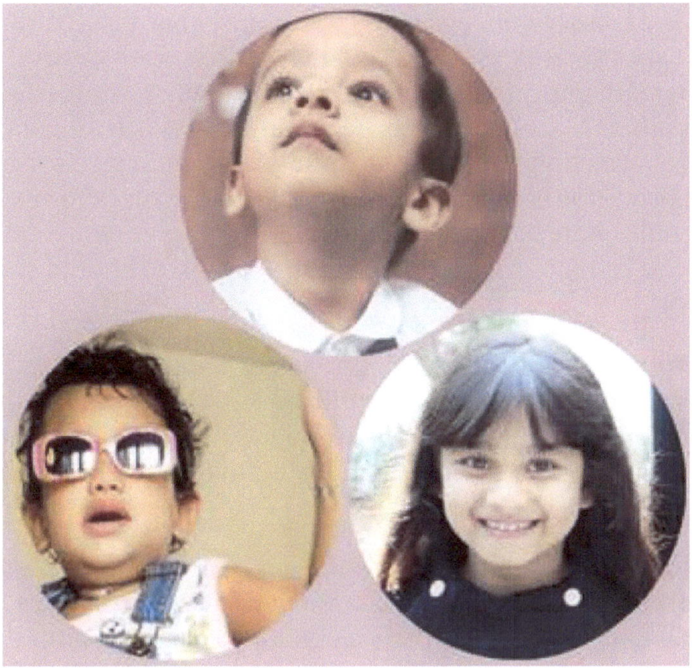

Fig. (14). The Childhood Shows the Man as Morning Shows the Day".

Concept of Dental Home

- The Dental Home concept has been promoted by the AAPD to provide dental treatment to infants, children, and adolescents, including children with special health care needs, under one roof.
- It allows the personnel involved in the oral health care management of children like parents, dental surgeons, dental professionals, and non-dental professionals to take part in the execution of dental treatment for children.
- At the same time, various specialists who are commonly involved in the management of medically, physically, psychologically, and mentally challenged children are available at a single centre, thereby reducing the need for lengthy referrals, delays and inconvenience to parents and children with special needs [7].
- The dental home is the ongoing relationship between the dentist and the patient, inclusive of all aspects of oral health care delivered in a comprehensive, continuously accessible, coordinated, and family-centred way. The establishment of a dental home begins no later than 12 months of age and continues through childhood and adolescence.
- By establishing a Dental Home and taking preventive steps recommended by the pediatric dentist, parents can avoid their children contracting early childhood

caries, which is extensive devastating tooth decay that results in pain, failure to thrive, and in various cases, extensive and costly restorative work.

- Dental home is an important concept for the dental profession to embrace. Evidence supports the advantages of receiving early professional dental care and intervention that are complemented by anticipatory guidance for parents, as well as periodic supervision visits based on the child's risk of dental disease. The dental home could increase opportunities for preventive oral health services for children that can reduce disease disparities. The dental home is a concept that deserves support.

Habit counselling – children pick up some habits as they learn through socialization. Most of those habits should be inspired because they teach kids ways of life. However, certain of habits in infancy should be stopped as the child grows. These include thumb sucking, and using the pacifier. Some habits are not easy to stop.

Preventive dental care – children need preventive dental care more than anyone else. Their teeth are still developing, and their bone structures are changing. Preventive dental care makes sure their teeth are in perfect health through various stages. Preventive dental care includes services like fluoride treatment, dental sealants, space maintainers, *etc.*

Early diagnosis – another great benefit of pediatric dentistry is early diagnosis. In the medical world, detecting a problem early is the best way to curb it before it advances. Some oral problems like teeth misalignment, discolouration on teeth, gum recession, plaque build-up, among others, can be controlled early before they rise into complex problems.

Dental Conditions

- ***Fighting Dental Anxiety*** – dental anxiety and phobias are common among children. Particularly, if the child has gone through many medical interventions, it is hard to get them to go forward with others in the future. Visiting a dentist regularly is part of good oral health practice. It is a known fact that it is a tug of war to get the child to the dentist if he has anxiety and phobias. Pediatric dentists know their way around dental anxiety. They can help the children get comfortable with the idea of dental intervention.
- ***Overall health care*** – a paediatric dentist capable of a lot more than parents are aware. They are trained health experts who know a lot about the human body. With the mouth being the first contact point of things that get into the body, dentists participate in overall health care.

Why Pediatric Dentistry is Better for Children?

Professionals working in pediatric dentistry are dedicating themselves exclusively to children and are therefore better equipped to manage any problems occurring in their mouths. This will include tooth decay, cavities, delayed eruption, loss of baby teeth, and even wisdom teeth. These professionals are qualified to administer sedation to children to undergo invasive and intensive dental treatments.

Maintaining calmness is easy for pediatric dentists because they are working with children every day. They tailor their approach according to every patient's specific area of concern. Children feel more comfortable in the pediatric dentists' chair because of their experience in keeping children calm.

Pediatric dentists design their offices keeping young children in mind. They are equipped to provide treatment to children for any oral health issue to help them keep a smile on their faces.

CONCLUSION

Children are unique in their stages of development; hence there is a need for a separate dental speciality for children. Pediatric dentists have specific skills and expertise to treat oral diseases in infants, children, and teens. It is recommended that a child should have his first visit to the dentist when he turns one year old. Early engraining of oral hygiene habits will develop strong teeth and gums in the child throughout life. Paediatric dentist can be the child's best friend and can protect him from long-term problems and lifelong complications. By introducing early oral health education and applying preventive dentistry procedures, the pediatric dental patient can be insured for a lifetime of Excellent Dental health.

CONSENT FOR PUBLICATION

Not applicable.

CONFLICT OF INTEREST

The author(s) declare no conflict of interest, financial or otherwise.

ACKNOWLEDGEMENT

Declared none.

REFERENCES

[1] American Dental Association Commission on Dental Accreditation Accreditation standards for advanced specialty education programs in pediatric dentistry. Chicago, Ill 2018. Available at: https://www.ada.org/~/media/CODA/Files/ped.pdf

[2] American Academy of Pediatric Dentistry. Perinatal and infant oral health care The Reference Manual of PediatricDentistry. Chicago, Ill: American Academy of Pediatric Dentistry 2020; pp. 252-6.

[3] Guideline on management of the developing dentition and occlusion in pediatric. Dentistry American academy of pediatric. Dentistry reference manual 2020; 32: pp. (6)10-1.

[4] Gelbier S, Kupietzky A, Tsai AT-P. History of the International Association of Paediatric Dentistry: A 50-year perspective. Int J Paediatr Dent 2019; 29: 387-402.
[http://dx.doi.org/10.1111/ipd.12492]

[5] Pediatric Dentistry Timeline. Available at: http://mouthmonsters.mychildrensteeth.org/ pediatric-dentistry-timeline/

[6] Bhaskar V, McGraw KA, Divaris K. The importance of preventive dental visits from a young age: systematic review and current perspectives. Clin Cosmet Investig Dent 2014; 6: 21-7.
[PMID: 24672258]

[7] Policy of Dental Home Oral Health Policies. AAPD -Reference Manual 2019.

CHAPTER 2

Emotional Development of a Child

Raghavendra M. Shetty[1,*], **Trisha Gadekar**[2] and **Aditi Pashine**[3]

[1] *Department of Clinical Sciences, College of Dentistry, Ajman University; Center of Medical and Bio-allied Health Sciences Research, Ajman University, Ajman, UAE*

[2] *Department of Pediatric Dentistry, Mamata Dental College, Khammam, Telangana, India*

[3] *Associate Dentist, MyDentist, Aberystwyth, UK*

Abstract: The emotional development of a child is the progressive process of the child's ability to control their feelings. The emotions of the child are expressed through facial expressions. Emotions in a child are influenced by their inborn temperament depending on the inherited genes. Crying, laughing, anger, fear, anxiety, or phobia represent different types of emotions. The impact of dental anxiety and fear often leads to avoidance or delay of dental treatment. Moreover, such individuals are difficult to treat and have behavioral problems further resulting in an unpleasant dental experience. All these factors lead to worsening oral health, which often requires complicated dental procedures. Hence, it becomes difficult for the patient to get out of this vicious cycle. Management of such patients is critical and requires careful handling and assessment. Various behaviour management techniques and advanced specialist care in the dental setting can assist fearful patients in attaining optimum oral health and significant overall improvement towards dentistry.

Keywords: Anxiety, Assessment Scale, Emotion, Fear.

INTRODUCTION

The emotional development of children and adolescents is symbolised by a vast variation according to age, maturity, intellectual development, temperament, experience, family background, and cultural background. These factors play a vital role in influencing the child's development and underlying emotions.

Crying, laughing, and anger represent the physiological response of the emotions, whereas fear, anxiety, or phobia represents physiological causes of emotions. Fear and anxiety are considered evolutionary mechanisms essential for human existence. While every human being is afraid and anxious, it may be difficult to

* **Corresponding author Raghavendra M. Shetty:** Department of Clinical Sciences, College of Dentistry, Ajman University; Center of Medical and Bio-allied Health Sciences Research, Ajman University, Ajman, UAE; Tel: +971 67056364; Fax: +971 67438888; E-mail: drraghavendra77@gmail.com

manage and understand another person's similar emotions. Usually, adults are aware of their fear and anxiety and often times, they have identified ways to regulate and control their anxiety, whereas it is a complex and sensitive issue while dealing with a child's fear and anxiety, especially in a dental setting. This is primarily due to its unknown nature and, secondly, due to difficulty in tackling the situation in the unique dental environment. Though pediatric dentists possess expertise in building and instilling a positive attitude toward dentistry during childhood, neutralizing a child's fear and anxiety requires proper implementation of behaviour shaping and management knowledge. They must be able to recognize the underlying reasons and provide an effective foundation for effective oral health care throughout an individual's life.

Assorted studies have suggested that avoidance of dental fear and anxiety often leads to poor oral health care. Hence, the primarily step towards successful dental treatment in children is to know the emotional development of the child and the recognition of dental fear and anxiety.

EMOTION

American Psychological Association defines emotion as a complex reaction pattern involving experiential, behavioural, and physiological elements by which an individual try to deal with a personally significant matter or event. Emotional experiences have three components: a subjective experience, a physiological response, and a behavioural or expressive response.

Types of Emotions in Children

1. Subjective Responses – These responses may vary with various kinds of expressions of the same emotion or different emotions.

Ex- Some children may be scared of sitting in a dental chair and would be fearful while some will be very much excited to get their check-ups done.

2. Physiological Responses – It results due to stimulation of the autonomic nervous system and may be expressed as fear, anxiety, or phobia.

3. Behavioural Responses – It is the actual expression of the emotion. Here the child's expression would exactly be the same as he/she is feeling inside, like crying, laughing, anger, disgust, *etc.*

Emotional Development in Children

Bridge, in 1932, gave a model of emotional development which considered distress and delight as the basic manifestation of emotion which is present since birth. In the next few months, primary emotions (positive and negative) can be noticed such as happiness and sadness, surprise and disgust, fear, and anger. With social interaction and personal experience, more complex emotions are seen, such as love and jealousy, empathy, shame, guilt, and so on. As per the model, "the emotional reactions are generalized and poorly organized to a single or more type of situations during early weeks of life where it takes more definite form to specific situations as the child ages," thus leading to gradual development and maturation of different emotions such as anger, fear, affection, joy, *etc.* According to this model, the development of fear occurs during 5-6 months of life (Fig. **1**).

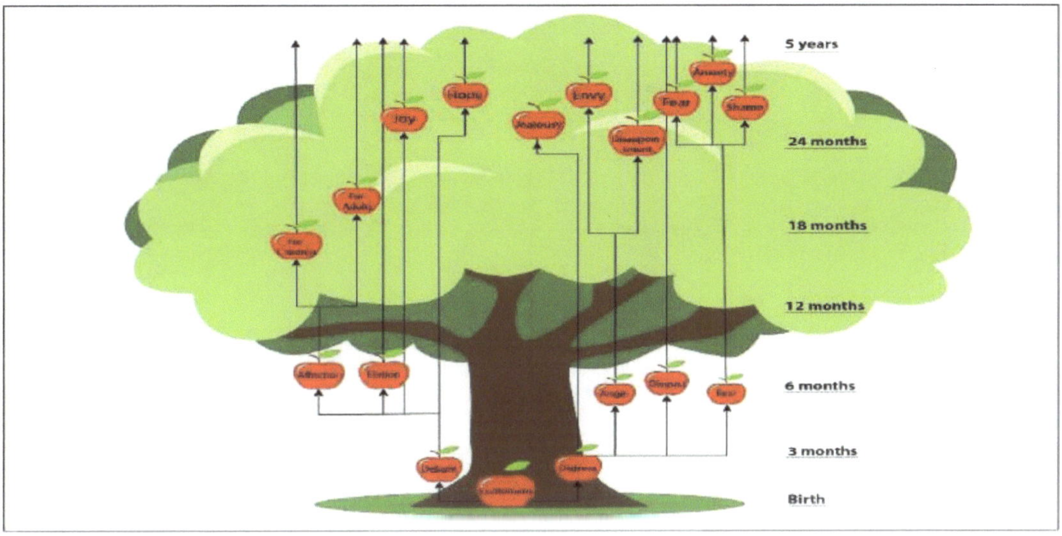

Fig. (1). Bridge's Classic Model of Emotional Development.

However, later a different approach known as the differential emotions theory suggested expressions of various emotions present even during the first months of life. Most recently, an upgraded differentiation model of emotional development was put forth by Widen and Russell in 2008 (Fig. **2**). This is a two-dimensional model with one axis depicting the degree of a person's arousal and another one the degree of pleasure/displeasure. In this model, fear shows high arousal with displeasure.

There are three important components of emotional development: (i) the expression of emotion, (ii) the understanding of emotion, (iii) the regulation of emotion. Any emotion, whether positive or negative, is conveyed through the face, voice, hands, and physiological reactions. To understand one's own emotions and to understand those of others are two different entities with a close correlation. It is astonishing to know that understanding another person's emotions add to a better knowledge of one's behaviour. The regulation of emotion has various components, including physiological (sympathetic and parasympathetic system), socialization, coping, *etc.* As the child ages, various changes occur in all three components of emotions depending on internal and external conditions. When a situation arises where an individual is unable to maintain an emotional balance, it may lead to the development of psychopathology, including anxiety disorders.

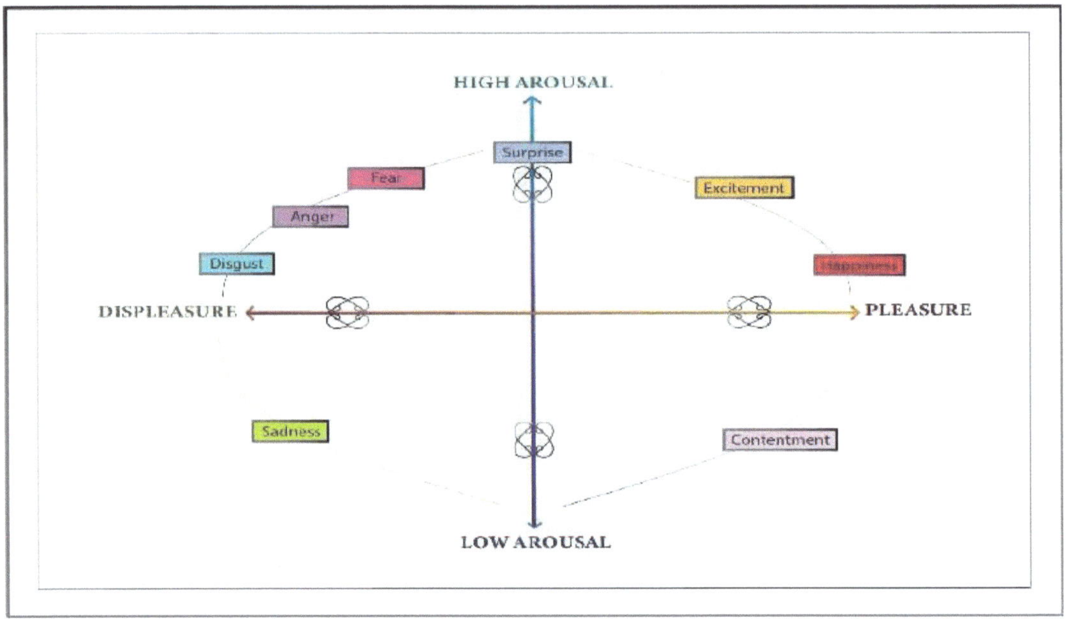

Fig. (2). Widen and Russell Differentiation Model of Emotional Development.

Children evolve through definite stages of emotional & mental development. The child's behaviour patterns are constantly adapted. A myriad of emotions develops in the child from birth to adolescence (Fig. **3**). As the child learns to think and act as an individual, emotional development begins (Table **1**). Crying is often the beginning of seeking babies, as this eventuates in getting what they want. Here in this chapter, the discussion would be restricted to fear and anxiety, which are closely related.

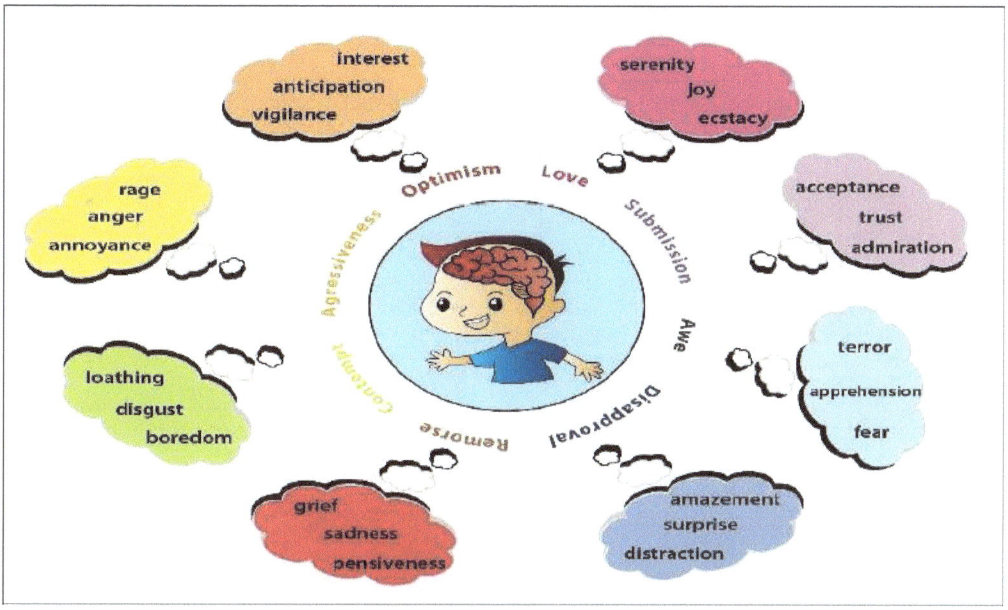

Fig. (3). Myriad of emotions in the child's mind.

Table 1. Overview of Emotional Development in the Child.

Age	Emotional Development	Clinical Implication and External Modifications	Pictorial Representation
0 to 6 months	• Crying is the primary emotion at this stage. • Sucking, grasping, and swallowing reflexes are seen. • Fear of the unknown, and fear of separation is present. • They are attracted to hand and face movements along with the mother's and father's voices. • A one-way conversation is based on gestures; noises are seen.	• Children are sensitive to loud noise and hence should not be introduced to loud environments. However, the light sound produced by toys can make them comfortable and feel happy in the environment. • Parental presence should always be there. • The child responds to friendly handling and smiles at people and therefore, 6 months would be the correct time to introduce the child to their first dental visit.	**0 to 6 months** 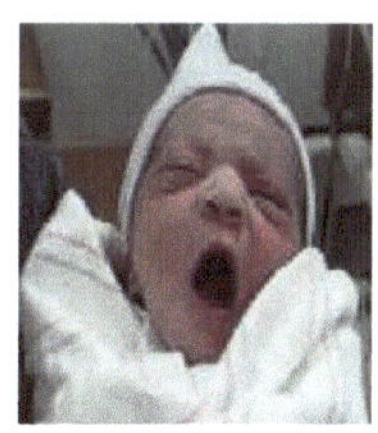

(Table 1) cont.....

Age	Emotional Development	Clinical Implication and External Modifications	Pictorial Representation
6 to 12 months	• Strong attachments in the child-parent relationship are seen. • Starts moving unsupported and independently. • Becomes more familiar with the surroundings, and they pick up small objects and explore the environment around them. • Fear of strangers is still present.	• Parental separation should not be attempted, while parental presence can work effectively. • Grip reflexes become strong, and hence the dentist can give the child toys to hold during the treatment or dental instruments to make them more comfortable with the environment.	**6 to 12 months** 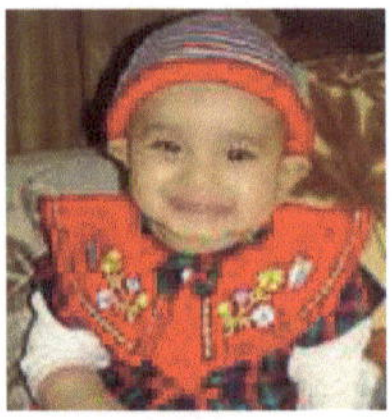
1 to 2 years	• Referred to as the exploratory period. • Fear of separation present • Intense curiosity is seen with a desire to explore everything around them, which may trouble the parents too. • Temper tantrums can be significantly seen in this age group. • Fear of bodily injury, fear of animals.	• Data Structuring by setting the rules • Careful introduction of positive and negative reinforcers. • Parental separation should not be attempted. • Parental and Sibling Modelling. • Intense curiosity – the child can be allowed to explore through the dental operatory and introduction to the instruments. • Tell Play Do and voice control can be used effectively.	**One to 2 years** 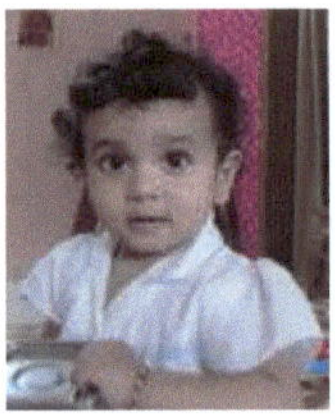
3 to 4 years	• Increase in contentment and individuality. • Emotional stability. • A sense of security with strangers develops. • Enjoy make-believe play. • Fear of bodily injury, Fear of animals, imaginary fear of ghosts, *etc.*	• Parental separation can be attempted. • Exploratory play technique, use of poetry and drawings can be done to manage the behaviour • Sibling modelling will help. • The presence of subjective and objective fear can be present and can be managed with euphemisms. • Audiovisual modelling. • Desensitization.	**3 to 4 years** 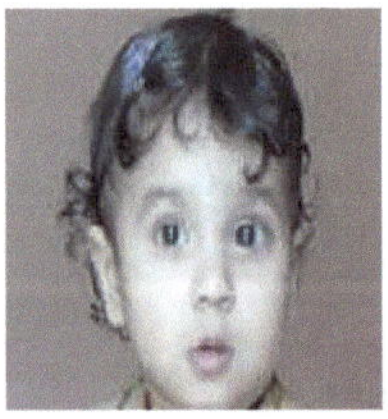
5 to 7 years	• Balance, self-containment, and independence is seen developing in the personality • The children display politely confident behaviour. • Increased self-confidence, friendly, able to cooperate in a disciplined way, and are more aware of gender characteristics. • Fear of bodily injury • Imaginary fear from ghosts *etc.*	• Parental separation can be attempted. • Tell Show Do will be effective. • Exploratory play. • Audio distraction. • Setting the rules during the treatment. • Data Structuring can be done. • Gender-related pictorial anxiety scales and tests would give wonderful results regarding the child's cooperation.	**5 to 7 years** 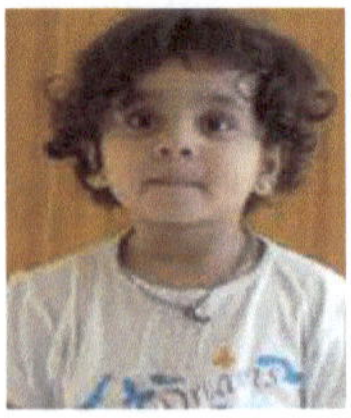

Commonly Seen Emotions in Children

Crying

The cry is the first emotion as it is present since the birth of an individual. Though, like other emotions, it is a mode of expression for a person but needs careful evaluation in a dental set-up. Elsbach in 1964, classified types of cries and reviewed them as the personality trait and if studied carefully, can assist in behaviour management of a child patient. Hence, in 1963, he classified cries into distinct categories (Fig. **4**).

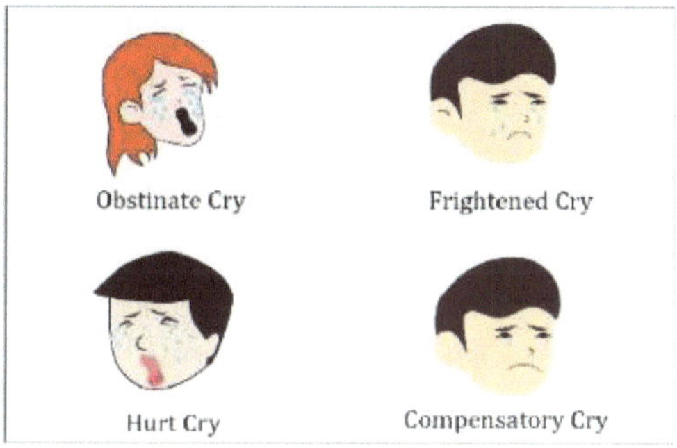

Fig. (4). Types of cries.

Obstinate Cry

The cry is loud, high-pitched, and characterized as a siren-like wail. The more disturbed the child, the louder and higher-pitched the cry. The child screams without any tears. It represents the child's external response to anxiety.

Management: One of the most difficult kinds to manage the crying child. Depending on the degree of obstinacy, the child needs to be managed. For a child showing mild features, voice control used along with parental absence (on consent) is usually helpful, while for a higher degree of uncooperative behaviour pharmacological methods have to be used.

Frightened Cry

Torrent of tears along with breath-catching sobs with fear is seen. Here, fear is the only reason for crying.

Management: In this type, parental presence is usually beneficial due to the emotional component associated with it. It helps keep them motivated. Dentists must remain empathetic with them, without the use of any force or firmness. Once a dentist is successful in gaining trust, such patients are easy to manage in successive appointments.

Hurt Cry

A small whimper is symbolic of such a cry. The child may show a single tear falling from the corner of the eye and running down the child's cheek without making any sound or resistance to the treatment procedure. Sounds like moaning or groaning might be accompanied by breathing difficulty. This means they are trying to cooperate at the expense of their comfort and trying to hide the pain.

Management: The only management is to alleviate the pain and assure the child. Also, reconfirm with the child about pain or any discomfort before proceeding further.

Compensatory Cry

A constant and continuous whining noise without tears and sobs comprises a compensatory cry. It is a slow and monotonous kind of sound. It is a coping mechanism for a child to overcome the fear, though he is trying to cooperate at the same time.

Management: they are usually young children and easy to handle. As they adapt to the situation, the cry lessens. Proper communication is important.

Anger

Anger is an outburst of emotions caused by a child's lack of skill in managing a situation. Infants and young children respond in a direct and primitive manner, but the responses become violent and more symbolic with development.

Fear

Fear is defined as 'the emotion of pain or uneasiness caused by the sense of impending danger, or by the prospect of some possible evil.' It is one of the primary emotional reactions to a perceived threat or danger. It is an unpleasant emotional state comprising of psychological and physiological reactions to an exogenous threat or danger involving agitation, alertness, tension, and mobilization of the alarmed reaction (fight-flight-fight mode). ***According to Dorland medical dictionary,*** fear is a painful feeling of impending danger, evil, or trouble. The common fear evoking dental stimuli includes anaesthetic administration, removal of teeth, and the sound of a drill.

Factors for Dental Fear and Anxiety

1. Direct conditioning (Past aversive experience in dental/medical set-up): Painful encounters in a hospital or dental office are the most frequent reason for dental fear and anxiety.

2. Indirect conditioning (Vicarious learning): Unpleasant experiences of family members or peers might also lead to the acquisition of dental anxiety, which creates a negative attitude towards dental treatment.

3. Endogenous factors: It has been well established that in some children, it may be related to heredity, age, gender, and general anxiety is frequently associated with dental anxiety and fear.

Carter *et al.* in 2014, suggested five pathways that are related to the development of dental fear and anxiety (Fig. **5**). However, numerous factors such as genetic vulnerability, negative affectivity/anxiety vulnerability, preparedness, cognitive biases, and operant conditioning also affect dental fear and anxiety.

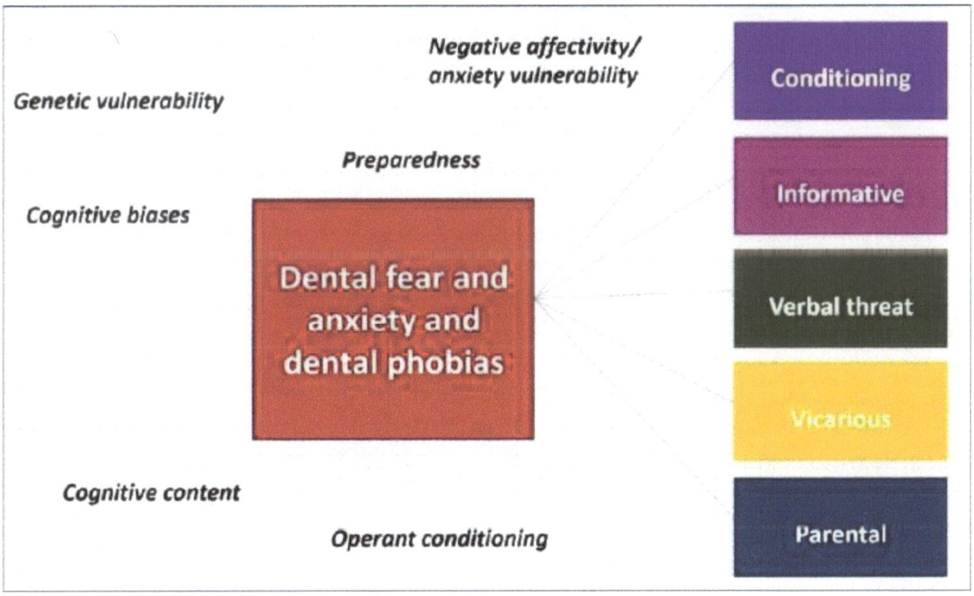

Fig. (5). Pathways of Development of Fear.

Types of Fear

It can be broadly classified as objective fear (active or real) and subjective fear (anticipated).

Objective Fear/real Fear

In terms of dental fear, this is often present in children with previous unpleasant dental experiences and/or repeated hospitalization (Fig. **6**). Such type of fear magnifies the apprehension leading to increased intensity of pain. This is the most basic example of objective fear directly taking the body into fear and adrenaline rush.

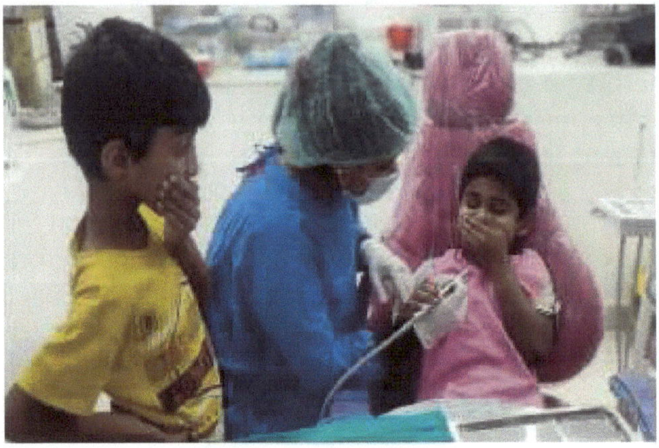

Fig. (6). Objective Fear.

Example: A child with previous dental experience and who initially took vaccination would have anxiety about the syringe. This type of fear can be successfully overcome by desensitization techniques and tell-show-do techniques.

Subjective Fear/anticipated Fear

It is based on feelings and attitudes suggested to an individual by others without personally experiencing them (Fig. **7**). The mental picture producing the fear is retained in mind and becomes magnified when they face it. Fear of dentistry in adults is more based on what they heard about it from their parents than anything else, which very well explains subjective fear. In a dental setup, a child might feel that it is always associated with a painful experience. Hence, this is a learned type of fear consisting of most of the responses of the innate fear pattern.

Example: Parents using the name of doctor/dentist to scare the child, parents inducing fear in the child by telling if you don't do a particular activity, we will take you to the doctor for the injection, leading to the child developing a subjective fear for LA syringes or sometimes the peer suggesting the pain of injection syringe. It is difficult to overcome and may need successive counselling.

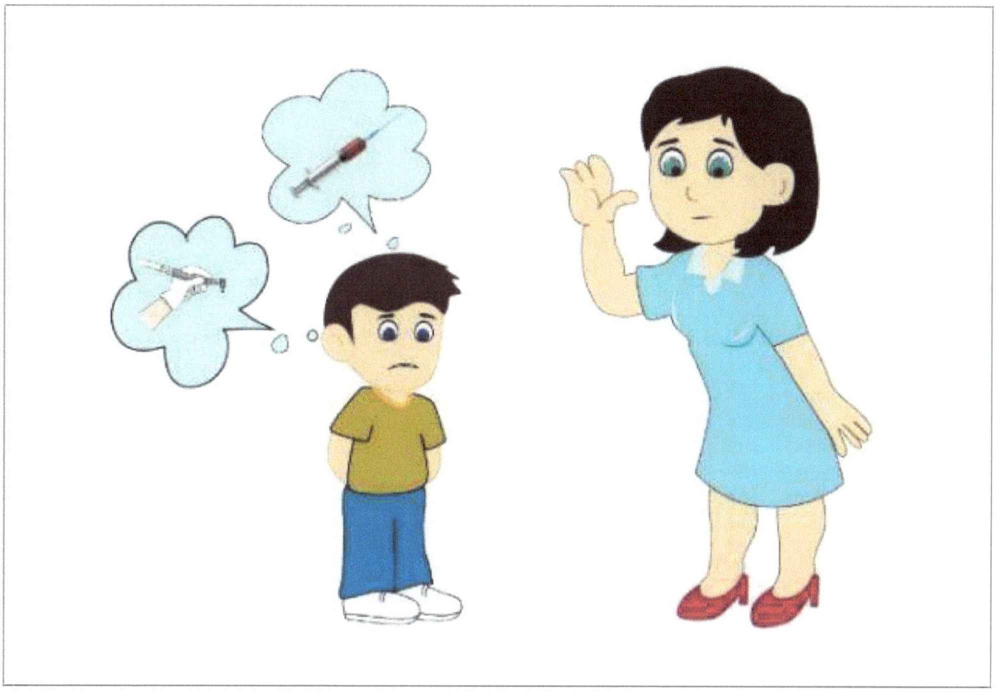

Fig. (7). Subjective Fear.

Though fear itself is an emotion, its expression might vary based on the circumstances and personality traits of an individual. It might be expressed in the form of:

a. ***Shyness***: in the form of crying, turning the head away from the stranger and clinging to a familiar person, running away, and hiding, talking as little as possible, blushing in older kids, stuttering, displaying nervous mannerisms like shifting one foot to another, pulling cloths, bending the head to one side, and coiling to look at the stranger.

b. ***Embarrassment***: usually seen in children older than 6 years with their social experience. A hurt cry can be seen in such child patients.

c. ***Worry***: it has no stimulus for arousal, but it is a product of the child's own mind. The child might think that dental appointments are very painful and will build an imaginary fear.

d. ***Anxiety***: anxiety and fear are interchangeably used terms with the slightest conceptual difference between them, which will be discussed later in the chapter (Table **2**). Fear often leads to an anxious state.

Table 2. Difference between Anxiety and Fear.

Anxiety	Fear
A complicated state of helplessness, a perceived inability to predict or control upcoming situations, and a state of readiness to counteract probable future threats. *Ex: A child's denial and continuous cry before going to a dental clinic where he had a past unpleasant experience.*	Motivational state is aroused by specific stimuli that give rise to defensive behaviour or escape. *Ex: A frightened child with the sight of a local anaesthesia syringe or an irrigation syringe in the first or second appointment who had pain in the previous appointment.*
Anxiety precedes an encounter with a feared object or situation. *Ex: Child getting anxious by the sight or sound of air rotor.*	Fear is a response to the actual or activated response to the object or situation. *Ex: A child being afraid after starting with cavity preparation using air rotor in the oral cavity.*
Generalized response to an unknown threat or internal conflict.	Focused or known external danger/ objective.
Unclear or uncertain origins. *Ex: A child getting anxious by seeing any medical person who is wearing a white apron thinking he is going to give injections/vaccination.*	Well-established origins. *Ex: A child being afraid about the LA syringe due to pain arising from the prick of it.*
Responses include worrying, hypervigilance, cognitive distortions, avoidant behaviour, and in extreme conditions, activation of the autonomic nervous system.	Responses include activation of the autonomic nervous system and defensive actions.

Anxiety

Anxiety is a complex emotion analogous to fear and arousal without any objective or real danger. It is defined as an unpleasant feeling in combination with a notion of impending doom or danger from within rather than from an outside environment. Dental anxiety denotes a condition of suspicion that something threatening might happen related to dental treatment and it is coupled with a feeling of losing control over it. It can also be considered as an evolutionary step to protect from far-off or imaginary threats.

Types of Anxiety

- **Trait Anxiety:** Life-long, stable condition of anxiety as a permanent feature of one's personality. Children are easily frightened and hypersensitive to stimuli.

- **State Anxiety:** These are acute transient circumstantial allied episodes of psychological and physiological alteration that do not persist beyond the provoking situation and are causally related to the specific moment.

- **Free Floating Anxiety:** Condition of diffuse chronic anxiousness of unknown reason. Diverse types of thoughts/emotions or events provoke anxiety.

- **Situational Anxiety:** Only seen in situations or related to specific objects.

- **General Anxiety Disorder:** This is characterized by a chronic persistent and pervasive feeling of anxiety no matter whatever the external situation may be.

Phobia

A phobia is defined as an irrational kind of fear leading to the conscious avoidance of a particular object, activity, or circumstance [1]. It represents a severe type of anxiety and is characterized by excessive and persistent anxiety concerning either discernible situations/objects (drilling, injections) or dental situations in general. Phobia is a clinical diagnosis and refers to a marked fear that interferes with a person's normal daily routine, whereas fear is not always extreme. According to Shelhan (1982), there are two types of phobias: either exogenous/non-endogenous and endogenous, based on internal or external factors.

***Exogenous or Non-Endogenous*:** Seen in the psychologically affected group due to the external environment. The etiological agent can be readily identified.

***Endogenous*:** Produced from within without any detectable stress situation. A severe cluster of symptoms is present.

Fear and Anxiety Assessment Scale

Fear and anxiety assessment marks a major step for effective dental treatment planning in a clinical setting. It can be done by either dental personnel and/or researchers. The completion of a questionnaire by the parent as a proxy measure is important due to the following reasons:

- Early identification and intervention of a fearful/anxious patient and to reduce its implications.
- To recognize any specific dental procedure that a child might be anxious/fearful about.
- To encourage effective communication and effective treatment planning.
- To evaluate the outcome of any specific behaviour shaping/management technique.

The Dental fear and anxiety assessment can be broadly classified into four categories based on the method of assessment:

a. Self-report assessment includes a dental subscale of the children's fear survey schedule (CFSS-DS), modified dental anxiety scale, children's dental fear picture test, drawings, *etc.*

b. Parental proxy-based assessment: parent version of CFSS-DS.

c. Observation-based assessment: clinical anxiety rating scale and uncooperative behaviour rating scale (CARS/BRS); Frankl behaviour rating scale (FBRS); behaviour evaluation scale (BES); behaviour profile rating scale (BPRS) and verbal skill scale (VSS).

d. Physiological assessment: stress markers, such as heart rate.

Various Dental Fear and Anxiety Assessment Scales are as follows:

Corah's Dental Anxiety Scale (CDAS)

Corah, in 1969 developed the CDAS, which is the most widely used scale and was originally based on a single question to measure psychological stress. It consists of 4 item Questionnaire with the first two questions regarding anxiety and the other two related to fear (Table **3**).

Table 3. Corah's Dental Anxiety Scale.

Corah's Dental Anxiety Scale
1. If you had to go to the Dentist tomorrow, how would you feel about it?
a. I would look forward to it as a reasonably enjoyable experience.
b. I wouldn't care one way or the other.
c. I would be a little uneasy about it.
d. I would be afraid that it would be unpleasant and painful.
e. I would be very frightened of what the dentist might do.
2. When you are waiting in the dentist's office for your turn in the chair how do you feel?
a. Relaxed
b. A little easy
c. Tense
d. Anxious
e. So anxious that I sometimes break out in sweat or almost feel physically sick
1. 3. When you are in the dentist's chair waiting while he gets his drill ready to begin working on your teeth. How do you feel?
a. Relaxed
b. A little easy

(Table 3) cont.....

Corah's Dental Anxiety Scale
c. Tense
d. Anxious
e. So anxious that I sometimes break out in sweat or almost feel physically sick
4. **You are in the dentist's chair to have your teeth cleaned. While you are waiting and the dentist is getting out the instruments which he will use to scrape your teeth around the gums, how do you feel?**
a. Relaxed
b. A little easy
c. Tense
d. Anxious
e. So anxious that I sometimes break out in sweat or almost feel

The Modified Child Dental Anxiety Scale (MCDAS)

It was developed by Wong and Humphris in 1998 and was based on CDAS. The MCDAS developed by Wong and Humphris includes eight questions to assess dental anxiety about a few dental procedures (Fig. **8**). The MCDAS includes questions regarding local anaesthesia, extraction, and general anaesthesia. The scores range from 1 (relaxed/not worried) to 5 (very worried). The total scores can range from a minimum of 5 (little or no dental anxiety) to a maximum of 40 (extreme dental anxiety).

Instructions:
For the next 8 questions I would like you to show me how relaxed or worried you get about the dentist and what happens at the dentist. To show me how relaxed or worried you feel please use the simple scale below. This scale is just like a ruler going from 1 which would show that you are relaxed to 5 which would show that you are very worried. So that: 1 would mean: relaxed/not worried; 2 would mean: very slightly worried; 3 would mean: fairly worried; 4 would mean: worried a lot; 5 would mean: very worried

Items

How do you feel about. . .

. . . . going to the dentist generally?
. . . . having your teeth looked at?
. . . . having your teeth scraped and polished?
. . . . having an injection in the gum?
. . . . having a filling ?
. . . . having a tooth taken out?
. . . . being put to sleep to have treatment?
. . . . having a mixture of "gas and air" which would help you to feel comfortable for treatment, but which cannot put you to sleep?

Fig. (8). Modified Child Dental Anxiety Scale (MCDAS).

Faces Version of The Modified Child Dental Anxiety Scale ($MCDAS_f$)

The five numerical value (Likert scale) was replaced by faces by Howard and Freeman in 2007 to improve the cognitive skills of the child in selecting the responses (Fig. **9**).

Dental Fear Survey Scale

It was originally developed as a 27-item scale by Kleinknecht and his colleagues, which was reduced to 20 items in 1984. It is a Likert-type questionnaire that uses representative five-point ratings of dental avoidance, somato-visceral arousal during dental treatment, and naturalistic and clinical behaviours involved in receiving dental care. Though DFS is being widely used as a measure of dental fear, the scale was not developed to produce a single fear score. Instead, it provided information on a wide variety of stimuli that may stimulate fear or avoidance reactions. Alamri *et al.* validated the Arabic version of the Dental Fear Survey Scale recently in 2019 [2].

Faces Version Of The Modified Child Dental Anxiety Scale ($MCDAS_f$)

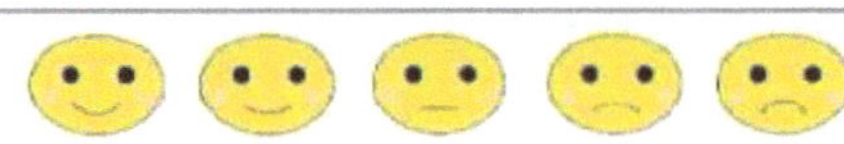

How do you feel about...					
...going to the dentist generally?	1	2	3	4	5
...having your teeth lookes at?	1	2	3	4	5
...having your teeth scrapd and polished?	1	2	3	4	5
...having an injection in the gum?	1	2	3	4	5
...having a filling	1	2	3	4	5
...having a tooth taken out?	1	2	3	4	5
...being put to sleep to have treatment?	1	2	3	4	5
...having a mixture of 'gas and air' which will help you feel comfortable?	1	2	3	4	5
...treatment but cannot put you to sleep?	1	2	3	4	5

Fig. (9). Faces Version of The Modified Child Dental Anxiety Scale (MCDAS).

Children's Dental Fear Picture (CDFP) Test

Introduced by Kleinberg *et al.* in 1994. It has three subtests: the Dental Setting Pictures (CDFP-DS), the Pointing Pictures (CDFP-PP), and a Sentence Completion test (CDFP-SC). Based on the assessment, a child was grouped into one of the three categories – fearful, non-fearful, or uncertain (Fig. **10**).

Venham's Picture Scale (VPS)/Venham's Picture Test (VPT)

Venham *et al.* in 1979, formulated a series of 8 paired drawings of the child *i.e.*, a non-fearful pose and a fearful pose. The patient is asked to pick for each pair which picture more accurately depicts his or her feelings at that time. Scores were calculated as a minimum of zero, and a maximum of eight (Fig. **11**). It is convenient for young children. The limitation is that the figures are dubious in portrayal and might be misleading at times.

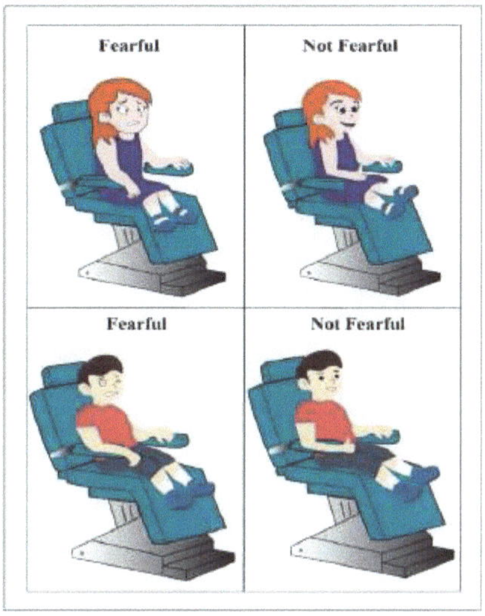

Fig. (10). Illustrations of pictures in CDFP.

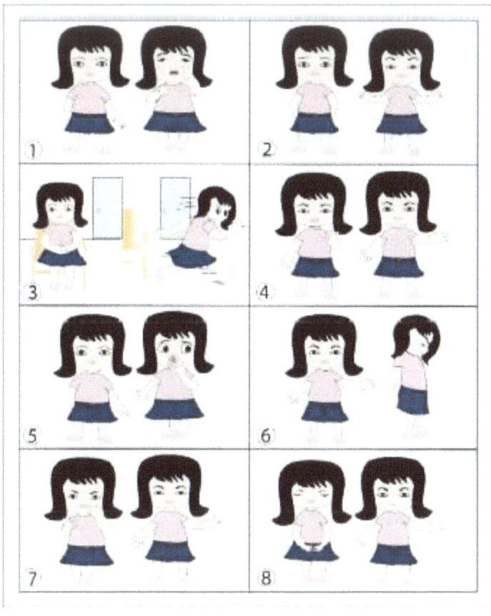

Fig. (11). Venham's Picture Scale.

DA5 Scale

Humphris *et al.* in 2002, prepared a card sort task that comprised five cartoon line sketch faces. These faces were fabricated for each individual which they saw alone in an individual room, and they were asked to play a game and help the interviewer. The cards were given in random order and the child had to put them in order of getting scared to getting happy. The order of anxiety was assessed according to the submitted order of cards by the child. The same process was followed for the next child.

Abeer Children Dental Anxiety Scale (ACDAS)

Date: Child's age: Gender: M / F Operator's name:

A. THE CHILD SELF-REPORT PART

I would like you please to tell me how relaxed or scared you feel at the dentist. please use the scale below from 1 to 3, and tick (✓) under the face that shows us **how you feel now.**

1- Happy 2- OK 3- Scared

How do you feel about:	1	2	3
1. Sitting in the waiting room?			
2. A dentist wearing a mask on his face?			
3. Laying flat on the dental chair?			
4. A dentist checking your teeth with a mirror?			
5. Having a strange taste in your mouth e.g. filling/gloves?			
6. Having a pinch feeling in your gum?			
7. The feeling of numbness (fat lip/tongue)?			
8. A dentist clearing your teeth by buzzy electricn arm that's spraying water?			
9. The sounds that you hear at the denitst?			
10. The smell at the dentist?			
11. Having a tooth taken out?			
12. Wearing a small rubbery mask on your nose to breathe special gas to help you feel comfortable during treatment?			
13. Having a pinch feeling on the back of your hand?			

B. THE CONGNITIVE PART

For Child: 14. Do you feel shy at the dentist? **1. Yes 2. No**

15. Do you feel shy beacuse of the look of your teeth? **1. Yes 2. No**

16. Are you worried about losing control at the dentist? **1. Yes 2. No**

C. THE CHILD ASSESSMENT

For Legal Gaurdian: 17. Has your child had previous dental treatment? **1. Yes 2. No**

18. How do you expect you child's behaviour today?
1. Happy 2. OK 3. Scared

For Operator : 19. At the end of the visit, what is your rating for the child's behaviour?
1. Happy 2. OK 3. Scared

Fig. (12). Abeer Children Dental Anxiety Scale (ACDAS).

Smiley Faces Program (SFP)

The Smiley Faces Program (SFP) was introduced by Buchanan in 2005. It is a four-item computerized dental anxiety scale, using faces as a response set, to assess dental anxiety in children. The use of computer graphics should help the child engage with the dental anxiety scale. The question is flashed up on the screen for 5 seconds and then the smiley faces with expressions follow up and the child needs to click on a face and the face enlarges itself and the score is given. The happy face becomes happier when clicked, while the sad face becomes sadder. In total, seven faces with different expressions are used in this scale.

Abeer Children Dental Anxiety Scale (ACDAS).

The scale was developed by Abeer *et al.* in 2014 and included a cognitive component for children and adolescents. It is made up of three parts (Part A, Part B, and Part C) with a total of 19 questions (Fig. **12**).

Facial Image Scale (FIS):

It consists of five faces ranging from very unhappy to happy. It is scored as one for the happy face and 5 for the very unhappy face (**Fig. 13**). It was developed by Buchanan in 2002.

Fig. (13). Facial Image scale.

Anxiety Thermometer

The patient is asked to point out the minimum to the maximum amount of anxiety on a thermometer ranging from 1 to 10 as a minimum to maximum anxiety (**Fig. 14**).

RMS-Pictorial Scale (RMS-PS)

RMS-PS was introduced by Shetty *et al.* in 2015. It consists of original photographs of a boy and a girl child. In each set, a row of five faces was arranged from happy to very unhappy (**Fig. 15**). The child patient is asked to choose the face which they feel about themselves during the assessment. The scale is scored from 1 (happy face) to 5 (unhappy face) [3]. The scale is reliable and valid, attractive, and easily interpreted by children. The scale delivers the feedback in a brief time regarding the anxiety of the child.

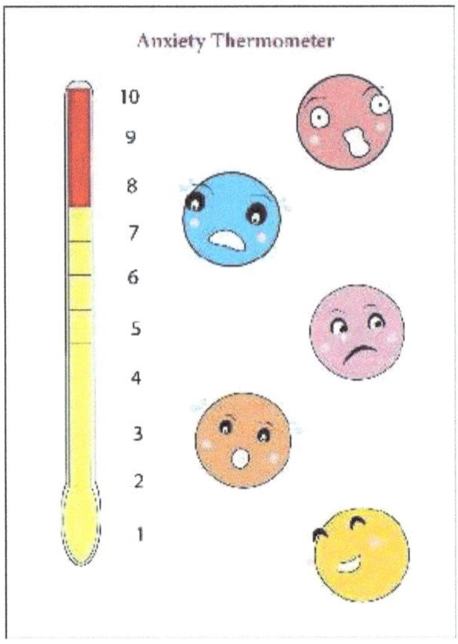

Fig. (14). Anxiety Thermometer.

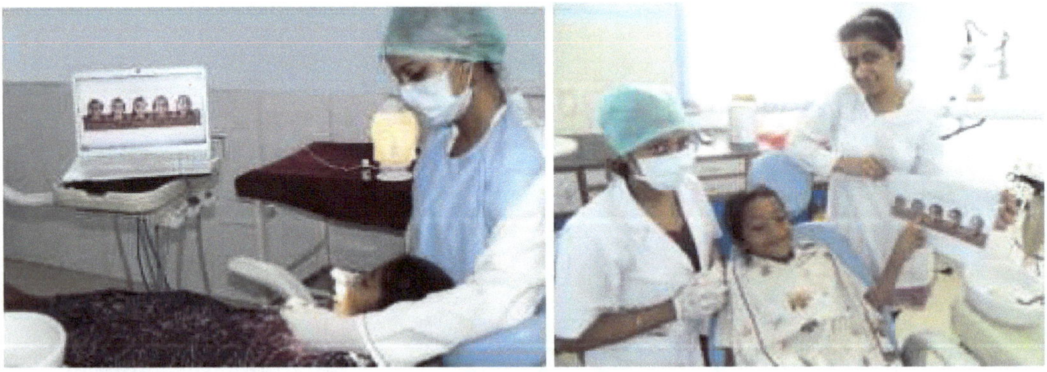

Fig. (15). RMS Pictorial Scale (RMS-PS) used to assess the anxiety.

Chhota Bheem Chutki (CBC) Scale

CBC scale introduced by Sadana *et al.* (2016) consists of two cards (one for boys and the other for girls). Chhota Bheem, the cartoon character, was used to represent emotions in boys and the Chutki cartoon character was used to represent emotions in girls. Both the cards consisted of six cartoon emotions portraying happy to unhappy, where a score of one was allocated to a happy face and six to an unhappy face and running. Children could relate to them more as most of the children population are aware of these cartoon characters and could relate with the animated character [4].

RMS-Tactile Scale (RMS-TS)

RMS-TS was introduced by Shetty *et al.* in 2018. A modification of RMS-PS known as the RMS-Tactile scale **(Fig. 16)** was introduced in 2018 for visually impaired individuals. The children were asked to touch the faces on the scale and recognise what they felt. A row of five faces was fabricated in a 3D effect ranging from happy to very unhappy. The scale was calculated by giving a numerical value of one (1) to the happy face and five (5) to the very unhappy face [5].

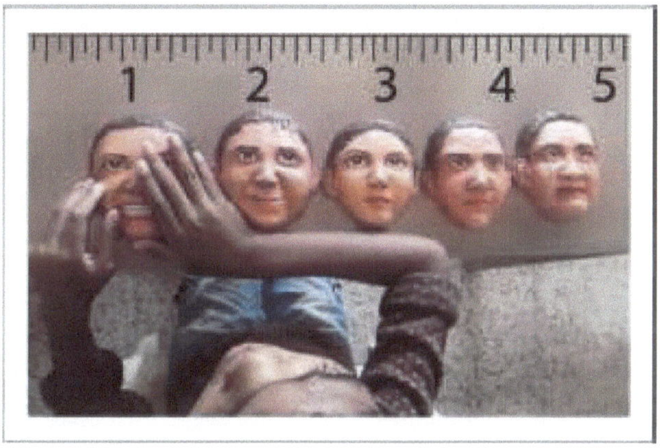

Fig. (16). Visually impaired child with RMS-Tactile scale.

Animated Emoji Scale (AES)

The AES (2019) includes five animated graphic emoji faces (interchange formats) showing different feelings ranging from score 1 (happy/laughing emoji) to 5 (very unhappy/sad and crying emoji) [6].

Animated Visual Facial Pain/Anxiety Rating Scale

Prasad gave the scale *et al.* in 2020, The scale consists of five faces with facial expressions ranging from happy to crying animated 3D clay faces where the score was 1 (absence of pain) for happiness while the score 5 (presence of severe pain) was for a crying 3D animated clay model [7].

CONCLUSION

The impact of emotions, especially dental anxiety and fear, often leads to avoidance or delay of dental treatment. It is important to assess the anxiety and accordingly choose the behaviour management/guidance technique for the positive cooperation of the child during the dental treatment and to provide a pleasant dental experience.

CONSENT FOR PUBLICATION

Not applicable.

CONFLICT OF INTEREST

The author(s) declare no conflict of interest, financial or otherwise.

ACKNOWLEDGEMENT

Declared none.

REFERENCES

[1] Garcia R. Neurobiology of fear and specific phobias. Learn Mem 2017; 24(9): 462-71. [http://dx.doi.org/10.1101/lm.044115.116] [PMID: 28814472]

[2] Alamri S, Alshammari S, Baseer M, Assery M, Ingle N. Validation of Arabic version of the Modified Dental Anxiety Scale (MDAS) and Kleinknecht's Dental Fear Survey Scale (DFS) and combined self-modified version of this two scales as Dental Fear Anxiety Scale (DFAS) among 12 to 15 year Saudi school students in Riyadh city. J Int Soc Prev Community Dent 2019; 0(0): 0. [http://dx.doi.org/10.4103/jispcd.JISPCD_196_19] [PMID: 32039074]

[3] Shetty RM, Khandelwal M, Rath S. RMS Pictorial Scale (RMS-PS): An innovative scale for the assessment of child's dental anxiety. J Indian Soc Pedod Prev Dent 2015; 33(1): 48-52. [http://dx.doi.org/10.4103/0970-4388.149006] [PMID: 25572374]

[4] Kaur J, Sadana G, Grover R, Mehra M, Gupta S, Sadana S. A novel Chotta Bheem–Chutki scale for dental anxiety determination in children. J Int Soc Prev Community Dent 2016; 6(3): 200-5. [http://dx.doi.org/10.4103/2231-0762.183108] [PMID: 27382534]

[5] Shetty RM, Gadekar TR. RMS tactile scale: An innovative tactile anxiety scale for visually impaired children. J Indian Soc Pedod Prev Dent 2018; 36(1): 76-81. [PMID: 29607844]

[6] Setty JV, Srinivasan I, Radhakrishna S, Melwani AM, Dr MK. Use of an animated emoji scale as a novel tool for anxiety assessment in children. J Dent Anesth Pain Med 2019; 19(4): 227-33. [http://dx.doi.org/10.17245/jdapm.2019.19.4.227] [PMID: 31501781]

[7] Prasad M, Nasreen A, Krishna A, Devi G. Novel Animated Visual Facial Anxiety/Pain Rating Scale-Its reliability, and validity in assessing dental pain/anxiety in children. Pediatr Dent J 2020; 5(3): 1-8.

CHAPTER 3

Psychological Development of a Child

H. Sharath Chandra[1,*], **M.H. Raghunath Reddy**[1] and **Vidya Iyer**[2]

[1] *SJM Dental College and Hospital, Chitradurga, Karnataka, India*

[2] *CSI College of Dental Sciences and Research, Madurai, Tamil Nadu 625001, India*

Abstract: Child psychology is an important part of paediatric dentistry, which acts as a guide for understanding children who are in different stages of physical, mental, emotional, and social development. Understanding the psychological development of the child helps in professional recognition of the child's needs, fear and anxiety at each stage which helps in better execution of behaviour management techniques. Child psychology provides an insight into principles of behaviour management that should be tailor-made for each child for effective and efficient dental treatment. This would enable the child to have a better and more pleasant dental visit, and also give the clinician a sense of professional satisfaction and reduce the fatigue in treating an uncooperative child.

Keywords: Child psychology, Behaviour management, Emotional development, Fear.

INTRODUCTION

Paediatric dentistry has evolved into a challenging speciality in which understanding the stages of psychological evolution of children is of utmost importance for correct diagnosis and achieving successful treatment. Understanding the psychology of the child helps in building a better relationship with the child and in gaining the child's trust which can eliminate fear and anxiety of dental procedures [1].

Psychologic growth and development of the child occurs gradually in a relatively predictable, logical and step-like sequential order which can be influenced by genetic, familial, cultural, inter-personal and intra-psychic factors. Psychological changes are examined in physical, cognitive, and social/emotional development across the lifespan. The Paediatric dentist needs to identify differences between

* **Corresponding author H. Sharath Chandra:** SJM Dental College and Hospital, Chitradurga, Karnataka, India; E-mail: sharathchandrah2012@gmail.com

each phase of a child's psychological development and the needs of the child at different levels to gain better compliance during the dental procedure.

Definition

Psychology is defined as a branch of science dealing with human and animal behaviour and related mental processes.

Child psychology is defined as the science that deals with the mental power or interaction between the conscious and subconscious elements in a child **(Kenneth Clark and George Miller, 1970).**

Importance of Child Psychology

- To treat the child more effectively and efficiently.
- To incorporate knowledge of cognitive and emotional development of the child.
- To improve patient compliance so that the dental procedure would be more comfortable for the child.
- Sense of calmness and security to the parent.
- It also brings a sense of professional satisfaction to the dental team, and it also becomes less stressful to treat an uncooperative child.
- Improves better promotion of child oral health [2].

Theories of Child Psychology

Classified into Psychodynamic and Behaviour learning theory (Fig. **1**):

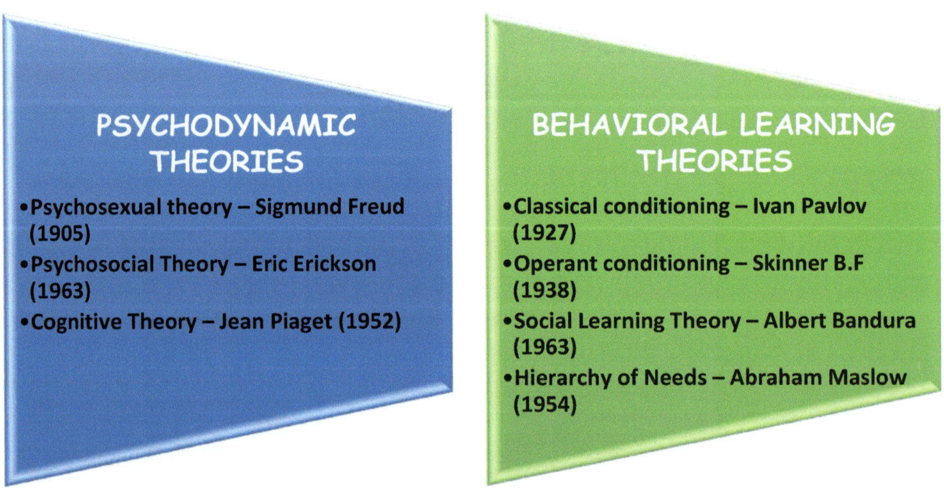

Fig. (1). Classification of theories of Child Psychology.

PSYCHODYNAMIC THEORIES

Psychosexual/ Psychoanalytic Theory

It was put forth by Austrian psychoanalyst and neurologist *Sigmund Freud*, who is often considered the first psychological theorist and pioneer of modern psychology. Freud emphasized the developmental aspects of personality and the decisive role of the early experiences during infancy and childhood in laying down the basic character structure of an adult person.

Freud developed a ***topographical model*** of the mental apparatus of the mind, which he divided into three systems based on awareness (Fig. **2**).

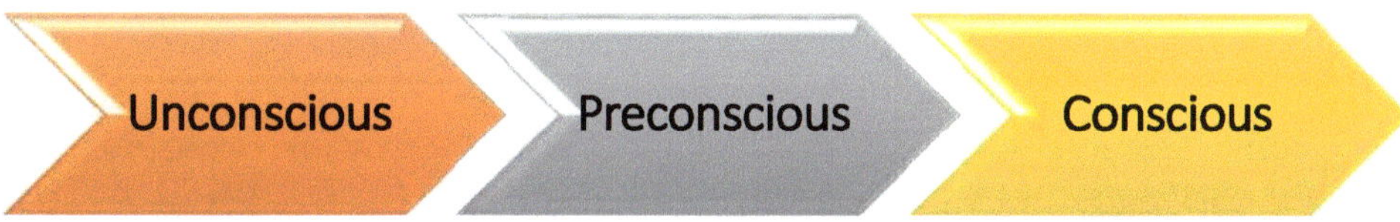

Fig. (2). Levels of awareness.

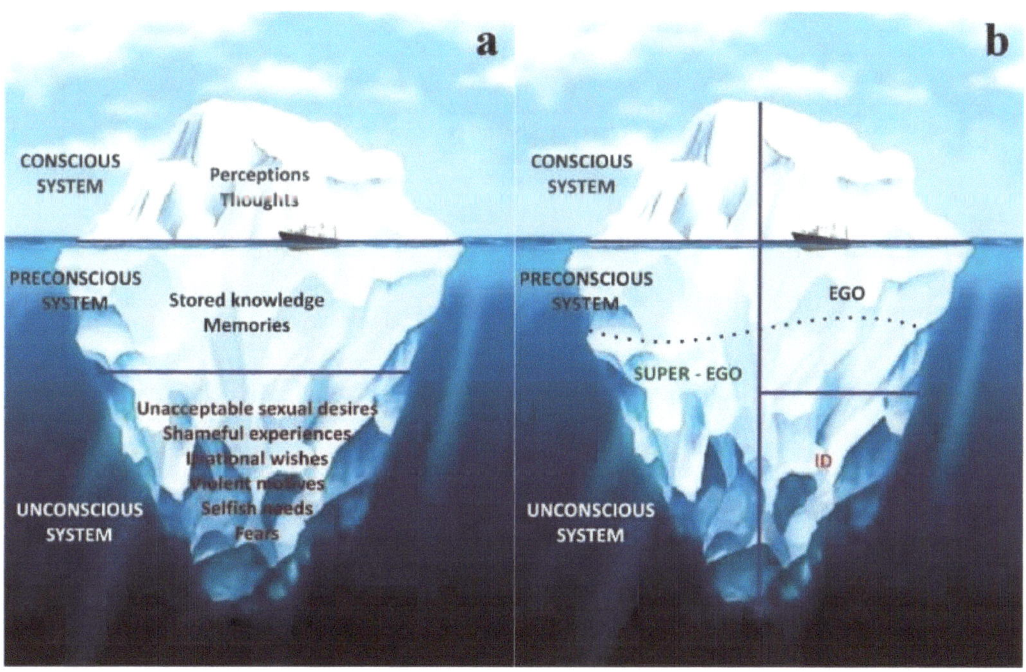

Fig. (3). a b. Freud's Topographical model.

He compared the mental process of the mind to an iceberg in water. The conscious mind is the only tip of the iceberg of what we see, which includes perceptions and thoughts; a person is aware of this system of the mind. But deep inside the mind, preconscious and unconscious systems are present, like below the water level iceberg is bigger than the tip of the iceberg. Thoughts stored in the preconscious system are brought to consciousness, whereas thoughts in the unconscious system influence the conscious system (Fig. **3a**).

Mental processes are either Unconscious or Conscious based upon the system they belong to. The unconscious system operates via the primary process, whereas Preconscious and Conscious systems operate via the secondary process. This topographical model was later included in Freud's revised structural model of personality, which comprises of Id, ego, and superego (Fig. **3b**).

To analyse Freud's developmental theories, his structural theory of mind should be addressed. It states that the psyche (personality) comprises three psychic structures: the Id, ego, and superego; also called the psychic triad (Fig. **4a, b**).

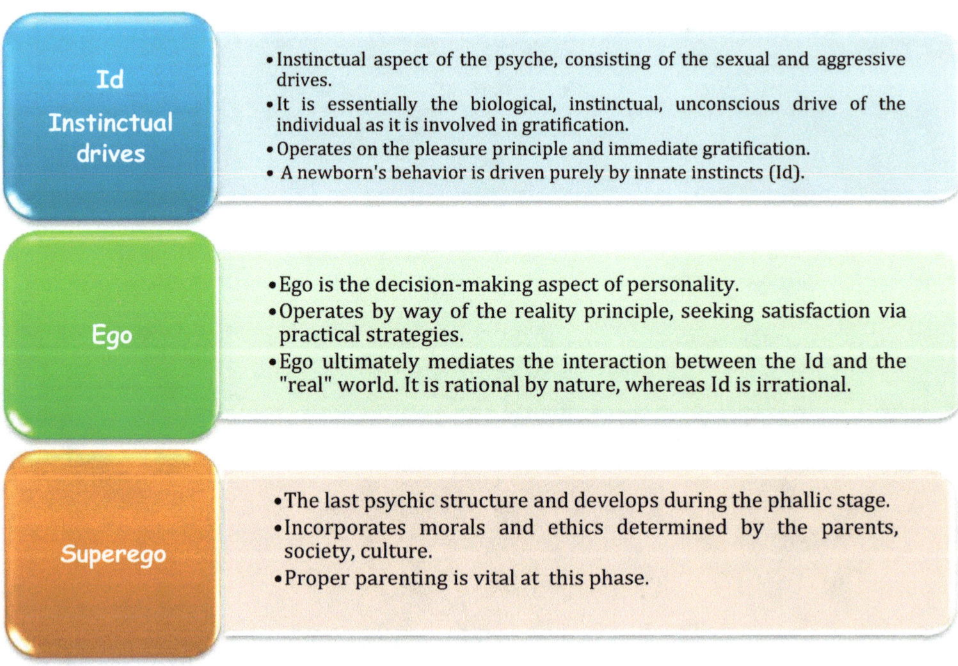

Fig. (4a). Psychic triad.

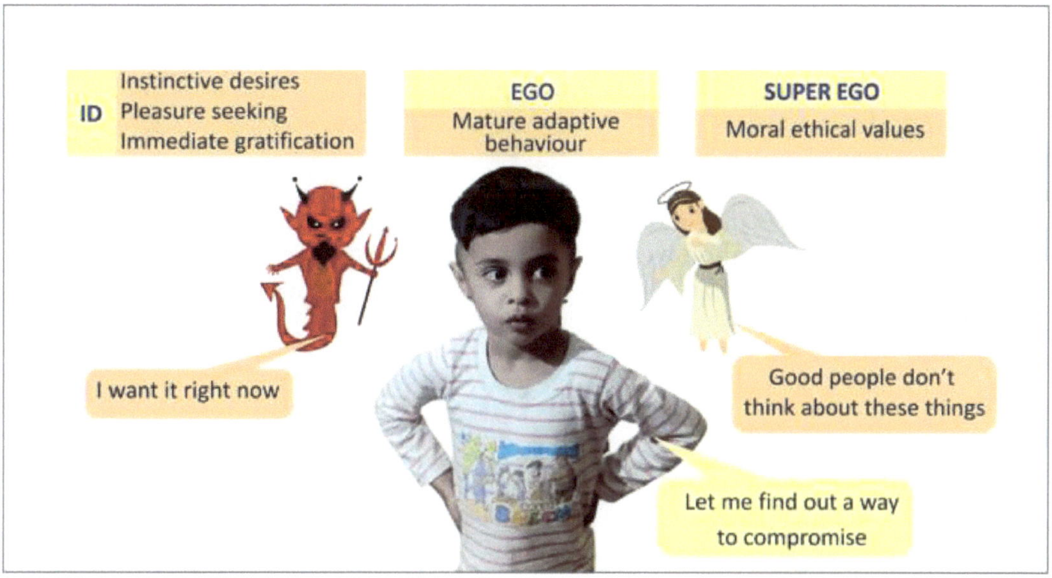

Fig. (4b). Psychic triad.

Psychosexual Development

Freud organised psychosexual development of personality into 5 stages (Fig. **5**).

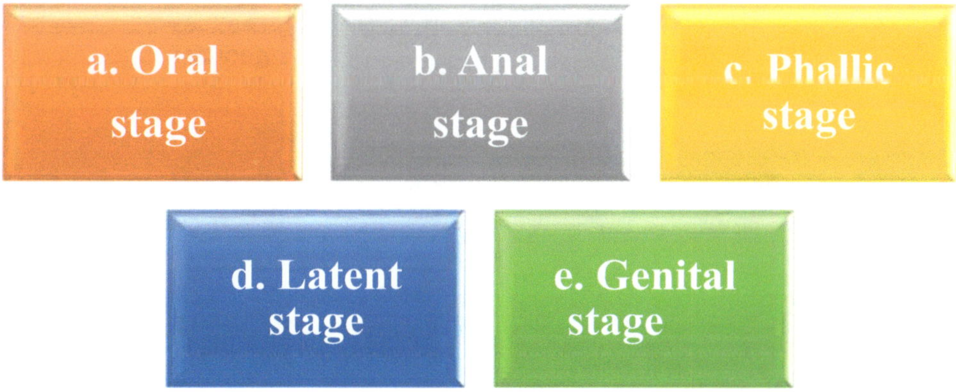

Fig. (5). Stages of Psychosexual development.

According to Freud, during the life span of an individual, they pass through a series of developmental stages which are dynamically differentiated and characterized by distinct modes of functioning.

Each stage is characterised by the concentration of different instincts or libido on different areas of the body, which are termed as ***Erogenous zones***. Freud regarded the instincts as a psychophysiological process, which has both mental and physical manifestations. The psychosexual energy or ***Libido*** is the driving force behind behaviour [3].

An erogenous zone is a part of the skin or mucous membrane which is extremely sensitive to irritation and, when manipulated in a certain way, produces pleasurable feelings and experiences, thus removing the irritation (Fig. **6**).

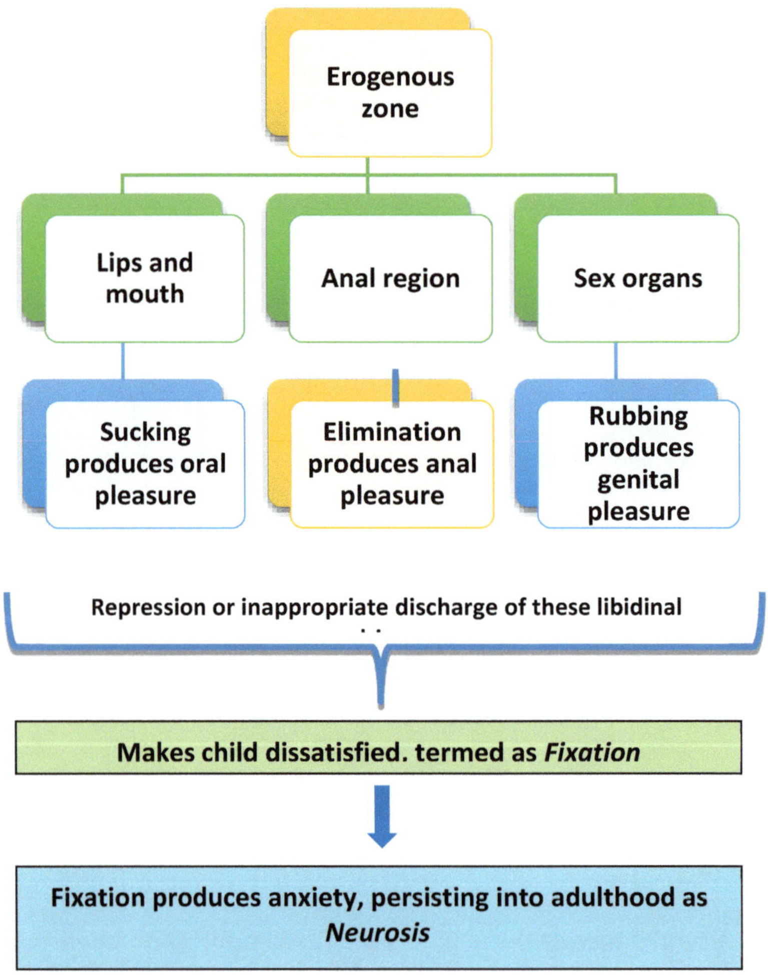

Fig. (6). Erogenous zones.

a. Oral stage: This stage starts from birth till eighteen months of age. The ***Erogenous zone*** is the mouth which is the primary means of interaction; ***gratification*** is achieved by oral stimulation, mainly by the sucking reflex and rooting reflex. The infant's need to seek pleasure is adequately met by sucking the breast of the mother and the child's dependence on the mother making her first love object which develops a sense of trust. Inadequate gratification leads to ***fixation*** of libidinal energy resulting in latent aggressive or passive tendencies. Oral fixation may result in the development of certain deleterious habits like thumb sucking, nail-biting, alcoholism, smoking *etc.* in future ages.

b. Anal stage: This stage starts from 18 months till 3yrs of age. The ***Erogenous zone*** is the anal region, ***gratification*** is achieved by the expulsion of faeces which removes discomfort and produces a feeling of relief.

Parents who utilize praise and rewards for using the toilet at the appropriate time obtain positive outcomes and help the children feel capable, productive, and creative adults.

During toilet training, the child faces increased chances to be reprimanded by parents or caretakers, feeling of inadequacy and an increased negative perception about parents or caretakers if he fails to perform appropriately. In this stage, fixation can exhibit anal expulsiveness (Whimsical disorganization) or anal retentiveness (Incessant orderliness).

c. Phallic stage: This stage starts from 3yrs till 6yrs of age. The Erogenous ***zone*** is the genitals, and children seek gratification by rubbing it. Urination is an important activity as it helps the child to integrate its gender identity. A boy identifies himself as a boy; similarly, a girl identifies herself as a girl initially from the process of urination.

The child's fantasy life is set up in this stage with the development of the Oedipus complex in boys and the Electra complex in girls, which are recreations of the phallic stage. With the emergence of these complexes, the child possesses a sexual attachment for the parent of the opposite sex and a hostile feeling toward the parent of the same sex (Fig. **7a & b**).

Freud advocates that the differences in the resolution of Oedipus and Electra complexes are the basis for many psychological differences between the sexes. At this stage, infantile sexuality tends to end because of social consequences and the realization of an unattainable love object.

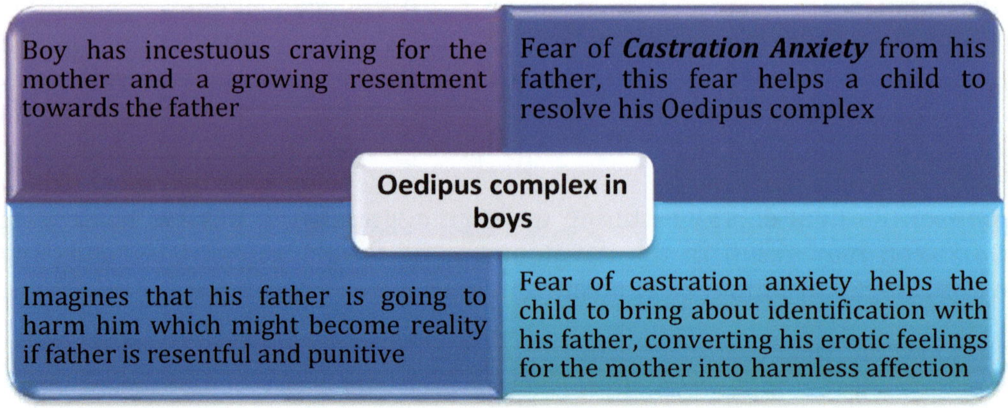

Fig. (7a). Oedipus complex.

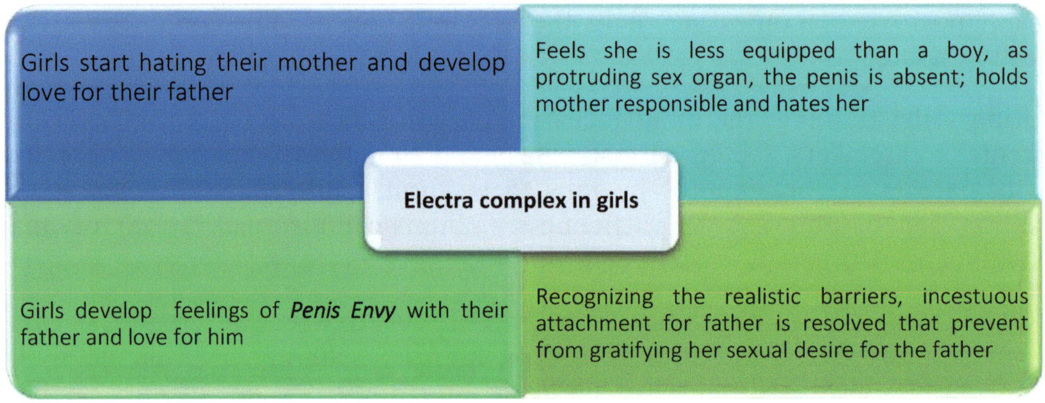

Fig. (7b). Electra complex in girls.

d. Latent stage: This stage starts from 6yrs to 12 yrs of age. There is no erogenous zone in this stage and sexual feelings are dormant. The child uses all his energy in academics, sports recreational activities and tends to build social relationships. The child diverts all his attention to being competent and proving himself, thus attaining self-confidence (Fig. **8**). Id's energy is suppressed, and the development of ego and superego takes over. Dysfunction at this stage results in immaturity and the inability to form healthy relationships as an adult.

e. Genital stage: This stage starts with the onset of adolescence. Sexual feelings reappear with new intensity and are more mature. An individual's ego develops fully and there is a transformation from a pleasure-seeking, self-loving child to a reality-oriented and socialized adult. Sexual attraction, genuine heterosexual relationships, socialization, group activities, vocational planning, and preparations for marrying and raising a family begin to manifest, getting established by the end of adolescence. Any dysfunction during this period, the child or young adult will be unable to develop meaningful, healthy relationships.

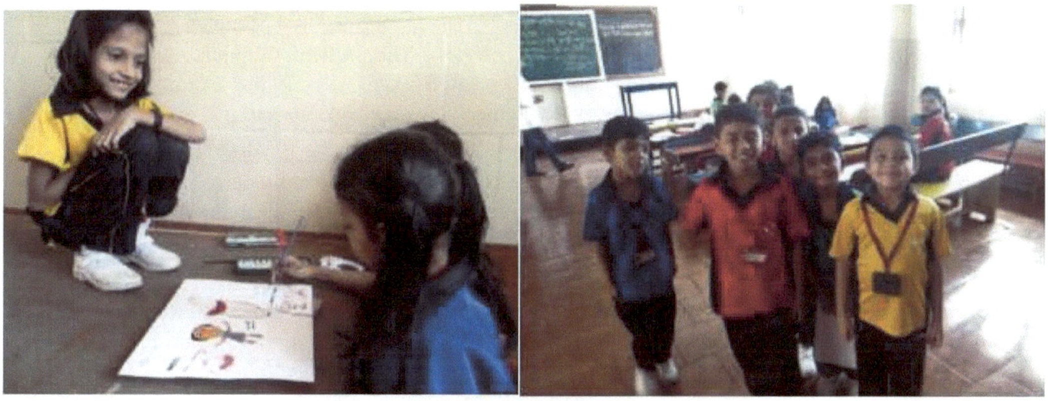

Fig. (8). Child building social relations and getting involved in recreational activities.

Ego finds a way out by unconscious resources in resolving conflicts with Id and superego to protect against anxiety and internal stress created by instinctual drives. Anna Freud, daughter of Sigmund Freud, defined and analysed a few major defence mechanisms (Table **1**).

Table 1. Ego Defence.

Ego Defences	Example
Repression: Burying of memories that are in the subconscious system to avoid disturbing or painful thoughts entering the conscious mind.	Repression and pushing down aggressive thoughts about same-sex parents as seen in Oedipus complex.
Denial: It involves a refusal to accept reality or to perceive it or even its existence, thus blocking external events from awareness.	Student denies bad performance in exams even after failing exams.
Projection: Individual ascribes his unwanted thoughts, motives, and feelings, especially which are aggressive and sexual fantasies or thoughts, onto another person.	The student projects his bad performance at school onto the teachers.
Displacement: Deflection of an aggressive impulse onto a powerless substitute target which can be an object or a person.	A Student performing badly at school comes back home and kicks his toy.
Sublimation: It is like displacement, but in this displacement of unacceptable emotions into more constructive and socially acceptable behaviour rather than destructive activities.	Displeasure occurred in the oral stage of development may lead to thumb-sucking or nail-biting in the future.

(Table 1) cont.....

Ego Defences	Example
Identification with the aggressor: It involves an individual who adopts the behaviour of a person who is more powerful and hostile towards them. He realises himself as a victim and identifies with the aggressor to gain empathy for the aggressor.	Stockholm Syndrome, where hostages or victims establish an emotional bond with their captors or abusers to gain their empathy and overcome their behaviours.
Rationalization: Making an impulse or an event less threatening by cognitive distortion of "the facts". It is often done fairly on a conscious level when they provide themselves with excuses.	The student rationalizes copying in the exam saying the exam paper was too tough to answer.
Reaction formation: Individual goes beyond denial and behaves in the opposite way to which he or she thinks or feels, converting unwanted or dangerous thoughts, and impulses into the opposite way.	When the individual is not able to control their temper, he starts to laugh loudly.
Regression: Reverting to a behaviour that is immature considering their age of development.	Throwing temper tantrums as an adult when they do not get things their way.
Introjection: Individual shows unconscious imitation.	Child enacts and dresses up like a superhero

Psychosocial Theory

It was introduced by the psychologist and psychoanalyst Erik Erikson, which is built upon Sigmund Freud's psychosexual development theory by drawing parallels in childhood stages and expanding it to include the influence of social dynamics as well as the extension of psychosocial development into adulthood.

Erikson divided human psychosocial development into eight stages called Crisis which are influenced by biological, psychological, and social factors throughout the lifespan. The Crisis needs should be resolved in order, for an individual to develop socially and emotionally. The outcome of the stage is determined by the child's environment and the caregiving strategies or experiences to which children are exposed.

As the individual grows, different stages arise, and they face new decisions and turning points during childhood, adolescence, and adulthood. Each stage is represented by two opposing psychological tendencies.

- Positive/syntactic
- Negative/dystonic.

Ego virtue/strength or maldevelopment arises respectively from these opposing psychological tendencies. If the virtue/ strength is adopted, it can help resolve the current decision or conflict and facilitate subsequent stages of development. The opposite is true if the maldeveloped quality is adopted [4] (Figs. **9** & **10**).

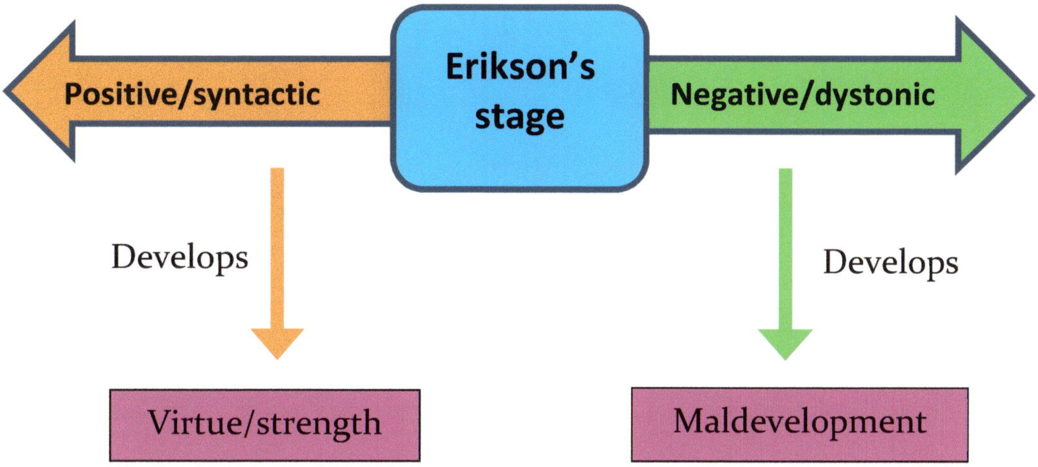

Fig. (9). Schematic representation of Erikson's stage.

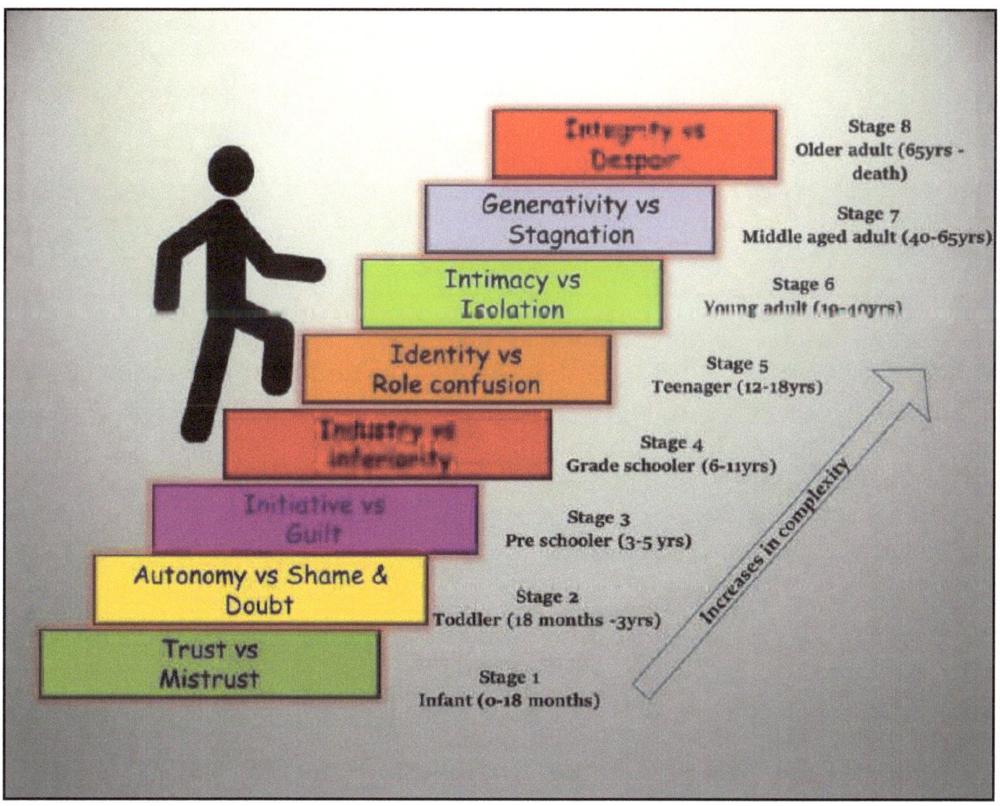

Fig. (10). Stages of Erik EriksonsPsychosocial Theory.

Stages of Erik Erikson's Psychosocial Theory (Fig. 10)

Stage 1: *Seen in Infant (0- 18 months)*

Crisis: Trust *vs* Mistrust

What happens in this stage: The child develops a sense of belief in the environment, especially parents or caregivers and develops a strong bond to meet his or her basic physiological needs like hunger and social needs like love and affection. If the needs are met infant develops a sense of trust. If parents/caregivers are inconsistent, rejecting, or emotionally unavailable, it leads to feelings of mistrust (Fig. **11**).

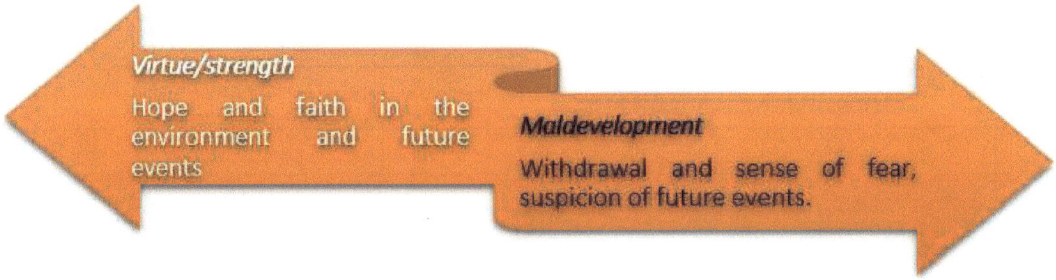

Fig. (11). Favourable and unfavourable outcomes of Stage 1.

Dental Implications

- Children of this age have separation anxiety.
- Any dental treatment at this age should be provided preferably in the presence of parent or caregiver by lap-to-lap technique or child sitting on the lap of parent on a dental chair so that child develops a sense of trust in the environment.
- In case the child develops mistrust, he becomes an uncooperative and frightened child in the future.

Stage 2: *Seen in Toddler (18 months -3 yrs)*

Crisis: Autonomy *vs* Shame & Doubt

What happens in this stage: Children tend to show will and want to do things for themselves, giving them a sense of independence. They tend to move away from mother and develop an individual identity. Toddlers tend to walk, talk, and use the toilet (control over sphincters) show determination for self-control and confidence. The child develops a sense of determination in doing what he/she can control and a sense of regret and sorrow for inappropriate use of self-control (Fig. **12**).

Stage 3: *Seen in Pre-schooler (3-5 yrs)*

Crisis: Initiative *vs* Guilt

What happens in this stage: Children tend to show greater autonomy, initiate motor and intellectual activities and show a keen interest in undertaking tasks. They tend to imitate the people they like, play with peers and other social interactions. Parent/ Caregiver should encourage, support, and guide the child's initiatives and interests. On successfully passing this stage, children feel capable and able to lead others, failure leads to self-doubt, a sense of guilt and a lack of initiative (Fig. **13**).

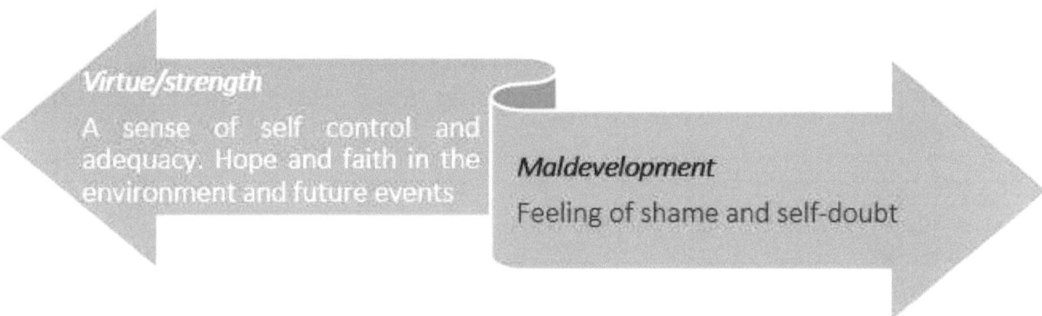

Fig. (12). Favourable and unfavourable outcomes of Stage 2.

Dental Implications

- Even though children develop a sense of autonomy and move away from their mother, they should not be separated from their mothers during dental visits as they might feel threatened.
- Parents should not be overprotective.
- The dentist should allow the child to sit on the dental chair on his own, on/off the dental chair light, provide options and make the child feel special.
- If the child fails in being autonomous during dental visits, reassurances from the parent and dentist will boost their confidence which will ensure cooperation in future visits.

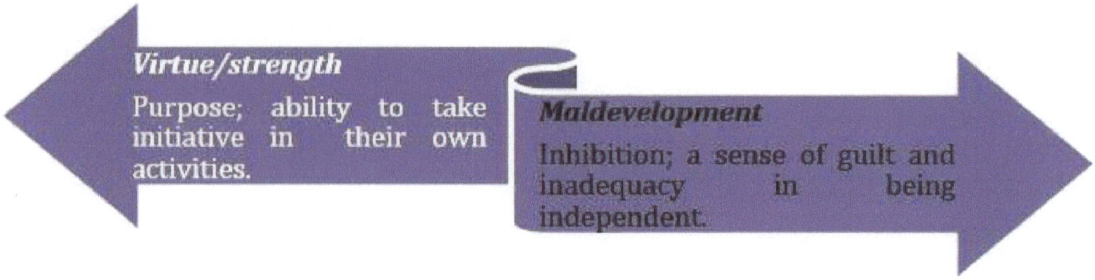

Fig. (13). Favourable and unfavourable outcomes of Stage 3.

Dental Implications

- A dental visit at this stage will be more curious for the child and parents should encourage them to view it as a new adventure.
- The dental team should teach the child and allow him to explore more about various things in the dental setup to overcome fear and anxiety.
- They should be given the task of maintaining oral hygiene and taught brushing techniques.

Stage 4: *Seen in grade-schooler (6-11 yrs)*

Crisis: Industry *vs* Inferiority

What happens in this stage: A child in this stage adopts an organised way of learning, inculcates the ability to work takes pride in work completion and accomplishments. Children tend to become industrious and master their skills. They build peer relations and set up a competition in the competitive world. Motivation and encouragement of children by parents and teachers develop a feeling of competence & belief in their skills. On the contrary, those who receive little or no encouragement will result in doubting their ability to be successful. Failure might result in a feeling of inferiority and low self-esteem (Fig. **14**).

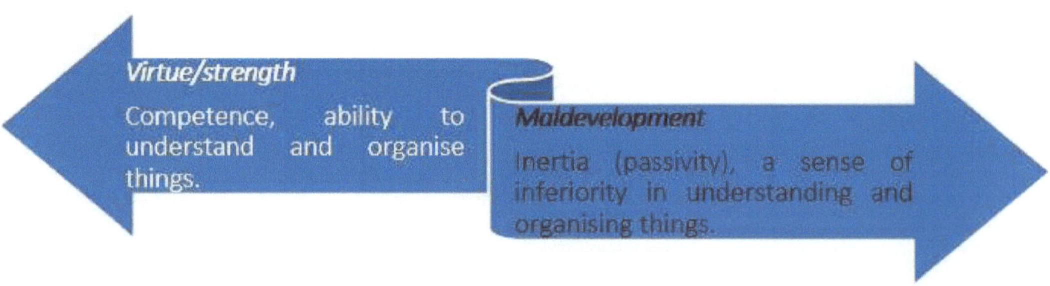

Fig. (14). Favourable and unfavourable outcomes of Stage 4.

Dental Implications

- Children at this stage try to learn and understand what is needed to please the dentist and parent. The desired behaviour should be positively reinforced by the dentist and parent, so the child is cooperative throughout the procedure.
- The dentist should set short term goals like using a triple syringe or air suction, where they take pride in work accomplishment.
- There is a decline of the influence of parents as role models and an inclination towards peer group influence, which can be utilised by the dentist for motivating the child about the esthetics and orthodontic correction of the teeth to look pleasing.

Stage 5: *Seen in Teenager (12-18 yrs)*

Crisis: Identity *vs* Role confusion

What happens in this stage: Children in this stage contemplate their previous experiences, and societal expectations, aspire to establish values and find themselves. They tend to isolate themselves from their parents and explore independence, relish being themself, thus creating personal identity. Peer group influence accentuates making them more confused, and they lack decision-making ability and choices. They will come out of this stage with a strong self-belief, a feeling of independence and control with proper encouragement and reassurances. On the contrary, if they remain unsure of their beliefs and desires, they will be insecure, which results in confusion about themselves and their future (Fig. **15**).

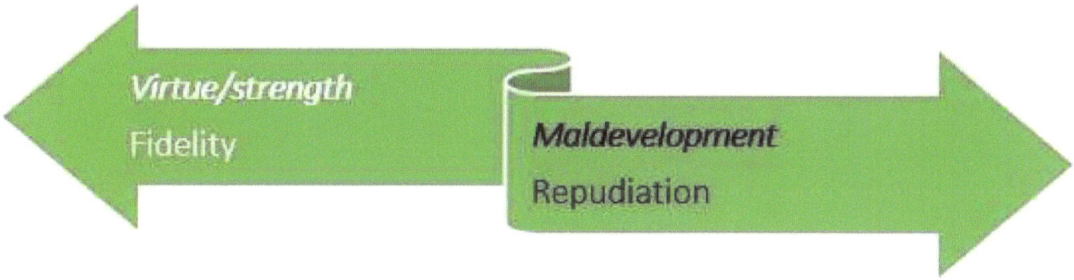

Fig. (15). Favourable and unfavourable outcomes of Stage 5.

Dental Implications

- A dental visit at this stage for any treatment is more dictated by peer influence rather than parental pressure.
- Most of the dental procedures would be orthodontic and aesthetic correction as they are more concerned about their appearance and being socially acceptable.

Stage 6: *Seen in Young adults (19-40 yrs)*

Crisis: Intimacy *vs* Isolation

What happens in this stage: Individuals at this stage tend to explore personal relationships, forming close friendships or long-term partnerships. Erikson's every step builds on skills learned in previous steps. Erikson believed that to develop intimate relationships, a strong sense of personal identity was important, failure of which develops fear of forming a committed relationship and are more likely to suffer emotional isolation, loneliness, and depression (Fig. **16**).

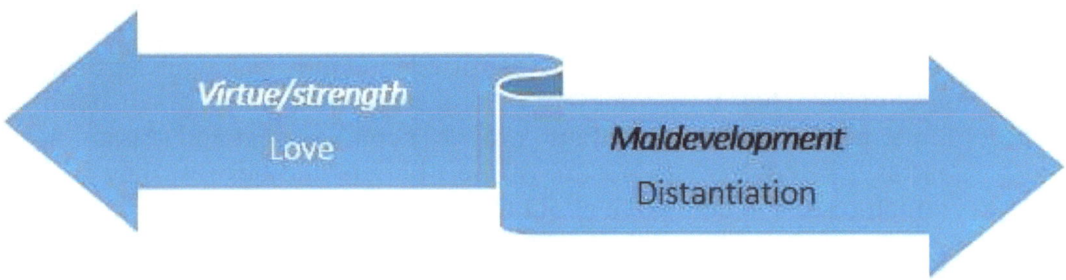

Fig. (16). Favourable and unfavourable outcomes of Stage 6.

Dental Implication

External appearances are dominant among the individuals in this stage as it is important to form an intimate relationship. Hence the individuals seek orthodontic correction of malocclusion and aesthetic correction of teeth.

Stage 7: *Seen in middle-aged adults (40-65 yrs)*

Crisis: Generativity *vs* Stagnation

What happens in this stage: Generativity is engaging oneself in establishing and guiding the next generation through parenting, coaching, or teaching. It is expressed through socially valued work and disciples, thus creating a living legacy. During adulthood, individuals strive hard to build their lives, focusing on career and family. Successful individuals in this stage will perceive that they are contributing to the world by being active in their home and community; failure at this stage will make them feel unproductive and uninvolved in the world. Stagnation develops in self-concerned people, isolation, and the absence of intimacy (Fig. **17**).

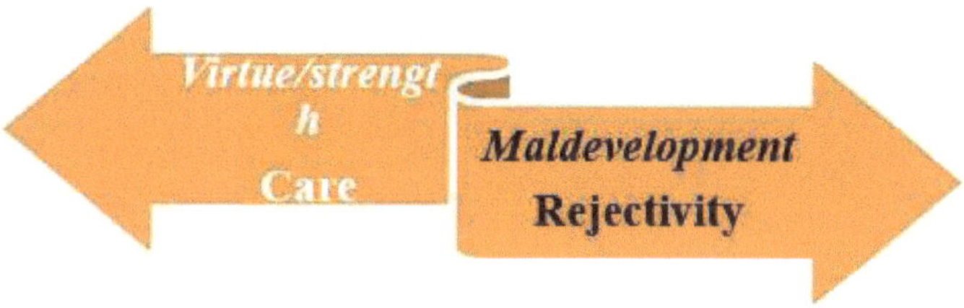

Fig. (17). Favourable and unfavourable outcomes of Stage 7.

Stage 8: *Seen in the older adults (65 yrs - death)*

Crisis: Integrity vs. Despair

What happens in this stage: This stage occurs during old age and is focused on reflecting on life by contemplating and acknowledging one's life accomplishments. Individuals who feel proud of their accomplishments will feel a sense of integrity and will attain wisdom, even when confronting death. Erikson stated healthy children would not fear life if their elders have integrity enough not to fear death. Those who are unsuccessful during this phase experience many regrets and will be left with feelings of bitterness and despair (Fig. **18**).

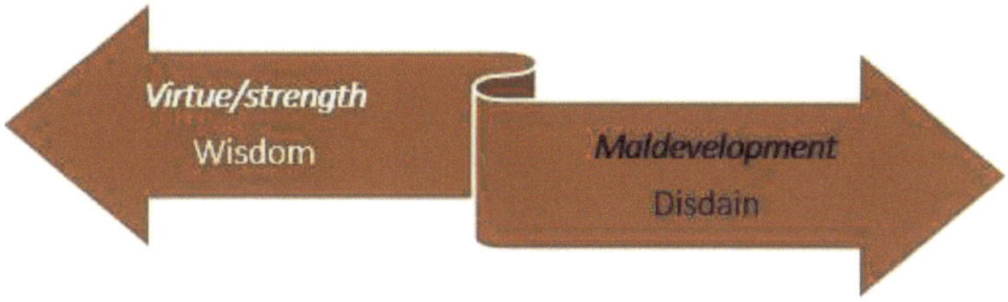

Fig. (18). Favourable and unfavourable outcomes of Stage 8.

Cognitive Theory

It was proposed by Swiss psychologist Jean Piaget who was the most popular psychologist of his era. According to Jean Piaget, the cognitive development of the child occurs as they pass through a series of stages, and at each stage, interaction between a child's innate abilities and environment occurs. Thus, helping the child to build knowledge and intelligence, which changes as the child grows.

Piaget put forward his assumptions about children's intelligence:

- Children think and see the world differently, their intelligence differs in quality rather than quantity compared to adults.
- Children are active learners and actively build up their knowledge about the environment.
- One must-see thing from a child's point of view to understand children's reasoning.

Piaget stated that infants at birth have a certain basic cognitive or mental structure genetically inherited and evolved, which he termed as Schema. Future learning and knowledge of the child are based on this mental structure called Schema [5].

Schema is defined as: "A cohesive, repeatable action sequence possessing component actions that are tightly interconnected and governed by a core meaning" according to Piaget (1952).

Hence schema is a building block or elementary unit of intelligent behaviour, which is a way of organising knowledge and helps individuals sculpt a mental representation of the world. With the progressive maturation of an individual's mental or thought processes, the number and complexity of schemata escalate.

Intellectual growth or building knowledge of an individual occurs by process of adaptation to the environment by three components [5] (Fig. **19**).

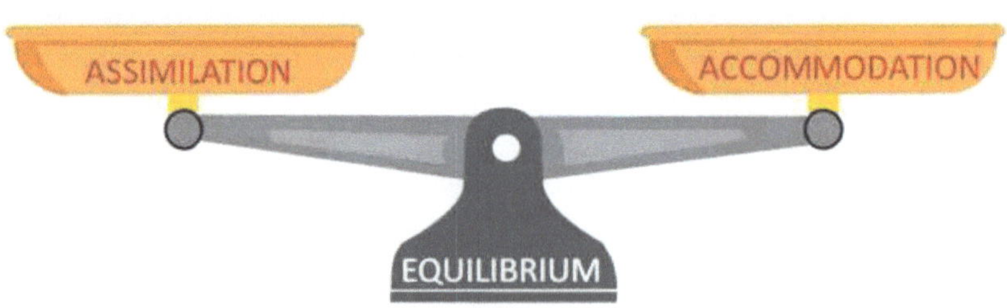

Fig. (19). Components of adaptation.

1. Assimilation

2. Accommodation

3. Equilibration.

1) Assimilation: It is the process of gathering new information to an already existing schema within the self. Assimilation does not change existing schema or perception; it only influences it.

e.g., a) Child sees a four-legged animal for the first time, mother tells it a doggy and child assimilates that information as 'a four-legged animal as doggy'.

b) Sees a flying thing, mother tells it a bird, and child assimilates it as 'flying things as bird'.

2) Accommodation: It is a process of modifying an already existing schema with new information. This may give rise to a new schema. The existing schema does not match the current situation or object; hence it must be modified with new information.

e.g., a) Child sees a cat and calls it a doggy as it is four-legged, mother tells it is not doggy and gives new information that it is a cat. The child assimilates this new information and modifies the existing schema.

b) Child sees a fly and calls it a bird, on modifying that it is a fly, child modifies existing schema.

This happens when the existing schema (knowledge) does not work and needs to be changed to deal with a new object or situation.

3) Equilibration: When any new information is assimilated, there is resistance to altering the existing scheme occurring through accommodation. This disagreement between assimilation and accommodation is resolved by equilibration, which draws evenness between them. Every individual seeks equilibration in their cognitive development, which helps them move from one stage to another in their intellectual growth.

Stages of Cognitive Development

According to Piaget, a child passes through 4 stages of cognitive development, and with every stage passing, the child's thoughts become more sophisticated and attain cognitive equilibrium [5] (Fig. **20**).

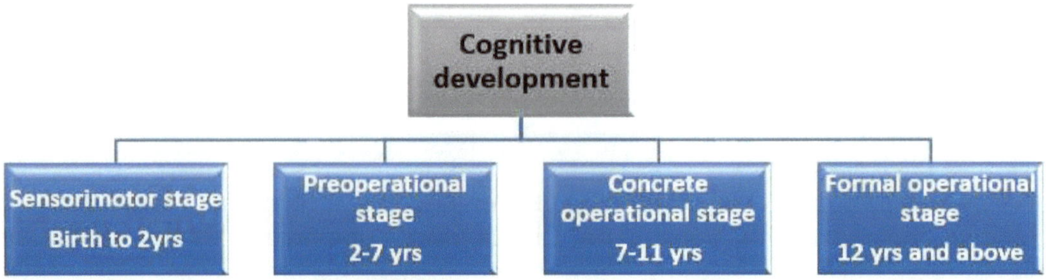

Fig. (20). Stages of Cognitive development.

a. Sensorimotor Stage (Birth to 2yrs)

Infant explores the world using sensory and motor abilities to develop a range of cognitive abilities. During the early stages of the sensorimotor stage basic reflexes, senses, and motor responses like sucking, grasping, looking, listening, crying, and moving his/her arms, predominately the trunk. Using these reflexes and responses the infants progressively attain knowledge and understand the environment. This stage is divided into 6 substages (Fig. **21**).

a. Simple reflex stage (birth to 6 weeks)
b. Primary circular reactions (6 weeks to 4 months)
c. Secondary circular reactions (4 and 8 months)
d. Coordination of secondary circular reactions (8-12 months)
e. Tertiary circular reactions (12 and 18 months)
f. Start of mental representation (18 months to 24 months)

This stage is considered as a period of rapid cognitive growth. The infant gains direct knowledge of the environment by using sensory reflexes, motor abilities and three adaptive processes. An infant also relates the result of the action performed through the assimilation and accommodation process, thus modifying the schema.

b. **Preoperational Stage (2-7 yrs)**

A child in this stage depicts objects by using words, and mental imagination and begins to think symbolically. The emergence of language occurs in this stage, the foundations of which are laid in the sensorimotor stage.

Thinking and language are better in this stage but their ability to think is still based on the child's judgement of the situation (intuitive), but not operational or logical or problem-solving. It is not how the world is, but it is how the child sees the world.

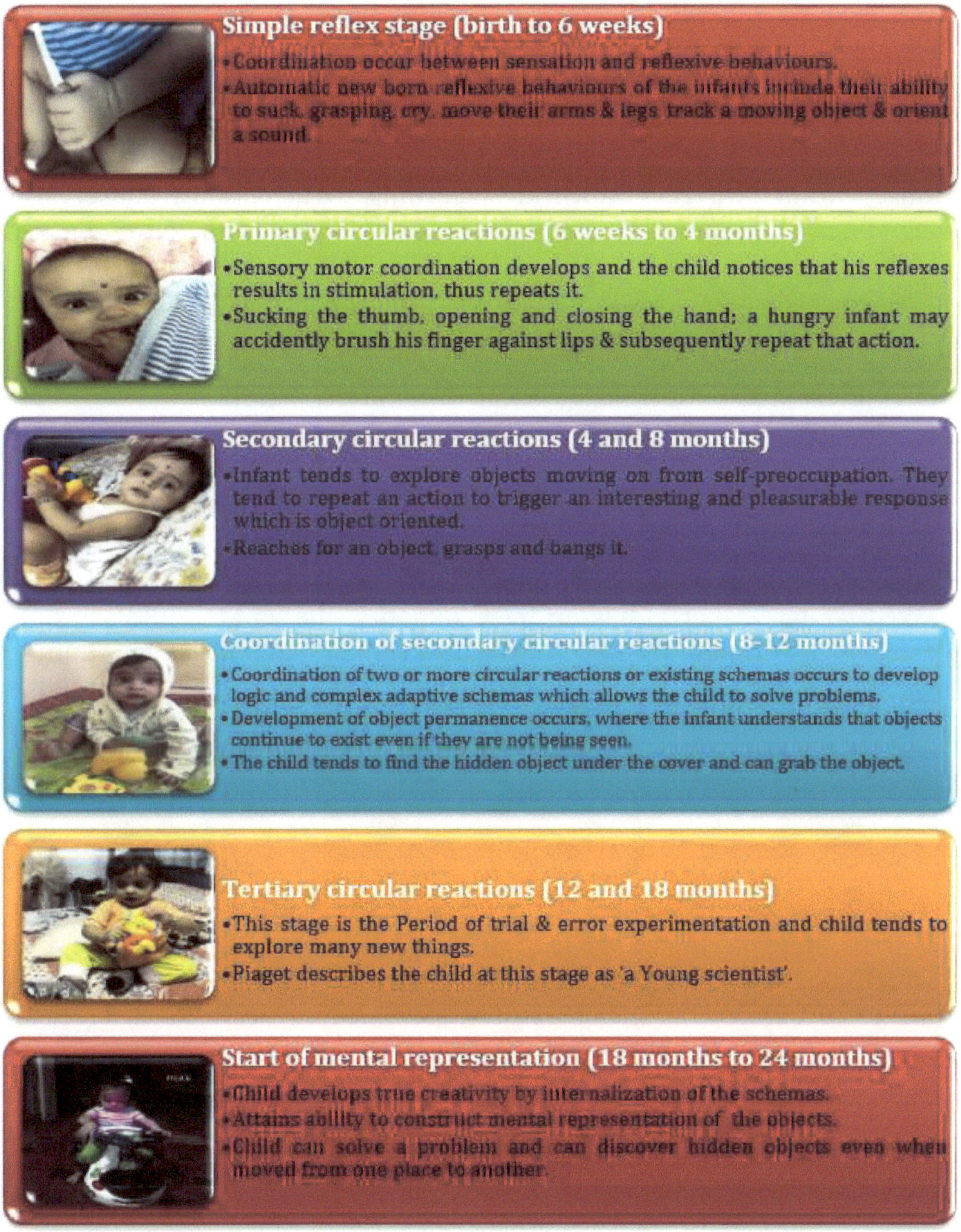
Simple reflex stage (birth to 6 weeks)
•Coordination occur between sensation and reflexive behaviours.
•Automatic new born reflexive behaviours of the infants include their ability to suck, grasping, cry, move their arms & legs track a moving object & orient a sound.
Primary circular reactions (6 weeks to 4 months)
•Sensory motor coordination develops and the child notices that his reflexes results in stimulation, thus repeats it.
•Sucking the thumb, opening and closing the hand; a hungry infant may accidently brush his finger against lips & subsequently repeat that action.
Secondary circular reactions (4 and 8 months)
•Infant tends to explore objects moving on from self-preoccupation. They tend to repeat an action to trigger an interesting and pleasurable response which is object oriented.
•Reaches for an object, grasps and bangs it.
Coordination of secondary circular reactions (8-12 months)
•Coordination of two or more circular reactions or existing schemas occurs to develop logic and complex adaptive schemas which allows the child to solve problems.
•Development of object permanence occurs, where the infant understands that objects continue to exist even if they are not being seen.
•The child tends to find the hidden object under the cover and can grab the object.
Tertiary circular reactions (12 and 18 months)
•This stage is the Period of trial & error experimentation and child tends to explore many new things.
•Piaget describes the child at this stage as 'a Young scientist'.
Start of mental representation (18 months to 24 months)
•Child develops true creativity by internalization of the schemas.
•Attains ability to construct mental representation of the objects.
•Child can solve a problem and can discover hidden objects even when moved from one place to another.

Fig. (21). Substages of sensorimotor stage.

This stage is divided into two substages:

a. Pre conceptual stage from 2-4yrs
b. Intuitive stage from 4-7yrs

The development of language and thinking in this stage is characterized by Egocentrism, Animism & Conservation [6, 7].

1) Conservation and reversibility: According to the law of conservation in physics, if any one aspect of measurable property changes, the other remains the same. This simple principle is applied to children with various experiments to see whether they understand such simple logic. But children of the preoperational stage lack conservation and reversibility.

Piaget conducted experiments on the conservation of volume, mass, number, length, quantity, area, and weight.

Volume: Classical Beaker Experiment

Two identical beakers of the same quantity of liquid are kept in front of the child and asked which beaker is having more quantity, the child would say both the beakers. The next liquid from one of the beakers is poured into a tall, thin beaker and asked the same question. The child would point out at the third beaker since the level of liquid is more (Fig. **22a**).

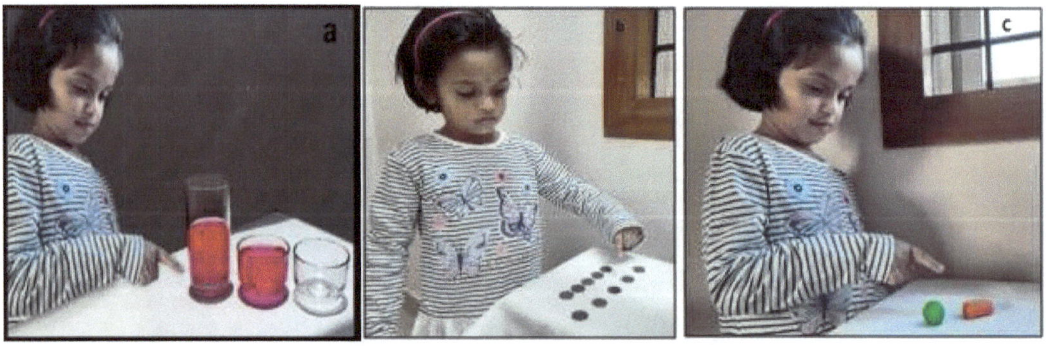

Fig. (22). a. Classical beaker experiment, **b.** Coin experiment, **c.** Clay experiment.

Number: Coin Experiment

Two identical rows consisting of the same number of coins are kept in front of the child and he/she would answer that both rows have an equal number of coins. The second row with the same number of coins are spread, and asked which row exhibits more coins, the child would answer as the second row since the length of the row is bigger (Fig. **22**b).

Mass: Clay Experiment

Two identical balls of clay are kept in front of the child, and then one of the clay balls is rolled into a sausage or flat pancake shape and asked which one is bigger. The child would answer sausage or flat pancake-shaped clay ball is bigger since the size of it is big compared to other clay balls (Fig. **22**c).

1. **Irreversibility** concept refers to a child's inability to mentally reverse the chain of events in conservation experiments.

e.g., The child could have rolled the sausage or flat pancake-shaped clay ball into the previous round shape, but they do not have the cognitive ability to do at this stage because of the concept of irreversibility.

1. **Centration:** Centration refers to a tendency the target attention only on one aspect of a situation or dimension while ignoring other dimensions or situations. The concept of cardinal numbers, conservation and reversibility, are based upon the concept of centration.
2. **Egocentrism:** It is the inability to take another's points of view or perspective and can only appreciate his/her perspective to a particular situation. Piaget assessed egocentrism through three mountain experiments.

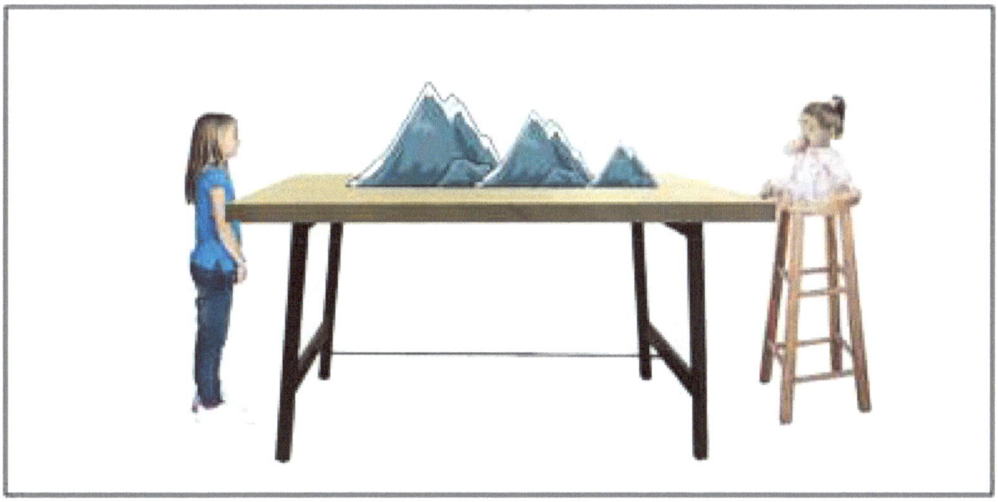

Fig. (23). Three mountain experiment.

Three mountains of different heights were placed on the table. A child and a doll are made to sit on either side of the mountains facing each other. The child is shown a series of photographs and asked which photograph matches the doll's view. The child would pick the photograph of what he/she sees from their side rather than the doll's view (Fig. **23**).

1. **Animism:** Tendency of the child to attribute properties of life to inanimate objects such as toys. Children tend to think that non-living things have life and feel that of a living person.

e. g. Children tend to eat along with their favourite doll and want to feed it; if the child gets grazed by a hit of the door, the child wants to hurt the door by hitting it back (Fig. **24a**).

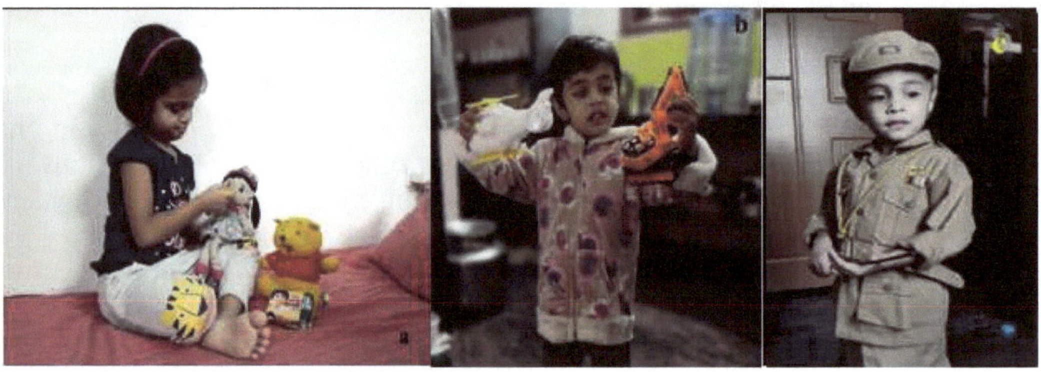

Fig. (24). a. Animism, **b.** Constructivism, **c.** Pretend play.

1. **Constructivism:** Children tend to think actively and are constantly trying to understand the world around them by observing, exploring, and touching the things in the environment (Fig. **24b**).
2. **Pretend play:** Children tend to pretend to be some other person and try to act like them (Fig. **24c**).

Clinical implications: Children tend to concentrate only on one aspect of the situation because of the concept of centration. Distracting the child during dental treatment by making him focus on the more pleasant, enjoyable aspects of the environment is very effective [5 - 7].

e.g., Talking about a favourite toy or cartoon character or using audio-visual distraction aids. Dental clinic ambiance should have intensely vivid colours with lots of toys around, a play area and an aquarium. So, the children tend to concentrate on a more striking and pleasing environment rather than fearsome instruments and the dental procedure.

Children tend to use symbols to represent objects and animism predominates. Hence use of euphemisms by Tell-Show-Do during the treatment procedure will be effective.

Egocentrism of the child should be put to good use during treatment. The child should be made manager of the saliva ejector and realise that treatment would stop & start on his hand signals, making him feel that he is the one controlling his treatment. Children should be allowed to make certain choices like which colour of the file or disposable drape, gloves to use *etc*.

Piaget termed children of this stage as young scientists. They should be taken to walk around dental clinics, making them know about various dental equipment, make them observe, touch, feel and use how it works. This makes them feel like a special person at that moment and helps to get acclimatised to the dental setup.

Pretend play predominates in this stage. Children are made to pretend like a dentist and are made to teach their favourite toy oral hygiene measures. This, in turn, makes the child follow those measures at home (Fig. **25**).

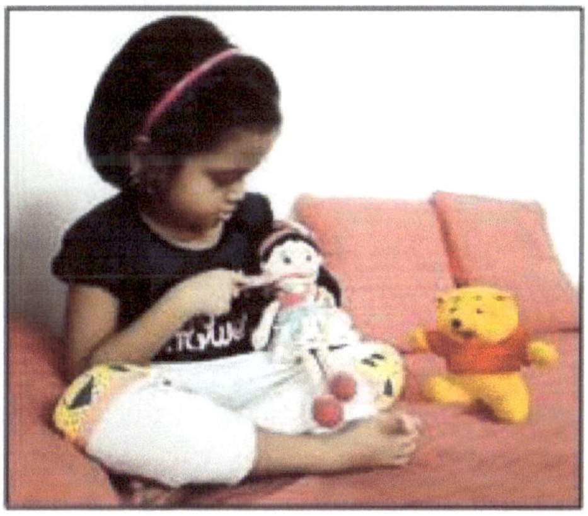

Fig. (25). Pretend play as dentist teaching oral hygiene measures.

Concrete Operational Stage (7-11 yrs)

According to Piaget, this stage is a major juncture in developing the cognitive ability of the child. Thinking becomes more logical or operational about a concrete situation and develops hypothetical concepts by reasoning.

Features of the stage

- Conservation
- Reversibility
- Decentration
- Seriation
- Transitivity
- Elimination of egocentrism

Conservation: A child in this stage understands the law of conservation that in a measurable property, even though one aspect of it changes, like appearance, the other aspect, like quantity, remains the same.

e.g., In the classical beaker experiment, a child understands that volume of the liquid is the same even though it is poured in a long and thin beaker.

In the coin experiment, a child understands that number of coins is the same even though the gap between the coins in the second row is increased.

Reversibility: The child understands that certain things which are changed can be reverted to their original state.

e.g., In the clay experiment child can reverse flat pancake or sausage-shaped clay into a previous round shape.

A child also understands that 5+5= 10 and 10-5= 5.

Decentration: It is the ability to concentrate on several aspects of objects or events simultaneously and understand the relation between the aspects, whereas children of the preoperational stage concentrate only on one aspect. The decentration feature helps to attain conservation in children.

e.g., In the classical beaker experiment, now the child understands the height of the beaker is also increased, the width of the glass is decreased. Hence the quantity of liquid is the same.

Seriation: Ability of the child to arrange objects methodically in order of quantified dimensions like weight or size.

Transitivity: It is the ability to understand the relation between different qualities or aspects of an object. (Fig. **26**).

Elimination of egocentrism: The feature of egocentrism that was seen in the preoperational stage is eliminated in this stage. Now the child can also think from others' points of view about a particular situation or aspect.

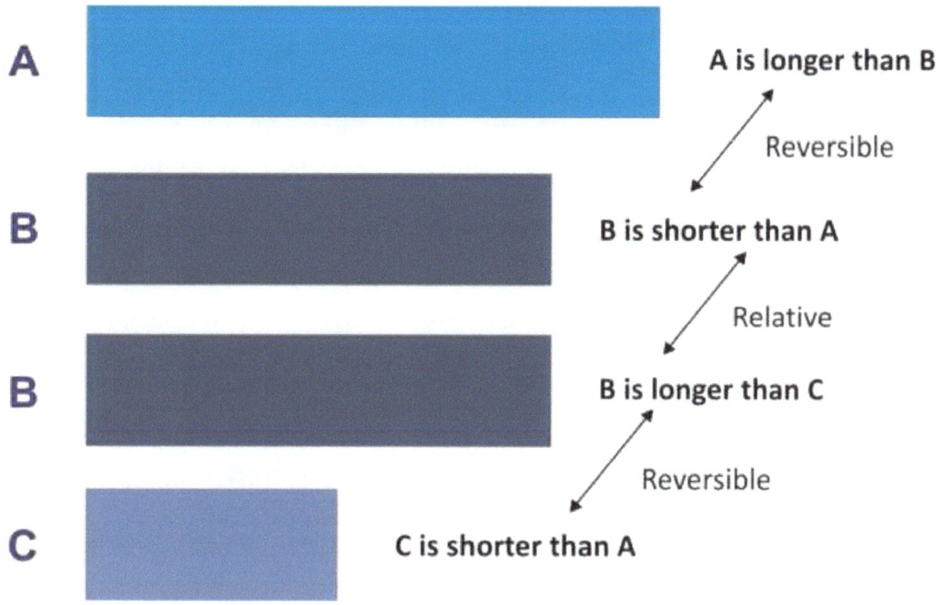

Fig. (26). Different lengths diagram.

e.g., Now the child can tell the view which doll can see in three mountain experiments.

Clinical Implications

- Concrete instructions can be given, like oral hygiene instructions for better maintenance of oral health.
- Maintenance of removable appliances and how to wear & remove it can be advised.
- Making the child get involved in the treatment. A mirror can be given to the child and make him understand how the treatment is being done.

Formal Operational Stage (12 Yrs and Above)

It is the final stage of cognitive development in which teens develop logic and abstract thinking. Individuals can formulate many potential solutions for a particular hypothetical problem or a situation in a systematic manner. Individuals develop scientific thinking and would solve problems with reasoning and logic.

Clinical Implications: Abstract thinking and peer influence have a huge role in this stage which can be utilised in motivating the teens for orthodontic and esthetics corrections.

BEHAVIOUR LEARNING THEORIES

Classical Conditioning Theory

It is proposed by Russian physiologist Ivan Pavlov is often referred to as Pavlovian conditioning. Classical conditioning theory involves linking together two stimuli to produce a new learned response in a person or animal [1, 8].

This theory was explained by Pavlov's classical experiments on the dog and is divided into three stages (Fig. **27**).

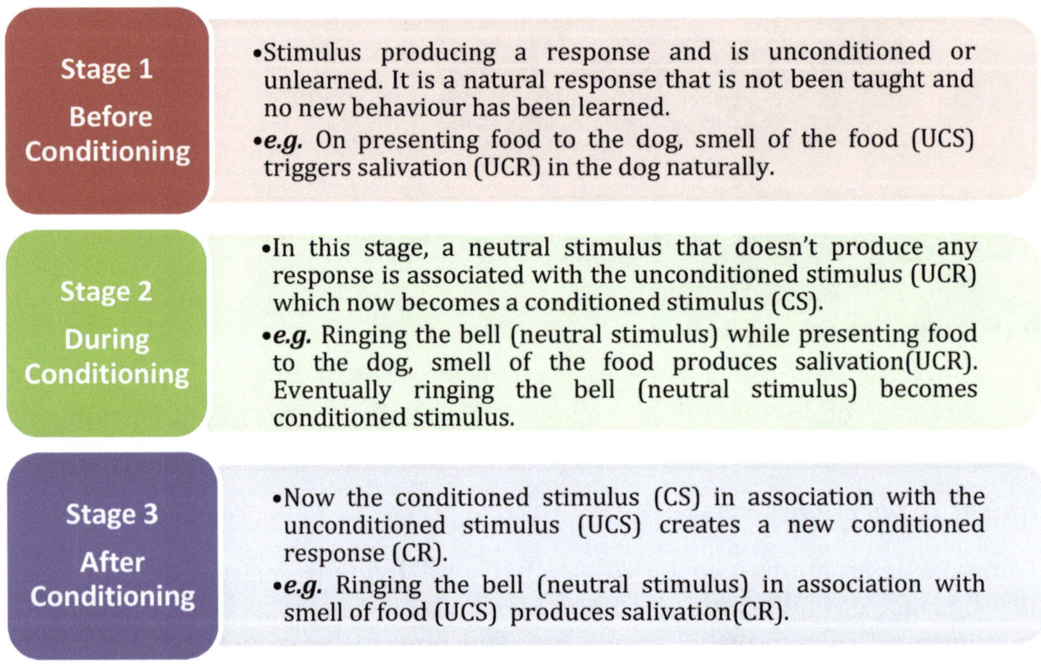

Fig. (27). Stages of Pavlov classical experiment.

Five key principles of Classical conditioning theory:

1. ***Acquisition***: It is the initial stage of learning when a neutral stimulus is paired with an unconditioned stimulus, and a response is elicited. On reinforcing this response, new behaviour is learned.

e.g., When presenting food to the dog, ringing the bell (neutral stimulus) along with the smell of food (UCS) produces a new behaviour of salivation only on ringing the bell.

2. ***Extinction:*** It is the disappearance or decrease of a conditioned response that occurs when a conditioned stimulus is no longer paired with an unconditioned stimulus.

e.g., When presenting food to the dog, the smell of food (UCS) is no longer paired with the ringing of the bell (CS) eventually, the salivation (CR) would disappear.

3. ***Spontaneous Recovery:*** It is the sudden reappearance of a conditioned response after a period of rest or stopping reinforcing a conditioned response.

e.g., If ringing the bell on presenting food is stopped, salivation would decrease. But after some period, if suddenly the bell is ringing, salivation would again increase.

4. ***Stimulus Generalization:*** It is the tendency of a stimulus, which is like a conditioned stimulus, to produce a response. This response is like a conditioned response.

e.g., Dog salivates when the bell is ringing with the smell of food, generalisation involves salivation by the dog to sounds like the ringing of the bell.

5. ***Stimulus Discrimination:*** It is the ability to differentiate between a conditioned stimulus and other stimuli that have not been paired with an unconditioned stimulus.

e.g., Dog discriminates, or it can differentiate the sound of a bell and other sounds. It would only salivate the sound of the bell ring, which is a conditioned stimulus.

Clinical Implications

The child, in his first dental visit, had unpleasant or bad experiences due to painful dental procedures (unconditioned stimuli) by the dentist with a white coat (neutral stimuli) acquires fear and cries (unconditioned response). Now an association between a white coat of the dentist and a painful experience is formed, resulting in conditioned stimuli. In the second dental visit, mere sight of a white coat (now conditioned stimuli) results in fear, and the child starts crying (conditioned response), even though no dental procedure is carried out [9].

Operant Conditioning Theory

It was given by ***BF Skinner***. He introduced a new term called Law of Effect - Reinforcement. Any behaviour is strengthened or repeated, which is reinforced or followed by pleasant consequences, and behaviour tends to die out or weakened, which is not reinforced or followed by unpleasant consequences. Hence a response becomes further stimuli.

Skinner identified three types of operant or responses following any behaviour of an individual.

- ***Reinforcers:*** These are responses that increase the probability of repeating certain behaviour. Reinforcers may be positive or negative.
- ***Neutral operant:*** Responses that neither increase nor decrease the probability of a behaviour being repeated.
- ***Punishers***: Responses that decrease the probability of a behaviour being repeated. Punishment weakens behaviour.

Skinner Described 4 types of Operant Conditioning [1, 9]

1. ***Positive reinforcement:*** Strengthening any behaviour by providing a stimulus that is pleasant and is rewarding to the individual.

e.g., Child should be positively reinforced for good behaviour during dental treatment so that child is more likely to repeat such behaviour in future visits. Positive reinforcers can be by verbal praise or by reward (Fig. **28**).

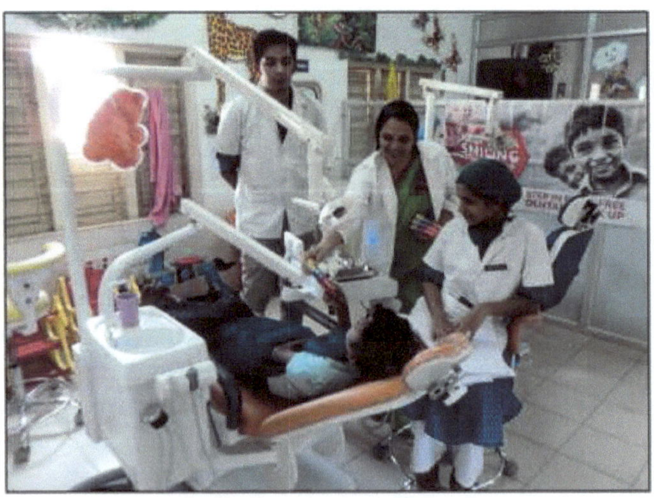

Fig. (28). Positive reinforcement.

2. ***Negative Reinforcement:*** It is the removal of unpleasant or adverse stimuli to strengthen desired behaviour, and the individual feels rewarded for the removal of such stimuli.

e.g., Momentarily withdrawing the treatment to make the child stop crying.

3. ***Omission or time out:*** pleasant stimulus is withdrawn after an unpleasant response or behaviour to strengthen the desired behaviour.

e.g., Taking out the favourite toy or any reward presented as positive reinforcement to stop the child from being uncooperative.

4. ***Punishment***: It is an aversive way of decreasing or weakening behaviour by presenting an unpleasant stimulus.

e.g., Momentarily sending the parent out of the treatment area to make the child stop throwing up temper tantrums, voice control and physical restraints.

Social Learning Theory

This theory was proposed by Albert Bandura. He acknowledged the other behaviour learning theories, Classical conditioning and Operant conditioning theories, for which he added his two ideas:

a. In between stimuli and response, mediation occurs
b. Observation learning, a process of learning behaviour through the environment

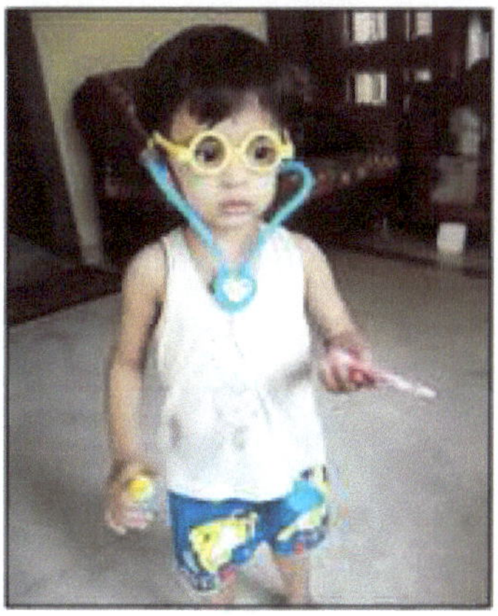

Fig. (29). Imitation.

Children come across many people around them; it can be parents, family members, peer groups, teachers at school or even characters they watch on TV. Children tend to encode and imitate the behaviour of those people who are called Models [10] (Figs. **29** - **31**).

First the child tends to observe and imitate the behaviour of people of same gender

Secondly, the child continuing to perform this behaviour is based on whether the behaviour is being reinforced by the people around them.
Reinforcement can be positive or negative, external, or internal

- **Positive reinforcement**: Praise or approval of a behaviour, children more likely to repeat the same in the future.
- **Negative reinforcement**: Punishment or disapproval of the behaviour, children tend to forgo or adopt different behaviour.
- **External reinforcement**: If the child wants approval by the parents or peers.
- **Internal reinforcement:** Feeling happy about being approved.

Third, the child tends to observe what happens to the other people with the desired behaviour they want to copy.

e.g., If the elder sister is getting rewarded to a particular behaviour, the child tends to copy that behaviour.

This is called **Vicarious behaviour**.

Fig. (30). Social Learning Theory.

HIERARCHY OF NEEDS

Hierarchy of Needs is a motivational theory in human psychology put forth by Abraham Maslow, which comprises a five-tier model of human needs. Human needs are depicted within a pyramid hierarchically.

From the bottom of the hierarchy upwards, the needs are physiological, safety, love & belonging, esteem and self-actualization. Needs at the bottom level in the hierarchy must be satisfied before individuals can attend to needs at a higher level in the pyramid. This five-stage model of human needs can be classified as Deficiency needs and Growth needs (Figs. **32** & **33**).

According to Albert Bandura mediation occurs by four processes

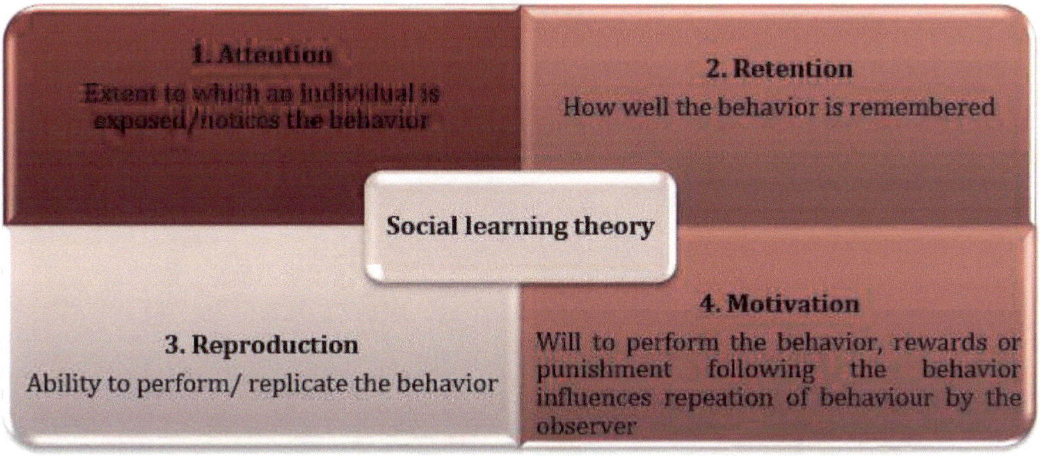

Fig. (31). Social Learning Theory.

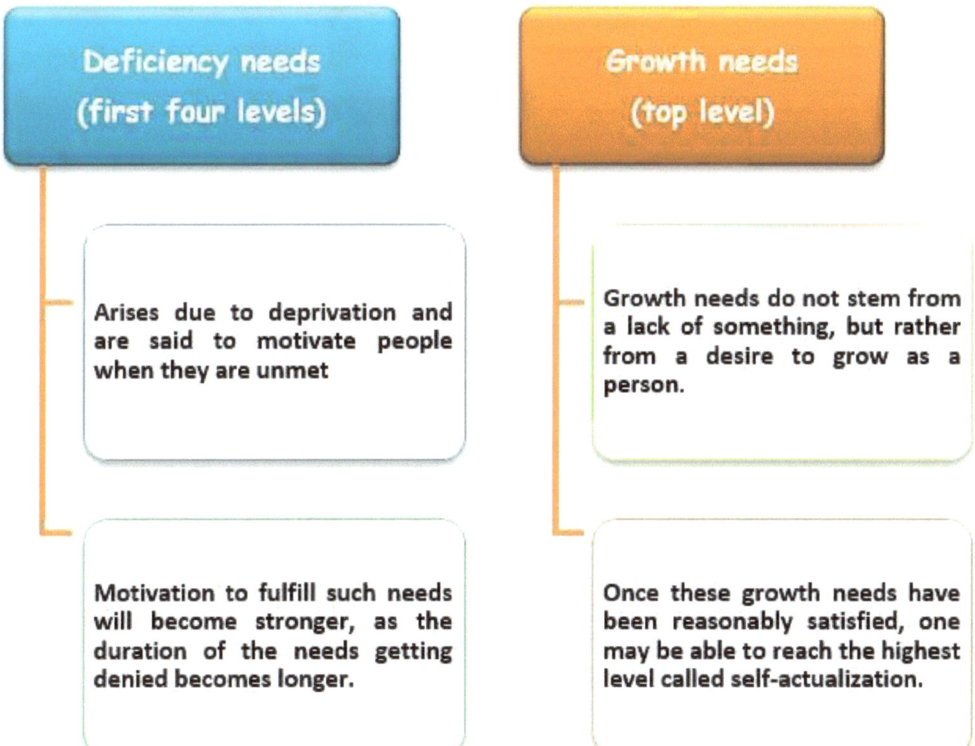

Fig. (32). Types of needs.

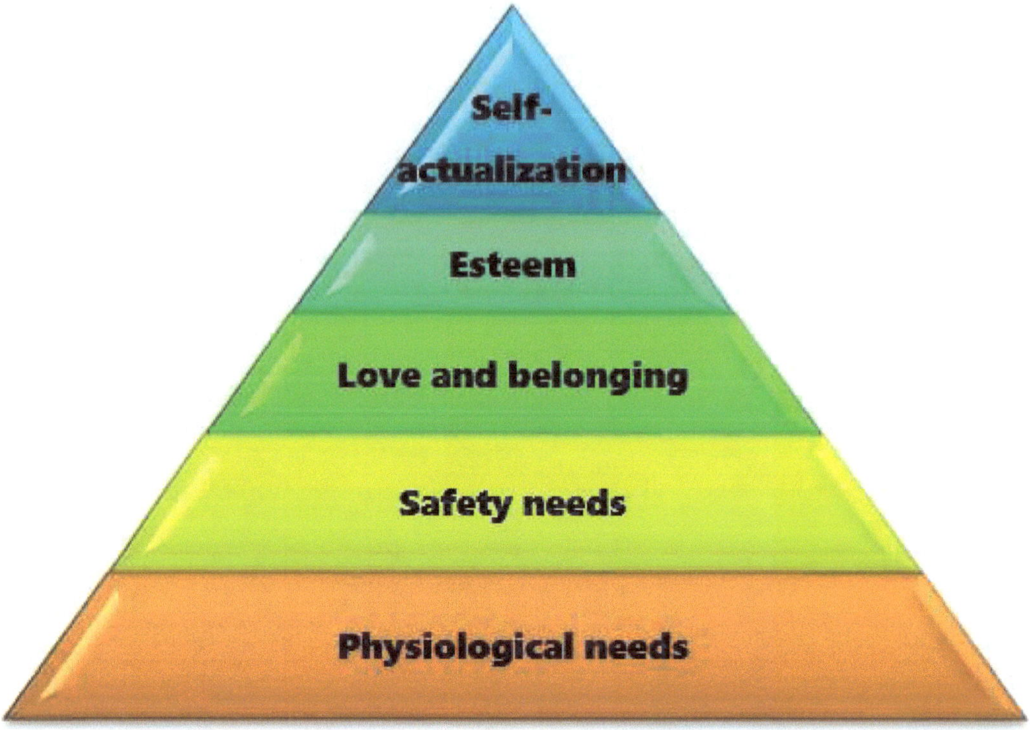

Fig. (33). Hierarchy of needs.

Physiological needs: For a human body to function normally and for survival, certain basic biological requirements are mandatory, called Physiological needs, without which all other needs become secondary.

e.g., Food, water, clothing, shelter, sleep, warmth, sex.

i. **Safety needs:** It is more of a psychological need which is a security of home and family, also stability, and freedom from fear.
ii. **Love & belonging/social needs:** It involves a feeling of belongingness, being loved and the need for interpersonal relationships.

e.g., Trust and acceptance, friendship, love, intimacy, being part of family or society

Esteem needs: Needs of reputation & respect, mastering their skills and competency.

Self-actualization needs: Very few people can reach up to this stage. It is a desire and having resources to become more and more capable by maximizing their potential. Self-fulfilment, urge for personal and professional growth, peace and build-up of strong ethics.

Dental Implications: Parent's attitude towards child oral health care and willingness for various dental procedures is based on the stage of the hierarchy of needs they belong to.

CONCLUSION

Fear and anxiety are often considered universal barriers rendering dental treatment to children by paediatric dentists. Child psychology is a crucial part of paediatric dentistry, and thorough knowledge of the psychological development of a child helps to understand the child better, and identify his fears and perceptions. Psychological behaviour management helps the helps the pediatric dentist to instil a positive dental attitude in children.

CONSENT FOR PUBLICATION

Not applicable.

CONFLICT OF INTEREST

The author(s) declare no conflict of interest, financial or otherwise.

ACKNOWLEDGEMENT

Declared none.

REFERENCES

[1] Carter AE, Carter G, Boschen M, AlShwaimi E, George R. Pathways of fear and anxiety in dentistry: A review. World J Clin Cases 2014; 2(11): 642-53. [http://dx.doi.org/10.12998/wjcc.v2.i11.642] [PMID: 25405187]

[2] Porritt J, Marshman Z, Rodd HD. Understanding children's dental anxiety and psychological approaches to its reduction. Int J Paediatr Dent 2012; 22(6): 397-405. [http://dx.doi.org/10.1111/j.1365-263X.2011.01208.x] [PMID: 22221141]

[3] Lantz SE, Ray S. Freud developmental theory.StatPearls. Treasure Island, FL: StatPearls Publishing 2021. Updated 2021 Feb 7 Internet.

[4] Orenstein GA, Lewis L. Eriksons Stages of Psychosocial Development.Stat Pearls. Treasure Island, FL: StatPearls Publishing 2021. Updated 2020 NOV 22 Internet.

[5] Heo J, Han S, Koch C, Aydin H. Piaget"s Egocentrism and Language Learning: Language Egocentrism (LE) and Language Differentiation (LD). Journal of Language Teaching and Research 2011; 2(4): 733-9. [http://dx.doi.org/10.4304/jltr.2.4.733-739]

[6] Asokan S, Surendran S, Asokan S, Nuvvula S. Relevance of Piaget's cognitive principles among 4-7 years old children: A descriptive cross-sectional study. J Indian Soc Pedod Prev Dent 2014; 32(4):

292-6.
[http://dx.doi.org/10.4103/0970-4388.140947] [PMID: 25231036]

[7] Hugar SM, Kukreja P, Assudani HG, Gokhale N, G Assudani H, Gokhale N. Evaluation of the Relevance of Piaget's Cognitive Principles among Parented and Orphan Children in Belagavi City, Karnataka, India: A Comparative Study. Int J Clin Pediatr Dent 2017; 10(4): 346-50.
[http://dx.doi.org/10.5005/jp-journals-10005-1463] [PMID: 29403227]

[8] Kryukov VI. Towards a unified model of pavlovian conditioning: short review of trace conditioning models. Cogn Neurodynamics 2012; 6(5): 377-98.
[http://dx.doi.org/10.1007/s11571-012-9195-z] [PMID: 24082960]

[9] Mallineni SK, Rajasekhar S, Nuvvula S. Knowledge and attitudes of dental graduates regarding the application of child psychology during the behavioral guidance of children: A cross-sectional survey of dental students. SRM Journal of Research in Dental Sciences 2018; 9(2): 53-7.
[http://dx.doi.org/10.4103/srmjrds.srmjrds_10_18]

[10] Do C. Applying social learning theory to children with dental anxiety. J Contemp Dent Pract 2004; 5(1): 126-35.
[http://dx.doi.org/10.5005/jcdp-5-1-126] [PMID: 14973566]

CHAPTER 4

Non-Pharmacological Behaviour Management

Raghavendra M. Shetty[1,*], **Aditi Pashne**[2] and **Trisha Gadekar**[3]

[1] *Department of Clinical Sciences, College of Dentistry, Center of Medical and Bio-allied Health Sciences Research, Ajman University, Ajman, UAE*

[2] *Associate Dentist, My Dentist, Aberystwyth, UK*

[3] *Department of Pediatric Dentistry, Mamata Dental College, Khammam, Telangana, India*

Abstract: Behaviour guidance, earlier known as behaviour management, of the child, is an essential part of paediatric dental practice. Various techniques are used by the dental health team for effective and efficient dental treatment of the child. At the end of the treatment, it is necessary to instil a positive dental attitude in the child's behaviour. The phrase 'behaviour management' has been replaced by 'behaviour guidance' in recent days, but both phrases are used as synonyms in most studies. Various behaviour management/guidance techniques can be used independently or in combination to ensure an efficient and effective dental treatment in the child patient. This chapter describes various behaviours of the child and appropriate non-pharmacological behaviour guidance techniques which can be employed by the dental health team for a successful dental treatment, thereby instilling a positive dental attitude in the child.

Keywords: Behaviour guidance, Behaviour management, Non-pharmacological.

INTRODUCTION

As per the American Psychological Association dictionary of psychology, behaviour can be defined as "an organism's activities in response to external or internal stimuli, including objectively observable activities, introspectively observable activities, and nonconscious processes."

According to Wright (1975), "Behaviour management is the means by which a dental team effectively and efficiently performs treatment for a child and at the same time, instils a positive dental attitude." It is of utmost importance to understand this definition, as firstly, as per this, any of the approaches (even if it involves drug use) would be considered as behaviour management, provided it fulfills other criteria of proving effective (*i.e.*, no compromise with the quality of

* **Corresponding author Raghavendra M. Shetty:** Department of Clinical Sciences, College of Dentistry, Ajman University, Center of Medical and Bio-allied Health Sciences Research, Ajman University, Ajman, UAE; Tel: +971 67056364; Fax: +971 67438888; E-mail: drraghavendra77@gmail.com

Satyawan Damle, Ritesh Kalaskar, Dhanashree Sakhare & Abdulkadeer Jetpurwala (Eds.)

treatment) and efficient (*i.e.*, providing maximum facilities and treatment accomplishment with time). The last and most important part is fostering a positive attitude over the whole course of dental treatment. And as per the famous McElroy's statement, "*Although the operative dentistry may be perfect, the appointment is a failure if the child departs in tears.*"

Behaviour Modification is defined as an attempt to alter human behaviour and emotion in a beneficial way and in accordance with the laws of learning.

Behaviour Shaping is the procedure that slowly develops behaviour by reinforcing a successive approximation of desired behaviour until the desired behaviour comes into being.

Recently, the terminology of behaviour management has changed to behaviour guidance. According to the American Academy of Paediatric Dentistry (AAPD), "**Behaviour Guidance** is a continuum of interaction involving the dentist, the dental team, the patient and the parent, directed towards communication and education which ultimately builds trust and allays fear and anxiety."

The objectives of behaviour guidance as per AAPD (2020) are:

- To establish proper communication.
- To alleviate a child's dental fear and anxiety.
- To promote patient's and parents' awareness of the need for good oral health and the process by which it is achieved.
- To promote the child's positive attitude toward oral health care.
- To build a trusting relationship between dentist/staff and child/parent.
- To provide quality oral health care in a comfortable, minimally restrictive, safe, and effective manner.

Behavioural Classification

Various systems have been introduced for classifying children as per their behaviour, which can be an asset to managing them in the dental environment.

Wright's Classification (1975)

I. **Co-operative behaviour:** The child is relaxed with minimal apprehension that can be treated by behaviour guidance. Children develop a good rapport and are interested in the dental procedure. They laugh and enjoy being in the dental environment and allow the proper functioning of the dental team.

II. **Lacking co-operative ability:** This type of children contrasts with the co-operative children. They are usually young children, less than 2½ years, disabled, handicapped, or with major behaviour problems.

III. **Potentially co-operative behaviour:** This category has various sub-categories depending on the type of representing behaviour.

   i. **Uncontrolled behaviour:** Usually belonging to 3-6 years. They throw tantrums in the reception area. They are incorrigible, presenting with tears, crying out loudly, and physically lashing out of their limbs.
   ii. **Defiant behaviour:** They belong to the pre-school age group and present with stubborn or spoilt behaviour. However, they are highly cooperative once they develop trust.
   iii. **Timid behaviour:** They are highly anxious, shy, and they whimper but do not cry hysterically. They are overprotected children and require building confidence in themselves.
   iv. **Tense cooperative:** They have the varying type of behaviours.
   v. **Whining behaviour:** Children are complaining throughout the dental procedure.
   vi. **Stoic behaviour:** Mostly physically abused children, but they are cooperative. They passively accept dental treatment without any facial expression.

Behaviour Rating Scales

Frankl's behaviour rating scale was introduced in 1962 and later was modified by Wright in 1975 by adding symbols (+, -) to represent the severity (Fig. **1**). It is the gold standard for behaviour rating in the dental clinic and is the most widely used to date. This classification is functional, quantifiable, and reliable.

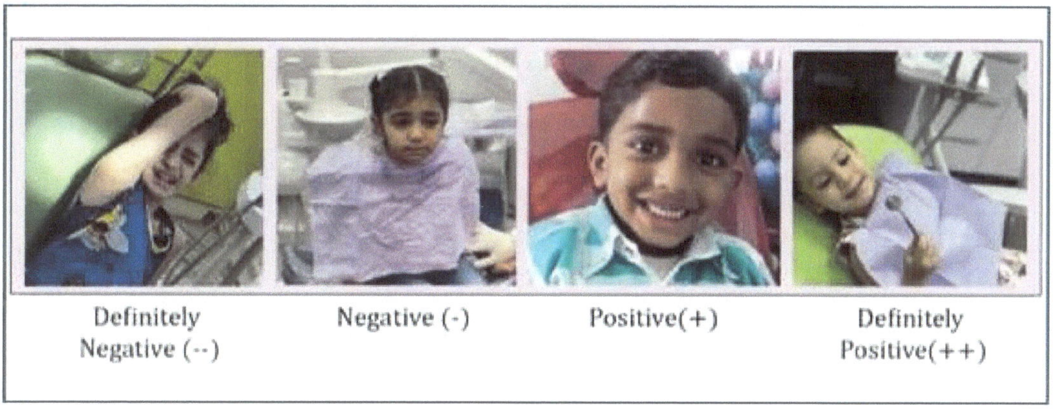

Fig. (1). Frankl's Behaviour Rating Scale.

Rating 1: definitively negative (--): The children refuse any kind of dental procedure. They are usually crying loudly, fearful, or displaying any other evidence of extreme negativity towards dental treatment.

Rating 2: negative (-): The children are reluctant to accept treatment. They are uncooperative, with evidence of a negative attitude, but not very pronounced.

Rating 3: positive (+): Such children accept treatment but are cautious while complying with the dentist's instructions.

Rating 4: Definitely positive (++): They have a good rapport with the dentist, accept the dental treatments, and are usually laughing and enjoying themselves throughout the appointment.

Effect of Dental Office Environment and Parental Presence

The dental office environment should be warm and homely. A comfortable environment helps the children be relieved of dental anxiety (Fig. **2a**), and the confidence of the child is achieved through counselling (Fig. **2b**). The dental operating environment should be made full of colours and with posters, TV and videogames, toys, storybooks, and comics. It should have a separate entry and an exit door. The dental auxiliary should be soft and gentle to the children and should greet them with a smile.

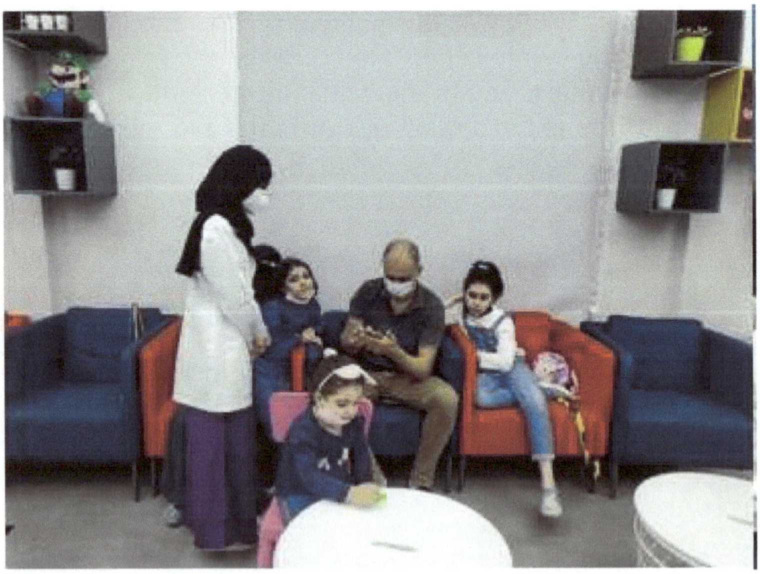

Fig. (2a). Dental Office Environment.

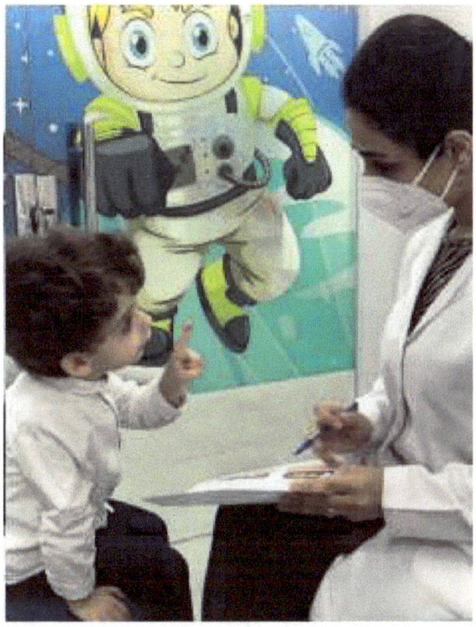

Fig. (2b). Gaining Child's Confidence.

The presence of a parent is a flexible rule and has to be used as per the requirement for successful patient management. Whether a parent should be present or not during the dental operation is a controversial matter as complete parental separation might cause emotional trauma to the young child, whereas sometimes the child might behave differently to gain parental sympathy.

Parental presence in the dental operatory is proven to be beneficial in younger children as it prevents separation anxiety and gains emotional support (Fig. **3**).

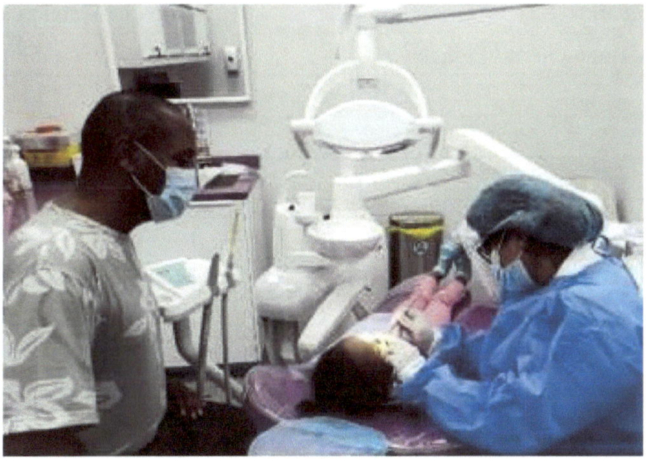

Fig. (3). Parental Presence in the Operatory.

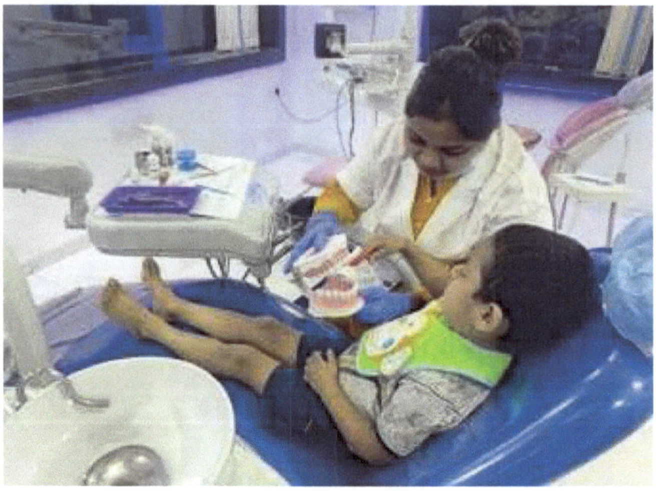

Fig. (4). Effective Communication.

Non-Pharmacological Behaviour Guidance Techniques

Most of the successful and well-proven techniques of behaviour guidance have their foundation in learning theories of behavioural science. More emphasis has been exerted on being empathic and communication skills in recent years. Depending upon the communication and empathetic behaviour skills of each dentist, individual difference during the application of these techniques might appear. Various classifications for non-pharmacologic behaviour management techniques are listed below Tables **1** and **2**.

Table 1. List of some important polymers and their roles.

Basic Behaviour Guidance	Advanced Behaviour Guidance
• Communication and communicative guidance	• Protective stabilization
• TSD	• HOME
• Desensitization	• Sedation and General Anesthesia
• Contingency management	-
• Modelling	-
• Voice control	-
• Distraction, Visual imagery, Nitrous oxide inhalation	-

Table 2. List of some important polymers and their roles.

Behaviour Shaping	**Behaviour Management of Children with Disruptive Behaviours**	**Other Behaviour Management Techniques**
a. Communication b. Behaviour shaping (modification) i Desensitization • TSD • Implosion therapy or flooding Technique ii. Modelling iii.Contingency management	a. Voice control b. Aversive conditioning • HOME • Physical restraints	a. Audio analgesia b. Bio-feedback c. Hypnosis d. Humor e. Assimilation and coping f. Relaxation g. Distraction h. Memory Restructuring i. Visual Imagery j. Use of Poetry and Drawing

Communication and Communicative Guidance

Chambers (1976) stated that communication is universally used for behaviour management in paediatric dentistry with both co-operative and uncooperative children. It is one of the primary strategies of behaviour management. It must be bi-directional *i.e.*; the dentist must carefully listen as well as be able to convey instructions and information properly to the patient. Though often confused to be the same, communication and voice control differ from each other. Communication can be considered as the first step toward behaviour management, whereas voice control is the first step to behaviour shaping.

Prerequisites for Effective Communication

- Communication should be comfortable, relaxed and highly attentive Fig (4).
- Eye contact is the primary medium of expression. However, gazing continuously should be avoided to prevent a frightening impact.
- Proper body posture. Slightly forward-leaning and speaking at the eye level with body-oriented towards the listener allows an amiable atmosphere.
- An enhanced communication requires proper silence in between *i.e.*, pauses to allow the listener to understand and facilitate conversation, especially during initial appointments.
- Always make sure communication should be from a single source otherwise, it might lead to confusion and dilemma for a child.
- Address the child by name, compliment them about their appearance, and try asking questions about their class, and their likes/dislikes. However, it should not be too intrusive at any time. Also, maintain a proper distance to allow a good and respectful interaction.
- Non-verbal communication can also be very effective. This includes

multisensory communication (Fig. **5**).

Guidance cooperation is the best model to describe the conversation in the dental clinic. This communication model was later modified into a 'child-centred approach' constituting permissive, empathetic, and personal verbal approaches. For children with special needs, augmentative, and alternative communication (AAC) helps overcome the conversation lag. It includes a picture exchange communication system (PECS), and various communication mobile apps like play the dentist [1].

Desensitization

The systematic desensitization technique was demonstrated by James and popularized by Joseph Wolpe (1975). Desensitization is traditionally used with a child patient with existing anxiety in the dental situation and to eliminate a dental phobia. It involves three steps:

1. Discussion about child's fear in a hierarchical order from least to the highest fearful situation in a dental clinic.

2. Teaching relaxation techniques/breathing exercises.

3. Introduction of a similar situation in the same ascending order *i.e.*, least to most fear-provoking.

Hence, simple, painless procedures (prophylaxis, fluoride application, pit, and fissure sealants) should be carried out during the initial visits, followed by the anxiety-inducing procedures which require local anaesthesia (pulp therapy, extraction). This systemic desensitization is effective as the child learns to substitute an appropriate or adaptive emotional response *i.e.*, relaxation, for undue or maladaptive response anxiety.

Recently, a computerized edition of systematic desensitization called CARL (Computer Assisted Relaxation Learning) and smartphone-based exposure treatment was introduced to help an individual with needle phobias.

Tell Show Do (TSD) Technique

Introduced by Addelston (1959), it is still considered to be the cornerstone of behaviour management as it is efficient, non-invasive, and comparatively easy to perform. It can orient the child gradually to anxiety-provoking stimuli (Fig. **6**). This is considered a type of desensitizing technique and is an approach by successive approximations. It is mostly indicated for the child's first visit, above 3 years of age (with cognitive development), and subsequent visits while introducing a new dental procedure to the apprehensive/anxious child.

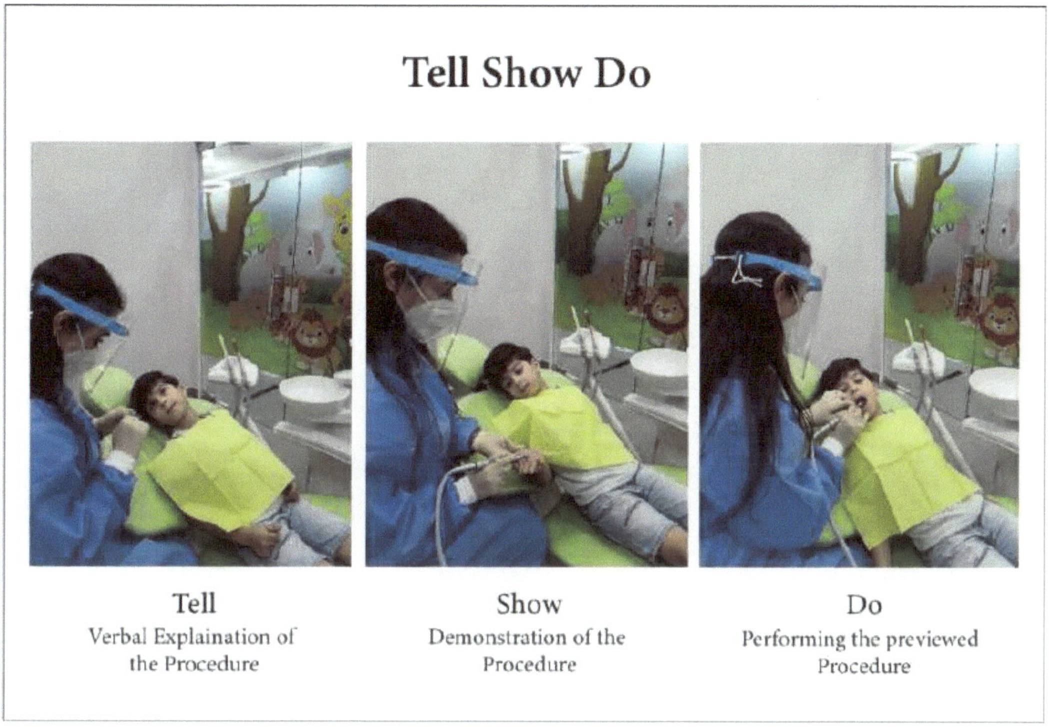

Fig. (6). Tell-Show-Do Technique.

Firstly, the dentist should use language that the child can understand and explain to the patient what will be done. The rule of thumb is, *"tell the child before you do it, while you are doing it, and after you are done with it."* This step is followed by a demonstration of the procedure to the child using a model or himself. Remember the multisensory approach – Child can SEE, TOUCH, SMELL, HEAR!! The final step is to proceed towards the dental procedure exactly as described.

Modification of TSD

***Ask-tell-ask*:** Ask, that is, inquiring and feelings about the visit. The next step is telling, which is explaining the dental procedure through demonstrations and simple, easily understood language appropriate to the child's cognitive category. Finally, ask which is to inquire again and confirm if the patient understands, and their experience of dental treatment.

***Tell-play-do*:** TSD was modified as Tell-Play-Do in 2017 for children aged 5-7 years. It is like tell-show-do but involves an additional component of allowing the child to play with dental equipment (Fig. **7**). As per the learning theory of Bandura, the child's anxiety toward the dental equipment is reduced; thereby, the child feels more comfortable and develops cooperative behaviour [2].

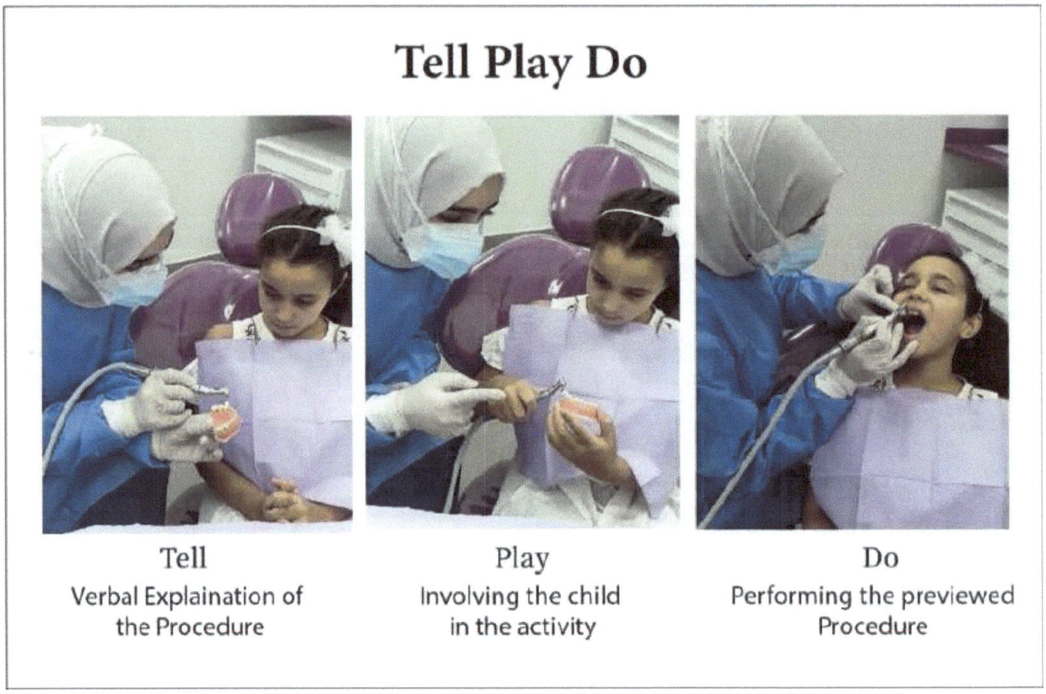

Fig. (7). Tell-Play-Do Technique.

Role Play and Drawings

We can ask the child to draw and colour paintings and involve them in role-play to relax themselves and decrease their anxiety which will benefit the pediatric dentist in carrying out the dental treatment (Figs. **8** and **9**).

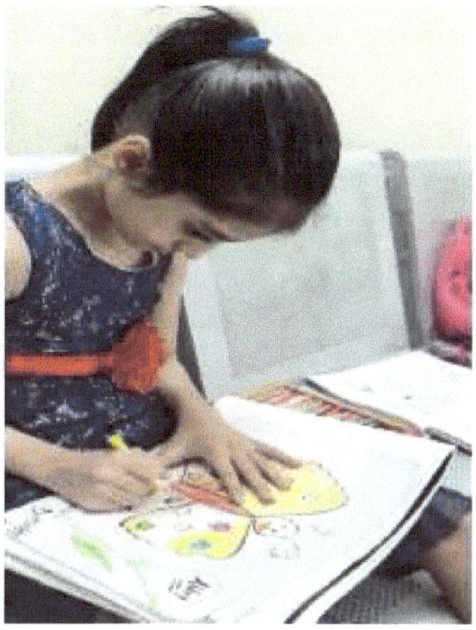

Fig. (8). Drawing and Colouring.

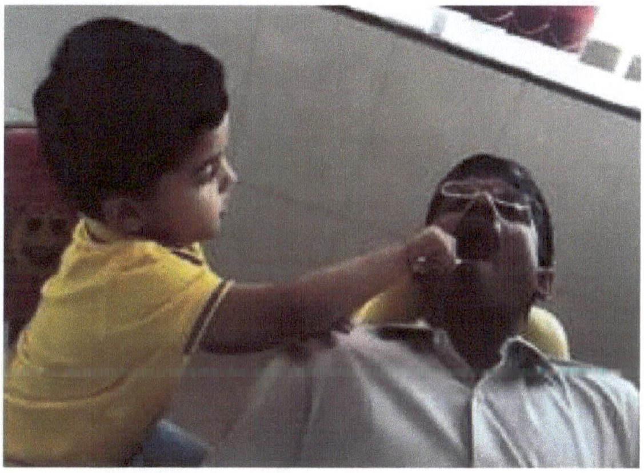

Fig. (9). Role play.

Flooding Technique or Implosion Therapy

In the 1960s, Thomas Stumpf propagated a technique called 'implosion therapy' to treat extreme fear or phobias. It refers to exposing the patient to the anxiety-provoking or fearing situation all at once and keeping in this situation till the anxiety and fear abate. Flooding in its original form involves forceful, prolonged exposure to the actual stimulus that provoked the original trauma (Fig. **10**).

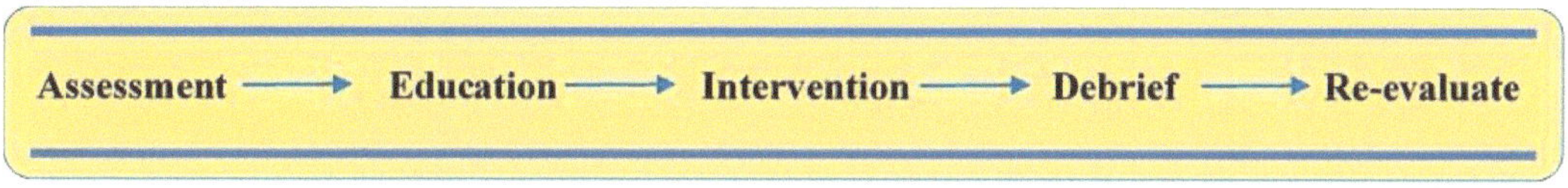

Fig. (10). Sequence of Implosion Flooding.

The difference between flooding and desensitization technique, according to Marks, 1972 is that both are two opposite ends of the approach to a distressing situation. The more surprising the confrontation is, the more prolonged its effect is, and the greater the accompanying emotion is, the more appropriate the label "flooding" for that procedure, whereas desensitization is step-wise exposure to the dental treatment as the child progressively moves to the more frightening or invasive treatment.

Contingency Management

This behaviour shaping technique which is based on Skinner's Operant Conditioning theory is a 'universally accepted technique' in behaviour management of a child. The dentist must always be genuine with reinforcement therapy. Reinforcement is based on learning theory in which a stimulus leads to a particular response (Fig. **11**).

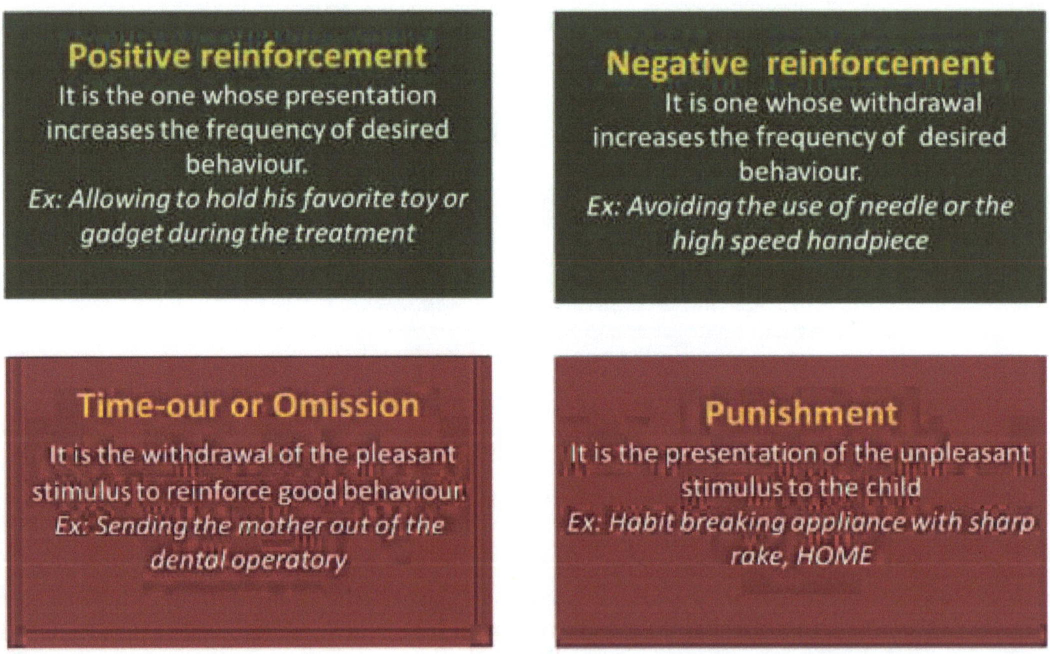

Fig. (11). Contingency Management.

Reinforcements can be of various types, as shown in Fig. (**12**).

Material reinforcers: Effective for children, such as teddies, toys and games, toothbrushes, and cartoon stickers.

***Social reinforcers*:** The patient should never be neglected on completion of the treatment. The best kind of reinforcers – praise, positive facial and verbal expressions, nearness, and physical contact – fall under this category.

***Activity reinforcers*:** Allow the child to watch his favourite cartoon or allow him to play his favourite game on the mobile.

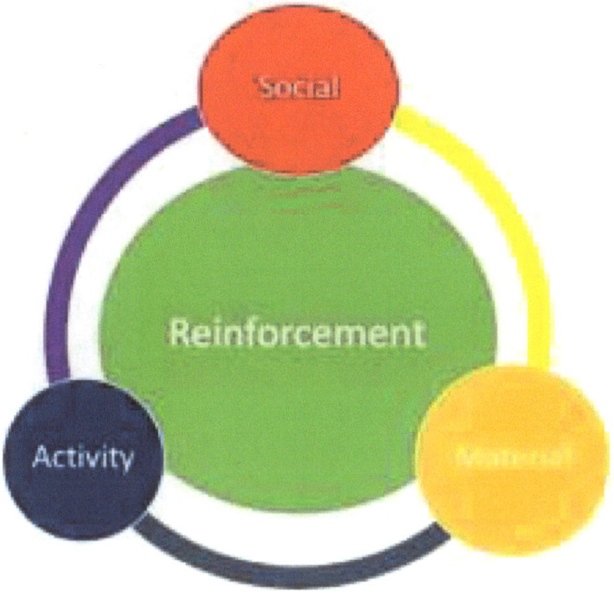

Fig. (12). Type of Reinforcers.

Modelling

The synonyms could include imitation, observational learning, identification, internalization, introjections, coping, social facilitation, contagion, and role taking.

This is based on Bandura's social learning theory. It is indirect learning *i.e.*, from others, maybe parents, teachers, peers, siblings, or the media. It is particularly effective when the model is perceived to be of similar status and gender. This technique is effective in young children during their first dental visit.

Types of Modelling

- Audiovisual (Televisions, handheld devices, computers). Filmed modelling is an economical and time-conserving approach.
- Live modelling by siblings or peers (Fig. **13**).

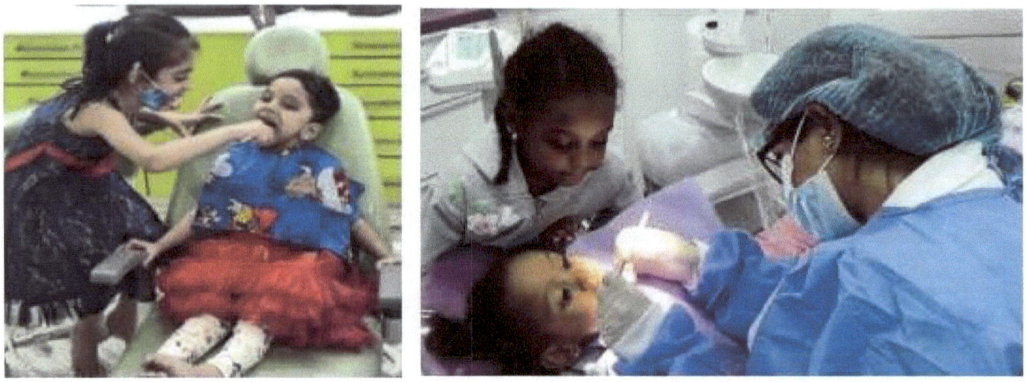

Fig. (13). Live Modelling.

Distraction

This is defined as diverting the patient's attention from what may be perceived as an unpleasant procedure. It can be either in the form of Fig. (**14**):

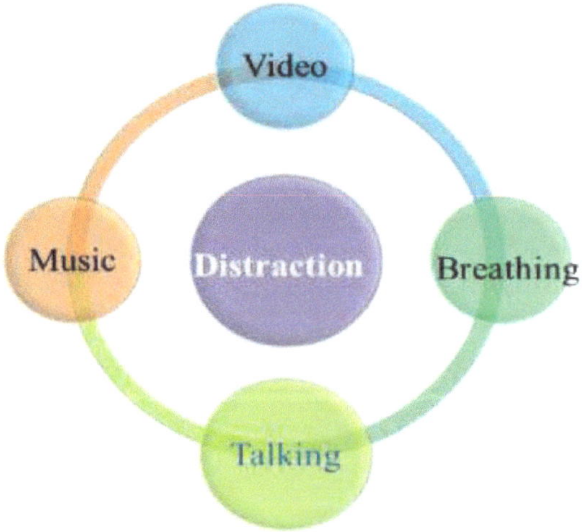

Fig. (14). Types of Distraction.

Active Distraction –Involves activity and overt participation of the child.

Passive Distraction –Passive forms of distraction, with the prerequisite that the child remains calm and quiet during a procedure initially with mild apprehension. Hence, distraction is achieved through patients' observation. Auditory and audiovisual techniques are the simplest forms of passive distraction used with young patients (Figs. **15** - **17**). Television, computer games, and 3D video glasses are used for both visual and auditory distractions [3 - 5].

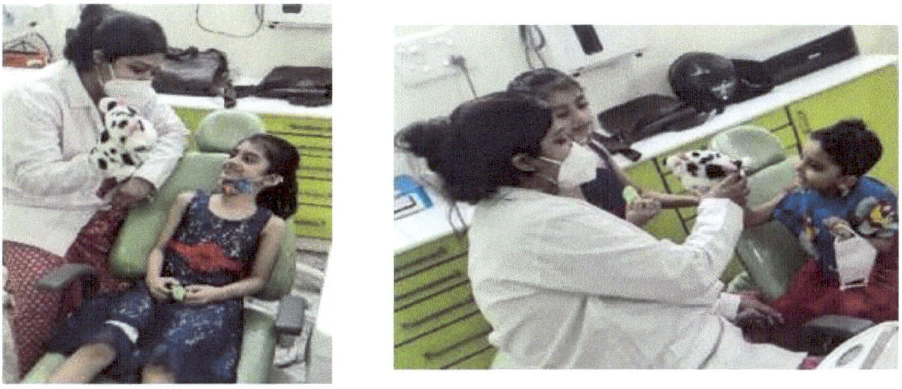

Fig. (15). Distraction technique using a puppet.

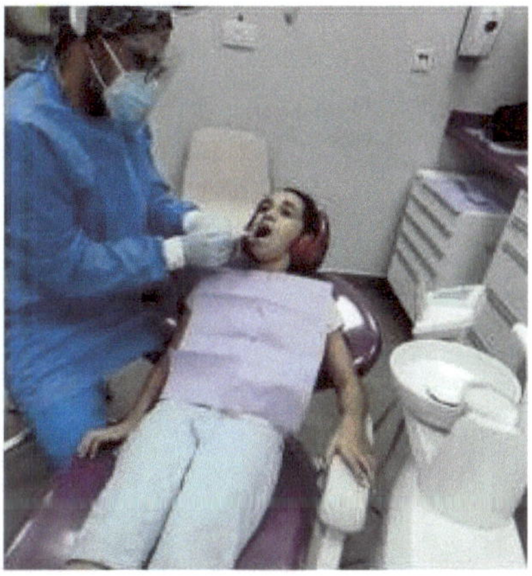

Fig. (16). Audio/Music Distraction.

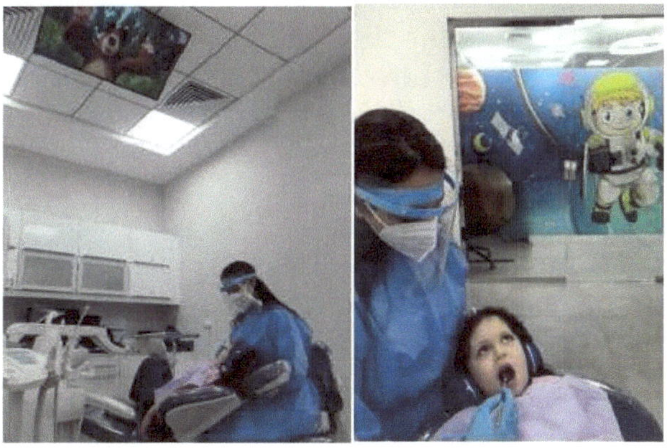

Fig. (17). Audio-Visual Distraction.

These distraction techniques can be routinely used during the administration of local anaesthesia in paediatric patients [6]. They are considered superior to passive distraction as they involve multisensory engagement, resulting in more effective interception of the pain stimulus. Guided imagery and relaxation are effective distraction techniques for decreasing pain and anxiety in paediatric patients. Huth *et al.* (2009) examined the effectiveness of a guided imagery program using a compact disc (CD) program and concluded that listening to the CD stimulated the imagination of the child.

Audio-Visual Distraction

Audiovisual distraction (Fig. **17**) may be more effective than traditional distraction methods, as it is more engaging by involving both visual and auditory senses [7]. Key concepts in AV distraction are imagination (helps in distracting children from the present situation), engagement (enables children's attention to focus on a single thing) and motivation (helps children to encourage getting treated for dental problems in the future). The audiovisual distraction is simple, economical, and effective in controlling dental anxiety in children and can be used for dental treatment under local anaesthesia [8].

Protective Stabilisation

The American Academy of Pediatric Dentistry suggested that the term 'restraint' should be substituted with 'protective stabilisation' [9]. Protective stabilisation is used to restrict the movement of the child's extremities, with or without the patient's permission, to decrease the risk of damage or injury during dental procedures. The main objective is to reduce or eliminate untoward movement. It also safeguards the patient, staff, dentist, or parent from injury. It facilitates the delivery of quality dental treatment. It is usually used for immediate urgent care where the child is unable to cooperate due to emotional or cognitive developmental levels, lack of maturity, or mental or physical conditions; sedated patients to help reduce untoward movement whereas contraindicated in medical, psychological, or physical conditions; physical or psychological trauma due to immobilisation; and practitioner's convenience.

The duration of stabilisation should be as small as possible, especially in a patient with severe disruptive behaviour, to avoid any physical or psychological trauma. Informed consent is mandatory during the use of protective stabilisation.

Types of Restraints

• *Molt mouth prop*: available in both adult and child sizes; allows accessibility on one side of the mouth but can lead to lip and palatal laceration and luxation of the teeth if not properly placed.

• *Rubber mouth prop/bite blocks*: These are available in various sizes to fit on occlusal surfaces. The bite blocks should have floss attached for easy retrieval. Recently, bite blocks have become available in various sizes with tongue depressors (Fig. **18**).

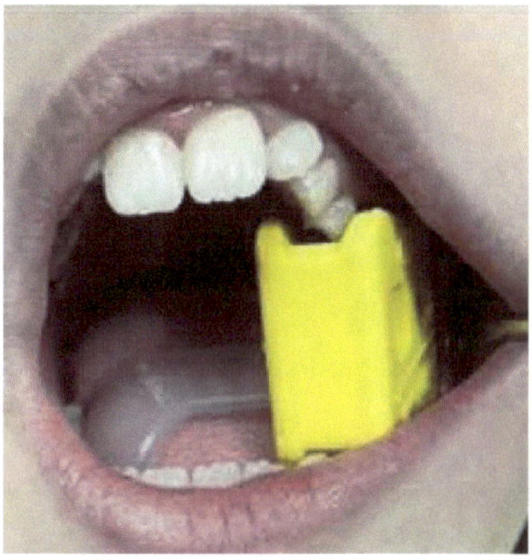

Fig. (18). Rubber mouth prop with tongue depressor.

• *Transparent bite block*: Modified bite blocks with an opening in the centre aid in the visibility of the working teeth and keep the tongue away from the working teeth (Fig. **19**).

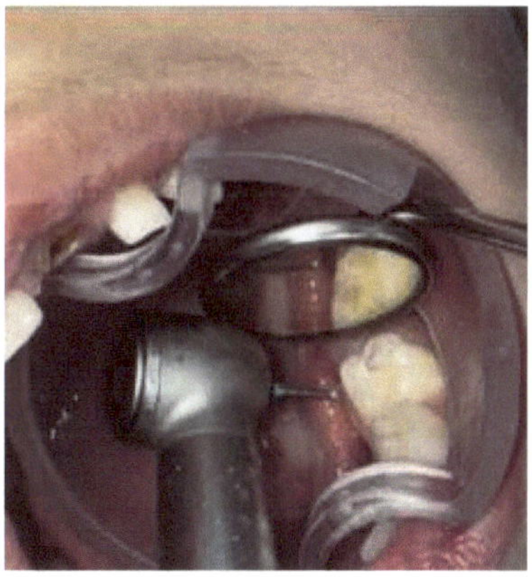

Fig. (19). Transparent bite block.

• *Papoose boards*: They have head stabilizers attached and are available in different sizes (Fig **20**).

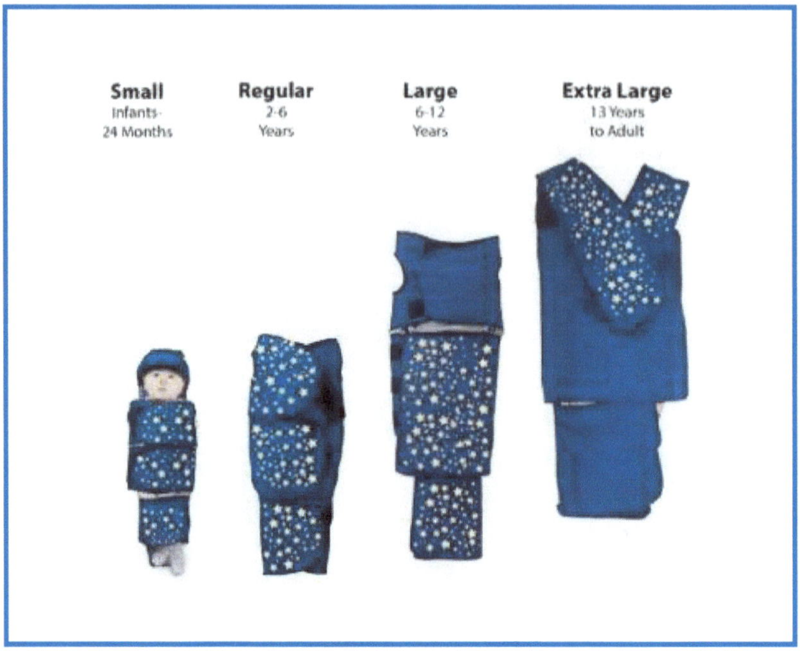

Fig. (20). Papoose Board.

• *Triangular sheets*: introduced by Mink; they help the patient sit upright during radiography. Generally difficult to use in small children and can cause airway obstruction. Hyperthermia can occur due to the use of papoose boards and triangular sheets.

• *Pedi-Wrap*: mesh fabric (to prevent hyperthermia) used for extremities – fastens the arms to the dental chair. It is usually used in patients with cerebral palsy.

• *Rainbow stabilizing wrap*: It is like the Pedi-wrap with a rainbow colour Velcro strap for stabilisation (Fig. **21**).

Audio Analgesia

Audio analgesia, or "white noise," is another method of pain reduction. This technique involves providing a sound stimulus of such an intensity that the patient finds it difficult to be attentive to any other thing. The is a kind of stimulus distraction, displacement of attention, and a positive feeling on the part of the dentist that can help.

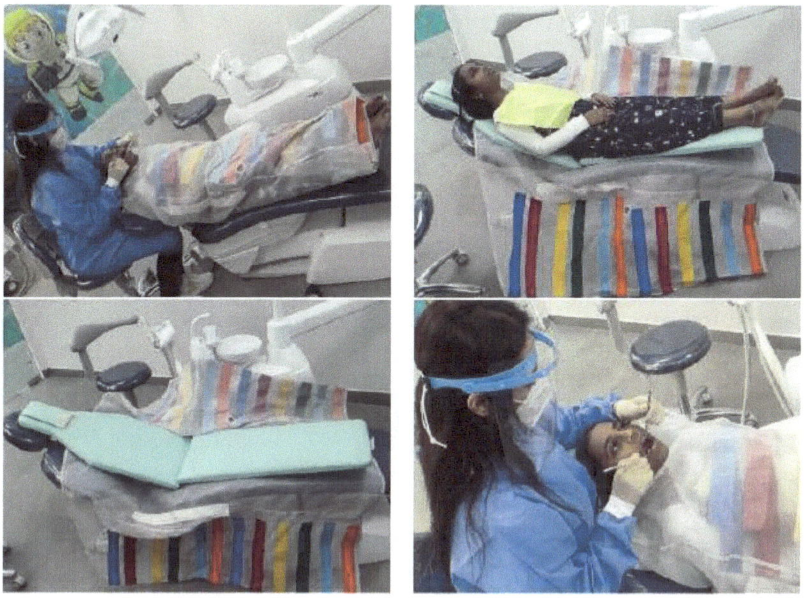

Fig. (21). Rainbow Stabilizing Wrap.

Lickliter described the procedure as one in which the patient wears earphones and controls his acoustic stimulation through a control box held in his lap. It has two control knobs, one for music and the other for a rushing, roaring sound derived from "white noise". At the beginning of the session, the patient selects the music he wants to hear – a stereophonic tape recording and adjusts it to a volume suitable for ordinary listening. When the dentist starts to work, or when his work causes any discomfort, the patient turns up the volume of the music. As soon as there is a trace or forewarning of pain, the patient turns the noise knob on.

It controls the level of the rushing, roaring "waterfall" sound. The overall sound pressure of the noise may be set as high as 116 decibels.

Hypnosis/ Psychosomatics/ Suggestion Therapy

It is defined as an altered state of consciousness without the use of pharmacologic agents. It is used to reduce nervousness and apprehension. It can be used to eliminate the hypnosis can enhance the efficacy of various treatment interventions and may be beneficial in managing anxious children.

Technique: Proper patient preparation; induction of hypnosis followed by deepening, and recovery with a post-hypnotic suggestion.

Cognitive Restructuring - Reframing

Memories associated with a negative or difficult event are restructured into positive memories using information suggested after the event has taken place.

Restructuring involves four components including visual reminders, positive reinforcement through verbalisation, concrete examples of encoding sensory details, and a sense of accomplishment. The objectives of memory restructuring are to restructure difficult or negative past dental experiences and improve patient behaviours at subsequent dental visits. It may be used with patients who had a negative or difficult dental visit, with not many contraindications.

Newer Methods of Behaviour Guidance

ATP Technique

Audio tactile performance technique (ATP) is a specially designed health education method, indicated especially for visually impaired children to improve oral hygiene, including Verbal Information and Tactile Sense. There is a time restriction for health education, and the process is continued for each child individually until they can perform it independently, correctly, and confidently.

Applied Behaviour Analysis (ABA)

ABA utilizes behavioural learning theory to modify behaviours through systemic experimentation. An ABA approach will involve studying the perpetuating factors of a particular behaviour along with the accompanying response. ABA methods involve functional analysis to teach specific skills accordingly. For example, ABA techniques can be used to teach oral hygiene habits to a child. Stepwise learning is done, followed by reinforcements.

Essential Oil Therapy – Aromatherapy

Aromatherapy is an alternative medical practice of using natural aromatic essential oils involving inhalation, absorption, or ingestion to enhance mood, reduce pain and improve cognitive function [10]. It involves the benefits of being a cost-effective, non-invasive therapy with minimal adverse effects. Recent randomized trials have proven the effectiveness of lavender oil in reducing dental anxiety in children. The pure concentrates of herbal plants (essential oils) can provide mental and physical aids when used properly and safely (Fig. **22**) [11]. The fragrance of aromatic oil at the dental reception area may elevate the patient's mood as well as calm down their anxiety. This practice of routine usage can help to improve the quality of dental treatments and make it less stressful for a dentist, child, and parent. Rose and lavender oil are used frequently to reduce dental anxiety.

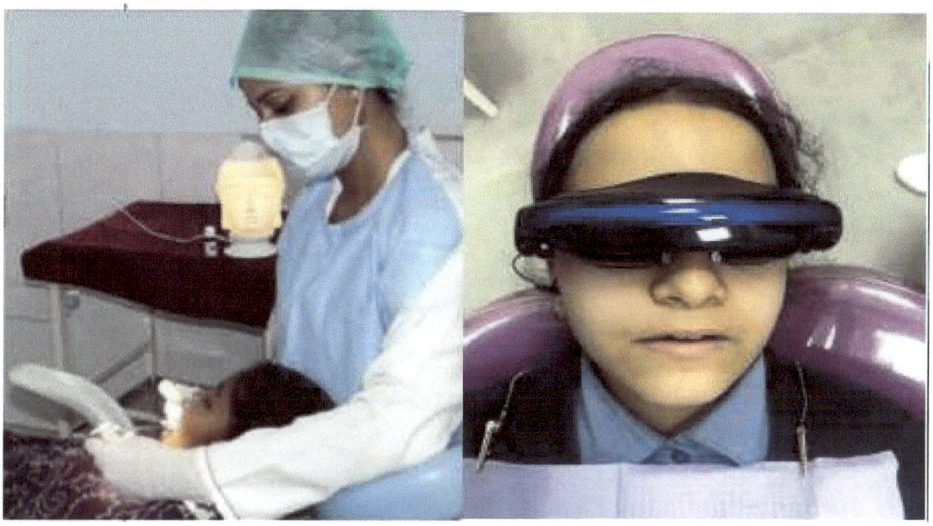

Fig. (22). Aromatherapy

Mobile Dental Application

Mobile and tablets are promising sources to deliver oral health care *via* various dental applications/software. They may act as tools for reducing dental fear and anxiety. An interactive session of using a mobile dental application pre-treatment and during the treatment reduces the child's anticipatory anxiety. RCTs comparing the mobile dental applications with conventional methods like TSD have revealed the mobile dental applications to be equally effective [12]. The drawbacks are concerns regarding increased smartphone usage and its adverse effects.

Virtual Reality-Based Distraction

Heim described virtual reality as interactive computer-based software that can involve children in the virtual 3D environment using VR goggles and headphones that completely obstruct the real/actual situation. It can be an effective tool for distracting during local anaesthesia injections, restorative procedures and extractions (Fig. **23**). It is contraindicated in medically compromised children, especially with epilepsy, migraine, and vestibular disturbances and in children with a previous history of nausea or dizziness following the use of a VR device. Currently, research is being focused on the effect of varying content being shown through the VR goggles in allaying dental anxiety [13].

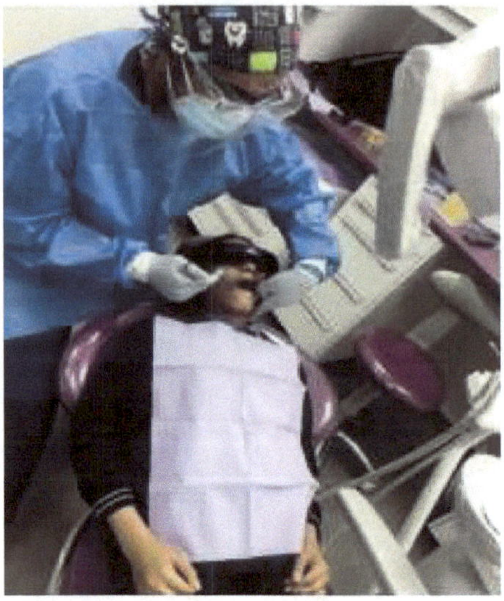

Fig. (23). Virtual Reality-Based Distraction.

WITAUL [Writing in the Air Using Leg] Technique

The WITAUL technique is one of the novel distraction techniques devised by Kamath in 2013. The technique involves raising the right leg in the air and writing hypothetically there. The WITAUL technique is easy for children above 4 years to explain and perform and requires no additional equipment. Alternative leg raising is found to be effective in reducing gag reflex in hypersensitive patients. This makes it versatile for use both in clinical and community settings.

Thaumaturgy

Isaac Bonewits has defined thaumaturgy as "the use of magic for non-religious purposes; the art and science of wonderworking." Thaumaturgy is a distraction technique since children in different age groups have differing cognitive development; hence, age-appropriate tricks can be used to distract the child's attention from unpleasant sensations associated with dental treatment. The distraction techniques using the thumb and light trick, book trick and item trick are effective in managing the behaviour of children of in various age groups, though the choice of technique is crucial in the treatment outcome [14].

Animal Assisted Therapy (AAT)

AAT has been studied extensively for various psychological disorders and relaxation therapies (Fig. **24**) [15]. The relationship of humans with animals, especially canine relationships, has been proven to be strong and beneficial in various areas. The addition of the therapy dog to an interprofessional team before sedation decreased anxiety levels and improved the behavioural outcomes of individuals with intellectual disabilities. Precautions include that the pet should be vaccinated, and the patient should not be phobic of the animals. It can be used especially in special-needs children, autism spectrum disorders and dementia.

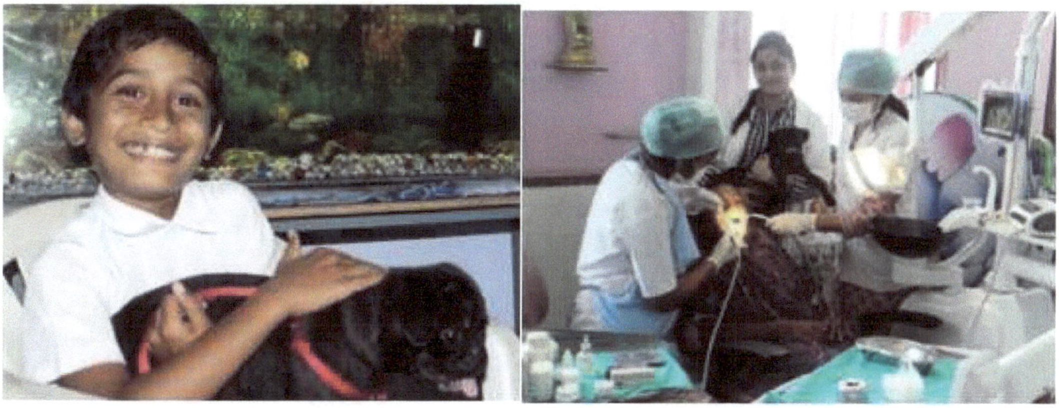

Fig. (24). Animal Assisted Therapy.

Robotic Approach

iRobiQ is an android robot resembling humans developed by Yujin Robot with a touchscreen and LCD on the front part of the body. This computerized panel can play animated/educational videos. It has multi-colour lights on its cheeks and eyes, and movable hands and wheels. With all these features, iRobiQ allows good communication with limited facial expressions such as disappointment, shyness, neutrality, surprise, and happiness. The procedure can be a useful adjunct to help reduce anxiety and make routine dental appointments fascinating. The robotic Approach can be used to motivate patients for good oral hygiene/preventive programs, confirming promising results in pain reductions and distress in children during dental treatment. However, the biggest disadvantage of the system is the high initial and maintenance cost of the robot [16].

Acupuncture and Acupressure

Acupuncture is an invasive approach in which needles are inserted at specific points in the body to treat a condition. It may provide an effective non-pharmacological approach to minimise the pain in children. Auricular acupuncture was found to be as equally effective as intranasal midazolam.

Acupressure is a non-invasive type of acupuncture and reduces general anxiety that is more appropriate for children. This technique involves the stimulation of acupoints through a wide variety of tools, including derma rollers or magnetic point stimulators. Avisa *et al.* (2018) concluded that acupressure could be a viable alternative to reduce dental anxiety in children undergoing scaling and restorative procedures [17].

CONCLUSION

Appropriate behaviour management techniques should be used to manage the child efficiently. A combination of techniques or behaviour guidance may be required to manage the child on the dental chair to perform the treatment and instill a positive dental attitude.

CONSENT FOR PUBLICATION

Not applicable.

CONFLICT OF INTEREST

The author(s) declare no conflict of interest, financial or otherwise.

ACKNOWLEDGEMENT

Declared none.

REFERENCES

[1] Zink AG, Molina EC, Diniz MB, Santos MTBR, Guaré RO. Communication Application for Use During the First Dental Visit for Children and Adolescents with Autism Spectrum Disorders. Pediatr Dent 2018; 40(1): 18-22.
[PMID: 29482677]

[2] Vishwakarma A, Bondarde P, Patil S, Dodamani A, Vishwakarma P, Mujawar S. Effectiveness of two different behavioral modification techniques among 5–7-year-old children: A randomized controlled trial. J Indian Soc Pedod Prev Dent 2017; 35(2): 143-9.
[http://dx.doi.org/10.4103/JISPPD.JISPPD_257_16] [PMID: 28492193]

[3] Liu Y, Gu Z, Wang Y, *et al.* Effect of audiovisual distraction on the management of dental anxiety in children: A systematic review. Int J Paediatr Dent 2019; 29(1): 14-21.
[http://dx.doi.org/10.1111/ipd.12430] [PMID: 30362187]

[4] Al-Khotani A, Bello LA, Christidis N. Effects of audiovisual distraction on children's behaviour during dental treatment: a randomized controlled clinical trial. Acta Odontol Scand 2016; 74(6): 494-501.
[http://dx.doi.org/10.1080/00016357.2016.1206211] [PMID: 27409593]

[5] Nuvvula S, Alahari S, Kamatham R, Challa RR. Effect of audiovisual distraction with 3D video glasses on dental anxiety of children experiencing administration of local analgesia: a randomised clinical trial. Eur Arch Paediatr Dent 2015; 16(1): 43-50.
[http://dx.doi.org/10.1007/s40368-014-0145-9] [PMID: 25256207]

[6] Abdelmoniem SA, Mahmoud SA. Comparative evaluation of passive, active, and passive-active distraction techniques on pain perception during local anesthesia administration in children. J Adv Res 2016; 7(3): 551-6.
[http://dx.doi.org/10.1016/j.jare.2015.10.001] [PMID: 27222759]

[7] Rath S, Khandelwal M, Rath S. Effectiveness of Distraction Techniques in Managing Pediatric Dental Patients. Int J Clin Pediatr Dent 2019; 12(1): 18-24.
[http://dx.doi.org/10.5005/jp-journals-10005-1582] [PMID: 31496566]

[8] Zhang C, Qin D, Shen L, Ji P, Wang J. Does audiovisual distraction reduce dental anxiety in children under local anesthesia? A systematic review and meta-analysis. Oral Dis 2019; 25(2): 416-24.
[http://dx.doi.org/10.1111/odi.12849] [PMID: 29498793]

[9] Best practices for protective stabilization for pediatric dental patients. Pediatr Dent 2017; 39(6): 260-5.
[PMID: 29179366]

[10] Cai H, Xi P, Zhong L, Chen J, Liang X. Efficacy of aromatherapy on dental anxiety: A systematic review of randomised and quasi-randomised controlled trials. Oral Dis 2021; 27(4): 829-47.
[http://dx.doi.org/10.1111/odi.13346] [PMID: 32267044]

[11] S PK, Aafaque S, S S, N N. Effect of Aromatherapy on Dental Anxiety Among Orthodontic Patients: A Randomized Controlled Trial. Cureus 2019; 11(8): e5306.
[http://dx.doi.org/10.7759/cureus.5306] [PMID: 31592362]

[12] Elicherla SR, Bandi S, Nuvvula S, Challa R, Saikiran KV, Priyanka VJ. Comparative evaluation of the effectiveness of a mobile app (Little Lovely Dentist) and the tell-show-do technique in the management of dental anxiety and fear: a randomized controlled trial. J Dent Anesth Pain Med 2019; 19(6): 369-78.
[http://dx.doi.org/10.17245/jdapm.2019.19.6.369] [PMID: 31942452]

[13] Shetty S, Katge F, Koticha P, Patil DP. Effectiveness of Virtual Reality Eyeglasses as a Distraction Aid to Reduce Anxiety among 6–10-year-old Children Undergoing Dental Extraction Procedure. Int J Clin Pediatr Dent 2019; 12(4): 297-302.
[http://dx.doi.org/10.5005/jp-journals-10005-1640] [PMID: 31866714]

[14] Agarwal M, Konde S, Sumaiyya S, Peethambar P. "Thaumaturgy"— A Novel Behavior-shaping Technique. Int J Clin Pediatr Dent 2020; 13(4): 318-21.
[http://dx.doi.org/10.5005/jp-journals-10005-1781] [PMID: 33149401]

[15] Cruz-Fierro N, Vanegas-Farfano M, González-Ramírez MT. Dog-Assisted Therapy and Dental Anxiety: A Pilot Study. Animals (Basel) 2019; 9(8): 512.
[http://dx.doi.org/10.3390/ani9080512] [PMID: 31370328]

[16] Kasimoglu Y, Kocaaydin S, Karsli E, *et al.* Robotic approach to the reduction of dental anxiety in children. Acta Odontol Scand 2020; 78(6): 474-80.
[http://dx.doi.org/10.1080/00016357.2020.1800084] [PMID: 32730719]

[17] Avisa P, Kamatham R, Vanjari K, Nuvvula S. Effectiveness of Acupressure on Dental Anxiety in Children. Pediatr Dent 2018; 40(3): 177-83.
[PMID: 29793563]

CHAPTER 5

Dental Caries: Etiology, Pathogenesis, and Caries Activity Tests

Armelia Sari Widyarman[1,*], **Enrita Dian R.**[2] and **Eko Fibryanto**[3]

[1] *Department of Oral Biology, Faculty of Dentistry, Universitas Trisakti, Jakarta, Indonesia*

[2] *Department of Pedodontic, Faculty of Dentistry, Universitas Trisakti, Jakarta, Indonesia*

[3] *Department of Conservative Dentistry, Faculty of Dentistry, Universitas Trisakti, Jakarta, Indonesia*

Abstract: Oral disease is one of the most significant global health concerns. Oral diseases have a monetary impact on people in developing countries. Disease can occur at any age and across a variety of demographic and socioeconomic conditions. Dental caries is a chronic microbial disease caused by a variety of factors, including the production of acid by bacteria *via* carbohydrate fermentation, which causes demineralization of tooth enamel, eventually leading to the loss of tooth structures and pulp infection. Caries is caused by an imbalance between tooth minerals and dental biofilms, which can develop over time in many people. Symptoms of dental caries begin with tooth pain and cavities and can lead to tooth loss. To prevent disease and maintain good oral health conditions, caries risk assessment is critical for controlling the progress of dental caries. Risk assessment is done by performing caries activity tests. Knowing the etiological factors associated with dental caries is important for clinicians and patients to prevent the disease from developing or halt its development and complications.

Keywords: Bacteria, Biofilms, Dental Caries, Oral Disease, *Streptococcus Mutans*.

INTRODUCTION

Oral diseases, which cause major health issues around the world, are economically affecting people of developing countries, as 10% of health expenditure is linked to dental care. These diseases can occur at any age and across all demographic and socioeconomic groups. Dental caries affects 2.43 billion individuals (36% of the global population) on their permanent teeth and affects 620 million individuals (9% of the global population) on their primary teeth. Latin America, the Middle East, and South Asia are regions with

* **Corresponding author Armelia Sari Widyarman:** Department of Oral Biology, Faculty of Dentistry, Universitas Trisakti, Jakarta, Indonesia; E-mail: armeliasari@trisakti.ac.id

Satyawan Damle, Ritesh Kalaskar, Dhanashree Sakhare & Abdulkadeer Jetpurwala (Eds.)

particularly high incidences of dental caries. According to the WHO, although there have been significant improvements in the oral health of the population in some countries, oral disease continues to occur in many individuals. The WHO has stated that poor oral health affects general health and quality of life, and that several oral diseases are associated with chronic systemic diseases. There are many debilitating symptoms associated with dental carics, including pain, mastication problems, aesthetic issues, and an inability to communicate due to damaged teeth or tooth loss [1, 2].

Etiology

Dental caries is a chronic microbial disease with numerous causative factors. Due to its acid production *via* carbohydrate fermentation by bacteria, it leads to the demineralization of tooth enamel, resulting in the loss of tooth structures. The major bacteria that cause dental caries are *Streptococcus mutans, Streptococcus sobrinus*, and *Lactobacillus* species. Many facultative and obligate anaerobic bacteria are also involved in the process, such as the *Actinomyces*, *Bifidobacterium*, *Eubacterium*, *Parvimonas*, and *Rothia* genera. Other bacteria may also take part in the formation of caries, such as *Streptococcus mitis*, *Streptococcus anginosus*, *Propionibacterium, Enterococcus faecalis, Scardovia, Prevotella*, *Selenomonas*, *Dialister*, *Fusobacterium*, *Pseudoramibacter*, *Veillonella, Atopobium, Granulicatella*, and *Leptotrichia*. On the oral mucosa, the predominant bacterial genera with a high concentration in dental plaque and gingival crevicular fluid and on the tonsils are *Bacteroides, Prevotella*, and *Porphyromonas* [3]. These bacteria can produce acid substances due to the high substrate availability on our teeth. The most common type of substrate is leftover foods that are not cleaned properly after eating. Bacteria can break down these remnants into simple sugars, which they then continue to ferment for their own use. If this goes untreated, acid is accumulated that causes the overall oral pH level to go down, and demineralization occurs [4]. From this description, we can define dental caries as an occurrence of disease caused by the over-accumulation of acid produced by plaque microorganisms, which brings about the destruction of the tooth structure.

Therefore, four key factors are required for dental caries to occur [5]:

- The tooth, acts as the host.
- The microorganism, acts as the causative agent (Figs. **1** and **2**).
- The substrate, acts as food for the causative agent.
- Time, required for the microorganism to ferment the substrate.

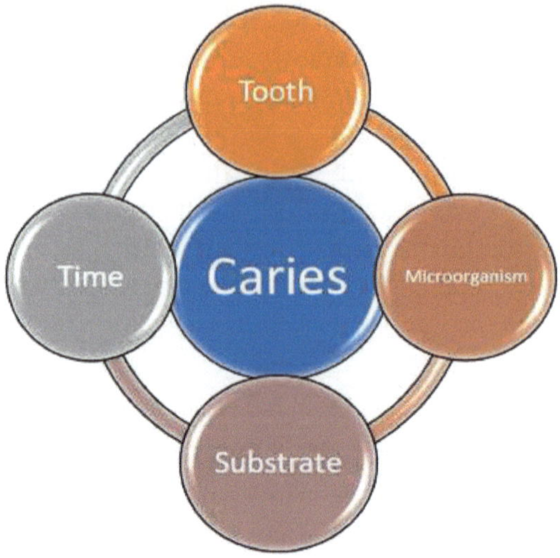

Fig. (1). Etiology of dental caries.

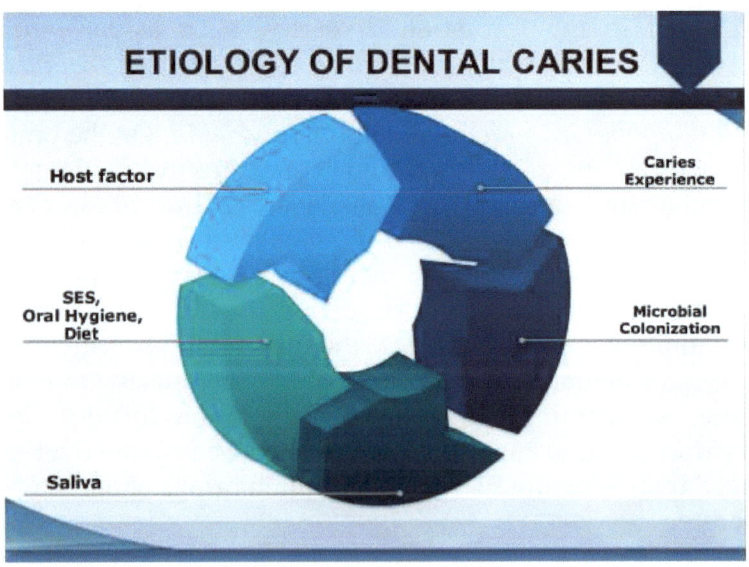

Fig. (2). Exhibiting etiological factors.

Pathogenesis

Dental Plaque and Biofilm

Dental biofilm is a polymicrobial community established within a solid-liquid interface, such as that formed by the oral microbiota on the surface of the teeth. Since it requires a liquid interface, the constant covering of saliva on teeth makes amassing biofilm a possibility. The extracellular polymeric substances (EPSs) become the pathological environment for cariogenic bacteria. Evidence shows that dental caries is caused by biofilms rather than infectious disease and begins when the biofilms cover the tooth surfaces. Dental biofilm is an active and complex environment embedded in EPSs. Biofilm starts to form when dental pellicle (glycoprotein film from saliva) covers thc tooth surfacc [6]. The initial microorganisms that colonize the biofilms and form the EPS are gram-positive bacteria, such *Streptococci* of the *mitis* and *mutans* species, which then attract other microorganisms [7].

Periodontal disease etiopathogenesis is normally associated with dental biofilms. The microorganism needs to be able to replicate and adhere a complex environment, such as gingival crevicular fluid and periodontal pockets, to survive. These microbial communities are known as plaque, which can be defined as numerous microorganisms that are embedded in an intercellular matrix. These microorganisms have their own metabolic, physical, and molecular interconnections. The microorganisms gain benefits from this consortium in terms of antimicrobial resistance, pathogenicity, development, and host defenses [8, 9]. The four stages of biofilm formation are 1) bacterial attachment to a surface, 2) microcolony formation, 3) biofilm maturation, and 4) the detachment (also termed dispersal) of bacteria, which may then colonize new areas, as shown in Fig. (**3**).

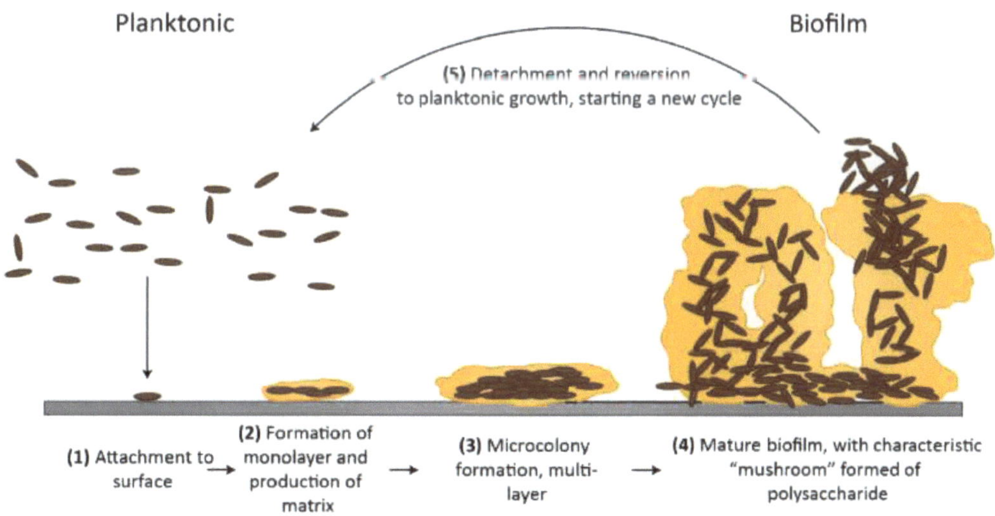

Fig. (3). Schematic representation of biofilm formation (Vasudevan 2014) [10].

The aggregation of cariogenic microorganisms in the biofilm leads to some changes in bacterial morphology. Some aerobic bacteria become facultatively anaerobic. The bacteria in the biofilm will replicate and become mature. Another essential characteristic of biofilm bacteria is quorum sensing, which involves the regulation of complex gene expression. These signals facilitate intercellular communication and lead to special characteristics arising in the biofilms [10].

The oral cavity is a complicated environment containing acid-producing and acid-resistant bacteria. There are 700 microorganisms in the human oral cavity and 200–300 bacterial species in dental plaque. Bacterial infection depends on the relationship between bacteria and the epithelium. The sticky material that covers the tooth surface is called dental plaque or a dental biofilm. The stickiness of plaque comes from dextran, which is sucrose fermented by *Streptococcus mutans.* This fermentation leads to enamel demineralization *via* lactic acid produced by *S. mutans.* These bacteria change sucrose into extracellular polysaccharides through glucosyltransferases (GTFs) and become another causal factor of dental caries in humans [11].

Moreover, this aids in the adhesion and accumulation of microorganisms on the teeth and protects the microorganisms from host immune defenses, increasing antibiotic resistance and altering gene expression. This contributes to the onset of enamel caries. A tooth cavity will develop if the dental plaque is not carefully removed. The mature dental plaque consists of a matrix of bacteria and polymers from the host, such proteins, DNA, and polysaccharides [12]. These molecules protect the bacteria against host defenses and improve their antimicrobial resistance. Several bacteria have resistance to acids and are associated with dental plaque, such as *Streptococcus mutans*, *S. mitis*, *S. constellatus*, *S. sanguis*, *S. salivarius*, *S. anginosus*, *S. gordonii*, *S. intermedius*, and *S. oralis* [13].

Sucrose is a main dietary source of dental caries, and many *Streptococcus* species possess extracellular enzymes that cleave the α-1 and α-2 glycosidic bonds of sucrose, producing glucose polymers (glucans and mutans) and fructose. These enzymes are known as glucosyltransferases (GTFs), and they are correlated with sucrose and caries. The biofilm accumulation from glucan-mutan polymers will eventually reach critical mass and cause the destruction of enamel. Therefore, this critical mass, which is closely related to glucosyltransferases and sucrose, is a biological causative factor of dental caries [14].

Demineralization Process

Dental caries is the localized destruction of dental tissue, which is caused by the fermentation of carbohydrates into acids produced by bacteria. Caries progresses slowly in many individuals and is triggered by the imbalance between tooth minerals and dental biofilms. The activity of microorganisms leads to changes in the pH of dental plaque due to acid production and the buffering action of saliva and tooth structures. It shows dynamic balance in the environment. If the pH drops below the critical value, the demineralization of enamel, dentine, or cementum will occur. Meanwhile, if the pH increases, remineralization will occur. The critical value of this pH phenomenon is affected by the bacterial maturation of carbohydrates, which drives the arrangement of an assortment of natural acids and a drop in pH. At first, H^+ will be taken up by buffers in plaque and saliva; when the pH proceeds to drop (H^+ increments), the liquid medium is drained of OH^- and phosphate particles, which react with H^+ to make H_2O and $(HPO)_4^{2-}$. Upon the exhaustion of these compounds, the pH can drop beneath 5.5, at which point the fluid stage gets to be beneath soaked regarding hydroxyapatite. Therefore, at whatever point the surface enamel is in contact with the microbial film, the metabolic activities inside this mass can cause variances and eventual drops in pH, which may result in the disintegration of the mineralized surface of the tooth [15]. This process occurs throughout the day. As a result, caries, or the repair and reversal of caries, develops over time. Three factors are listed in the classic definition of dental caries: the host, the bacteria, and the diet. Dental caries will take place if the tooth surface is colonized by cariogenic bacteria and if sucrose or refined sugar is available. The fermentation of carbohydrates by pathogens produces lactic acid and dissolves the hydroxyapatite crystal of the tooth, resulting in dental caries. The cavity is formed if there is imbalance between the demineralization and remineralization processes (Fig. **4**).

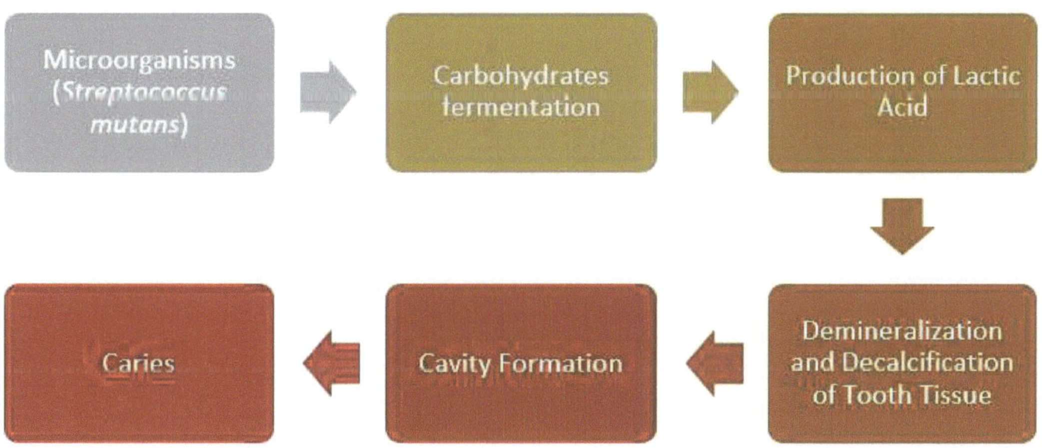

Fig. (4). Flowchart of dental caries pathogenesis.

Caries Activity Tests

The quantification of any one of the factors affecting dental caries could provide a marker of the risk for initiating, developing, or arresting the caries process. Even though dental caries is known to be a multifactorial disease, the vast number of caries susceptibility tests developed so far have been based on the microbiological aspects of dental caries. Caries risk assessment is critical for controlling dental caries. Caries assessment in primary dentition is important due to its relationship with the prevalence of caries in permanent dentition. Caries risk can be assessed by performing a caries activity test. These tests can provide information regarding the risk levels of caries for an individual patient and thus can provide information regarding the treatment needing to be given to that patient, both preventive and therapeutic. Even after therapeutic treatment, caries activity tests can be performed to maintain the success of dental restoration by observing and understanding behaviors towards decreasing the number of *S. mutans* and *Lactobacillus* species as part of dental counselling to reduce sucrose intake.

Microbiological parameters are used to test the caries activity. Caries activity tests have been developed to evaluate the acidogenic abilities of *S. mutans* and other aciduric bacteria in dental plaques related to the caries formation process. Practitioners have used the Cariostat device in caries activity tests for clinical purposes. According to earlier research, this method of determining the acidogenic potential of dental plaque is reliable for determining caries risk due to its high sensitivity and predictive ability. Below are several commonly used tests for detecting caries activity within an individual that are straightforward, simple, cheap, replicable whilst accurate, and that have clear backgrounds in the literature.

Definitions

Caries activity is defined as the occurrence of damage and the rate at which teeth are destroyed by the acid produced by plaque bacteria. It can also be defined as the sum of new carious lesions and the enlargement of existing carious cavities during a given time. Caries susceptibility is defined as the inherent propensity of the host and the target tissues to be afflicted by the carious lesions. Caries activity refers to the increment of active lesions (new and recurrent lesions) over a stated period. Caries activity is a measure of the speed of progression of a carious lesion.

A Caries Activity Test Helps to:

- Identify high-risk groups and individuals.
- Determine the need for personalized preventive measures and motivate the individual.

- Monitor the effectiveness of oral health education programs by establishing an initial baseline level of cariogenic pathogens as a basis for future evaluation.
- Ensure a low level of caries activity before starting any extensive restorative procedures.

- Serve as an index of the success of therapeutic measures by monitoring patient behavior towards reducing the number of *S. mutans* and *Lactobacillus* species as part of counseling to curtail sucrose intake.

Objectives

- To identify substantial risk groups and individuals.
- To determine the need for and extent of preventive measures.
- To determine the success of therapeutic measures.
- To motivate patients and monitor the effect of education programs related to diet counseling and oral hygiene procedures.
- Tests should have a sound theoretical basis.
- Tests should show maximum correlation with clinical status.
- Tests should be accurate with respect to duplication of results.
- Tests should be simple to perform.
- Tests should be inexpensive.
- Tests should take little time.

Uses

For a Clinician

- To determine the need for caries control measures.
- To act as an indicator of the patient's cooperation.
- To act as an aid in the timing of recall appointments.
- As a guide to the planning of expensive restoration procedures.
- To aid in the determination of prognosis.
- As a precautionary signal to the orthodontist in placing bands.

For the Research Worker

- As an aid in the selection of patients for caries studies.
- To aid in the screening of potential therapeutic agents.
- To serve as an indicator of the period of exacerbation and remission.

Ideal Requirements for Caries Activity Tests (Fig. 5)

Snyder has suggested that a suitable caries activity test should:

- Have a sound theoretical basis.
- Should have maximal correlation with clinical status
- Be accurate with respect to the duplication of results.

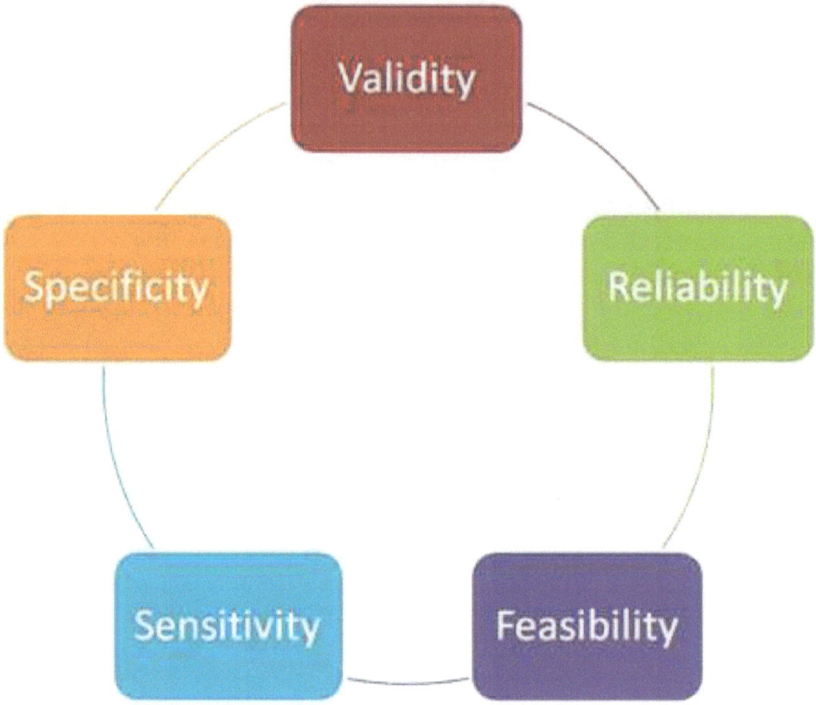

Fig. (5). Ideal characteristics of caries activity tests.

Be Simple & Inexpensive

The principle of this test is to measure the ability of microorganisms found in the saliva to produce organic acids from a medium containing a carbohydrate substrate with a pH indicator dye—Bromocresol green. Saliva is stimulated and collected in a calibrated plastic container. Subsequently, 0.2 ml of saliva is inserted into a petri dish or tube. A warm sterile medium (about 50°C) is then added to the corresponding petri dish or tube and homogenized. The petri dish or tube is allowed to harden *via* incubation at 37°C. It is assessed for color changes against a white background after 24, 48, and 72 hours of incubation, then compared with the uninoculated control petri dish or tube to qualitatively analyze the amount of acid generated by the bacteria. Color changes are divided into three groups, with each color indicating a different level of caries activity (Fig. **6**). This test meets some of the ideal test characteristics. Snyder and others have found a high correlation between the Snyder acid production test and *Lactobacillus* plate count.

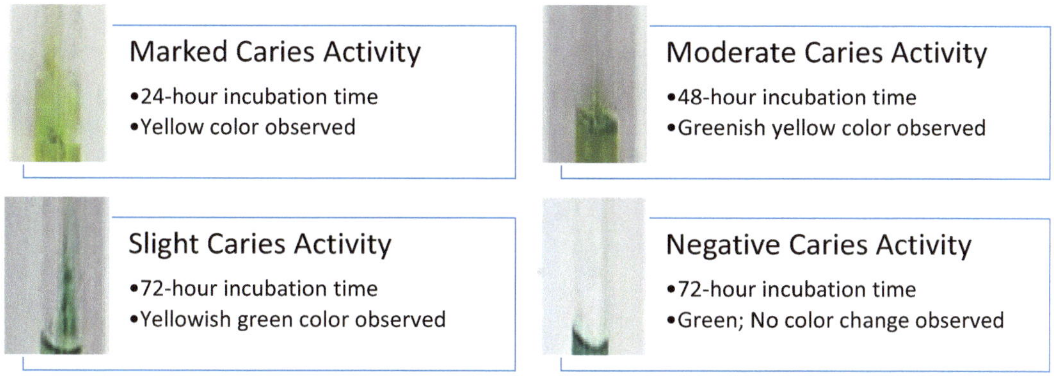

Fig. (6). Snyder's Test Result Interpretation (Tomer *et al.* 2019) [16].

a. Cariostat Test

Bromocresol green and purple are used as pH indicators. Plaque collection is performed before saliva collection for each subject. The plaque samples are collected *via* swabbing with a sterile cotton bud on the buccal surfaces of the maxillary first molars. Half of the plaque sample from the maxillary teeth is then inserted into the bromocresol green indicator, while the other half is inserted into the bromocresol purple. Both are subsequently incubated at 37°C for 48 h. The test tube is scored by comparing changes in both colors against a white background (Table **1**).

Table 1. Caries activity scores for Cariostat (Tomer *et al.* 2019) [16].

Score	Colour	pH
0	Blue	6.8
1	Green	5.2
2	yellow green	4.7
3	yellow	3.6

b. Lactobacillus Count Test (LBC)

This test, first introduced by Hadley in 1953, estimates the number of acidogenic and aciduric bacteria in the patient's saliva by counting the number of colonies appearing on tomato peptone agar plates after inoculation with a sample of saliva. The medium for the LBC test is Rogosa SL agar. A sterile wooden spatula is swabbed on each side of the mouth and pressed into the Rogosa agar medium. The medium is then incubated in an anaerobic jar at 37°C with an atmosphere of 85% nitrogen, 5–10% carbon dioxide, and 5–10% of oxygen. The milky white shapes on the Rogosa SL agar can be identified as colonies if they are round and convex with smooth borders and surfaces and are medium to large. Colony Forming Units (CFUs) are then measured on 1.5–2 cm of the circular area around the spatula impression (Fig 7), with 1 cm from the rounded tip. The number of microorganisms per ml saliva is the CFU (Table 2).

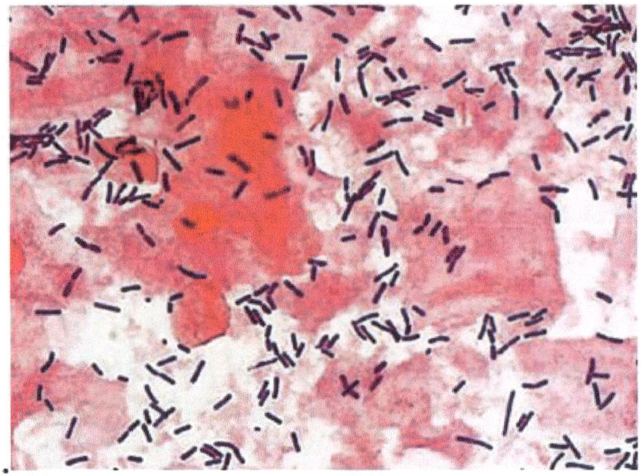

Fig. (7). *Lactobacillus* colony.

Table 2. ***Lactobacillus*** **CFU are classified by microbial count per ml of saliva (Tomer** ***et al.*** **2019) [16].**

Score	Category	-
0	0 colony	>10^4 CFU/ml saliva
1	1-20 colony	10^4 – $2x10^9$ CFU/ml saliva
2	21-40 colony	$2.1x10^5$ – $4x10^5$ CFU/ml saliva
3	41-100 colony	$4.1x10^5$ –10^6 CFU/ml saliva

CFUs: Colony forming units

Based on a recent study showing that LBC is associated with caries, a higher LBC count indicates an increase in caries rate and positive caries activity. At caries activity scores 1–3, there is a close relation between the Snyder test and LB count, however, there is no relation if the caries is inactive, or the caries activity score is 0. Both tests can be used to examine caries risk groups and make plans for future preventive treatments.

c. Fosdick Calcium Dissolution Test

This test measures the powdered enamel that is produced after being dissolved by acid, which is formed by the saliva of the patient mixed with glucose and powdered enamel. This test can display its results after four hours. As much as 25 ml of gum-stimulated saliva is collected, then put into a sterile tube with 0.1 g of powdered human tooth enamel inside. The tube is sealed and shaken for four hours at 37°C before being analyzed for its calcium content. Chewing gum is used to stimulate sugar production in the saliva. If paraffin is used, a concentration of about 5% glucose is added. As caries activity rises, so does the degree of enamel dissolution.

Dewar's Test

This test is like the Fosdick Calcium Dissolution test, but the pH is the variable being measured instead of the dissolution of powdered enamel. The final pH after four hours is measured instead of the amount of calcium dissolved. The lower the pH measured, the higher the caries activity is in that individual.

Caries Susceptibility Test is a simple, one-minute chair-side bacterial test for assessing patients' caries risk. CariScreen works by swiping a special swab with a reagent that reacts in the presence of adenosine triphosphate (ATP) over several teeth. Then, the swab is placed into a CariScreen testing meter (Fig. **8**).

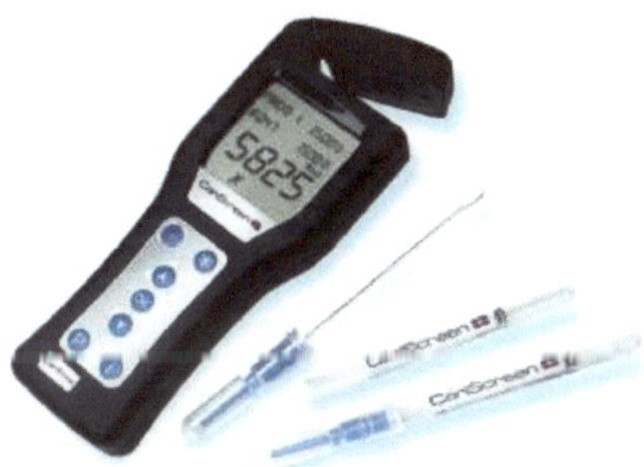

Fig. (8). CariScreen testing meter.

Procedure

• A bacitracin tablet is placed in buffered diluents and allowed to dissolve completely.

• The subject chews paraffin wax for 15–20 seconds, swallowing the saliva.

• While continuing to chew the wax, the subject expectorates approx. 1–2 ml of stimulated saliva directly into the diluents vial, which is then capped and gently mixed *via* repeated inversion.

• The dip slide coated on both sides with MSB agar (without bacitracin) is then immersed in the buffered diluents containing bacitracin and patient's saliva for a few seconds.

• A CO_2 tablet is placed in the empty dip slide vial, and two drops of water are added.

• The dip slide is replaced in its vial, and the cap is securely tightened.

The vial is placed upright for 48 hours at 37°C in an incubator and then allowed to stand at room temperature overnight.

• The colony density on the agar is compared with a reference colony density chart.

This test correlates strongly with actual laboratory methods of quantifying *Streptococcus mutans* by standard culturing. The colonies can be recognized when viewed through a magnifying lens by their opaque, highly convex appearance and irregular shape.

Advantages

The results will appear immediately.

This technology not only allows the dentist to measure the patient's risk for decay but also helps measure the progress of caries.

a. Swab Test
    ○ Developed by GRAINGER in 1965.

Procedure

- The procedure involves the sampling of the oral flora by swabbing buccal tooth surfaces.
- The sample is placed in the Snyder media.
- This is incubated for 48 hours, and the pH changes are read on a pH meter and correlated with caries activity.

Advantages

- This test has the advantage of not requiring the collection of saliva.
- The test is useful in predicting the caries increment, particularly in children with low or no previous caries experience.
    a. Salivary Reductase Test

This test measures the activity of the salivary enzyme reductase present in salivary bacteria.

Procedure

- Saliva is collected by having the patient chew paraffin and expectorate directly into the collection tube.
- The sample is then mixed with the dye Diaxo resorcinol.
- The changes in color are measured after 30 seconds and 15 minutes; these changes are taken as a measure of caries activity.

Advantages

- No incubation is required in conducting this test.
- This test provides quick results.

i)Oratest

This test was developed by Rosenberg in 1989.

Action

- Oratest is based on the rate of oxygen depletion by microorganisms in expectorated milk samples.
- Under aerobic conditions, the bacterial enzyme aerobic dehydrogenase transfers electrons or protons to oxygen.
- Once the oxygen is utilized by the aerobic organisms and an anaerobic environment is attained, methylene blue (a redox indicator) acts as an electron acceptor and is reduced to leucomethylene blue.
- The metabolic activity of the aerobic microorganisms is reflected by the reduction of methylene blue to leucomethylene blue.

Procedure

- The mouth is rinsed vigorously with 10 ml of sterile milk for 30 seconds, and the expectorate is collected.
- 3 ml of this is transferred to the screw cap tube with the help of a disposable syringe.
- To this, 0.12 ml of 0.1% methylene blue is added; the tube is then thoroughly mixed and placed on a stand in a well-illuminated area.
- The tubes are observed every 10 minutes for any color change at the bottom using a mirror. The time taken for the initiation of color change within a 6mm ring is recorded.
- The higher the infection rate, less time is taken for the change in color of the expectorate, reflecting higher oral microbial levels.

Advantages

- Less time-consuming.
- Economic.
- Non-toxic vehicle.
- Can be easily understood by auxiliary personnel.

Disadvantages

- Lack of specificity.

CONCLUSION

Knowledge of the etiological factors associated with dental caries is critical to prevent the disease from starting or to prevent its progression and complications. By doing so, the clinician may better work to prevent the growth of caries or provide treatment, while the patient will be better able to acknowledge the importance of dental caries and to maintain better oral health conditions. An accurate assessment of tooth vitality is of paramount importance in clinical practice. Although sensitivity testing is the de facto standard employed by most clinicians, it has acknowledged limitations. Careful consideration of diagnostic aids as well as Understanding their usefulness and limitations is essential if they are to be employed effectively in clinical dentistry.

CONSENT FOR PUBLICATION

Not applicable.

CONFLICT OF INTEREST

The author(s) declare no conflict of interest, financial or otherwise.

ACKNOWLEDGEMENT

Declared none.

REFERENCES

[1] Oral health [Internet]. [cited 2021 Apr 25]. Available from:. https://www.who.int/news-room/fac--sheets/detail/oral-health

[2] Richards D. Oral Diseases affect some 3.9 Billion people. Evid Based Dent 2013; 14(2): 35. [http://dx.doi.org/10.1038/sj.ebd.6400925] [PMID: 23792391]

[3] Kaur P, Singh S, Mathur A, *et al.* Impact of Dental Disorders and its Influence on Self Esteem Levels among Adolescents. J Clin Diagn Res 2017; 11(4): ZC05-8. [http://dx.doi.org/10.7860/JCDR/2017/23362.9515] [PMID: 28571250]

[4] Yadav K, Prakash S. Antibiogram profiles against polymicrobial pathogens among dental caries

patients at Janaki Medical College teaching hospital. Nepal Int J Appl Dent Sci 2015; 1: 156-62.

[5] Yadav K, Prakash S, Yadav NP, Sah RS. Multi-Drug Resistance of Bacterial Isolates among Dental Caries Patients. Janaki Medical College Journal of Medical Science 2016; 3(1): 37-44. [http://dx.doi.org/10.3126/jmcjms.v3i1.15374]

[6] Krzyściak W, Jurczak A, Piątkowski J. 2016.https://www.intechopen.com/books/microbial-biofilm--importance-and-applications/the-role-of-human-oral-microbiome-in-dental-biofilm-formation

[7] Lamont RJ, Koo H, Hajishengallis G. The oral microbiota: dynamic communities and host interactions. Nat Rev Microbiol 2018; 16(12): 745-59. [http://dx.doi.org/10.1038/s41579-018-0089-x] [PMID: 30301974]

[8] Jamal M, Ahmad W, Andleeb S, *et al.* Bacterial biofilm and associated infections. J Chin Med Assoc 2018; 81(1): 7-11. [http://dx.doi.org/10.1016/j.jcma.2017.07.012] [PMID: 29042186]

[9] Beceiro A, Tomás M, Bou G. Antimicrobial resistance and virulence: a successful or deleterious association in the bacterial world? Clin Microbiol Rev 2013; 26(2): 185-230. [http://dx.doi.org/10.1128/CMR.00059-12] [PMID: 23554414]

[10] Vasudevan R. Biofilms: microbial cities of scientific significance. J Microbiol Exp 2014; 1(3): 00014. [http://dx.doi.org/10.15406/jmen.2014.01.00014]

[11] Rathee M, Sapra A. Dental Caries.StatPearls. Treasure Island, FL: StatPearls Publishing 2021.http://www.ncbi.nlm.nih.gov/books/NBK551699/ Internet

[12] Karygianni L, Ren Z, Koo H, Thurnheer T. Biofilm Matrixome: Extracellular Components in Structured Microbial Communities. Trends Microbiol 2020; 28(8): 668-81. [http://dx.doi.org/10.1016/j.tim.2020.03.016] [PMID: 32663461]

[13] Johnston L, Vieira AR. Caries experience and overall health status. Oral Health Prev Dent 2014; 12(2): 163-70. [PMID: 24624396]

[14] Kawada-Matsuo M, Oogai Y, Komatsuzawa H. Sugar allocation to metabolic pathways is tightly regulated and affects the virulence of *Streptococcus mutans*. Genes (Basel) 2016; 8(1): 11. [http://dx.doi.org/10.3390/genes8010011] [PMID: 28036052]

[15] Abou Neel E, Aljabo A, Strange A, *et al.* Demineralization–remineralization dynamics in teeth and bone. Int J Nanomedicine 2016; 11: 4743-63. [http://dx.doi.org/10.2147/IJN.S107624] [PMID: 27695330]

[16] Tomer AK, Mangat P, Raina AA, *et al.* Diagnostic aids to detect caries-A review. IJADS 2019; 5(2): 16-20.

CHAPTER 6

Diagnosis of Dental Caries

Armelia Sari Widyarman[1,*], **Eko Fibryanto**[2] and **Tri Erri Astoeti**[3]

[1] *Head of Microbiology, Faculty of Dentistry, Universitas Trisakti, Jakarta, Indonesia*

[2] *Department of Conservative Dentistry, Faculty of Dentistry, Universitas Trisakti, Jakarta, Indonesia*

[3] *Department of Dental Public Health and Preventive Dentistry, Faculty of Dentistry, Universitas Trisakti, Jakarta, Indonesia*

Abstract: A balance between demineralization and remineralization is crucial for caries progression. Dental caries can progress if demineralization, which is associated with pathogenic factors, outweighs remineralization, which is linked to protective factors. In some sites, carious lesions are benign, whereas in others they progress and invade deep cavities. Dental caries can be classified according to the site where they occur and their size. Untreated carious lesions can lead to pulpal and periapical diseases. Treatment plan options are based on the diagnosis (pulpal or periapical).

Keywords: Demineralization, Dental Caries, Microorganisms, Remineralization, Substrate, *etc*.

INTRODUCTION

Dental caries is a common oral problem. In the absence of dental treatment, they can lead to tooth structure loss. Loesche stated that dental caries was associated with functional (mastication and pain) and nonfunctional issues (esthetics) and high treatment costs [1]. Dental caries is caused by host-related factors, such as tooth structure and diet (carbohydrate-rich) and microorganism-related factors, such as *Streptococcus mutans* and *Lactobacillus* spp. Host and microorganism factors are interrelated physically, functionally, and chemically. Other factors associated with dental caries are fluoride, saliva, individual behavior (laziness of maintaining oral health), education, dental health-related knowledge, income, and social class [1]. Hence, education also plays an important role in the risk of dental caries. Dental caries can progress when demineralization (pathogenic) factors outweigh remineralization (protective) factors. Acidic plaque (pH < 6.5) decreased salivary flow, impaired salivary buffer capacity, and poor oral hygiene

* **Corresponding author Armelia Sari Widyarman:** Head of Microbiology, Faculty of Dentistry, Universitas Trisakti, Jakarta, Indonesia; E-mail: armeliasari@trisakti.ac.id

Satyawan Damle, Ritesh Kalaskar, Dhanashree Sakhare & Abdulkadeer Jetpurwala (Eds.)

act as pathogenic factors. Saliva, sufficient calcium ions (Ca^{2+}) and phosphate ions (PO_4^{3-}) levels, good oral hygiene, fluoride, and antibacterial agents (*e.g.*, chlorhexidine and xylitol) act as protective factors. To determine the optimum treatment, a full dental examination must be undertaken to determine the location and severity of existing caries. The treatment options for carious lesions include surgical and nonsurgical options, depending on the caries progression (Fig. **1**) [2].

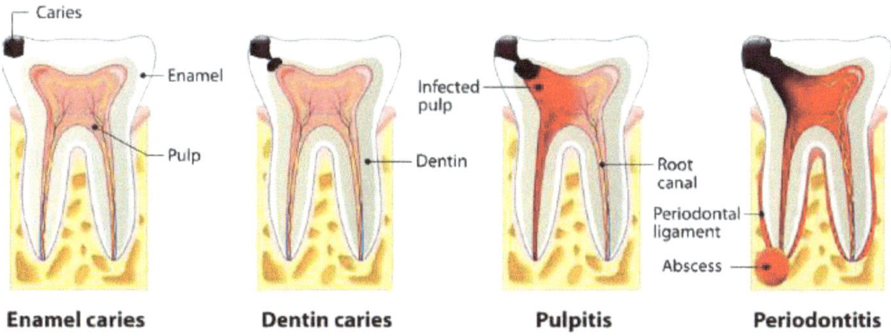

Fig. (1). Diagrammatic representation of dental caries progression [2].

Definitions

Dental caries is defined as a chronic oral disease caused by the bacterium *Streptococcus mutans*, which converts sugars into acid, causing tooth demineralization [3]. Demineralization is defined as mineral ions removal from hydroxyapatite hard tissues, while remineralization is defined as the restoration of mineral ions into hydroxyapatite hard tissues. Demineralization by *S. mutans* and other bacteria of inorganic structures and destruction of organic substances increase the risk of dental caries [1]. Unbalanced demineralization and remineralization of enamel and dentin cause dental caries (Fig. **1**). According to the World Health Organization (WHO), caries progression is a pathological process in which hard tooth tissue is softened, leading to cavity formation [3]. Based on the American Academy of Pediatric Dentistry Definitions, Oral Health Policies, and Clinical Guidelines, dental caries is the result of biofilm (plaque), mediated by saliva, with the biofilm inducing acid demineralization of enamel or dentin [3].

Four main factors are involved in tooth decay (Fig. **2**), namely [4]:

1. Tooth (host)
2. Substrate (fermentable carbohydrate)
3. Microorganisms (bacteria)
4. Time

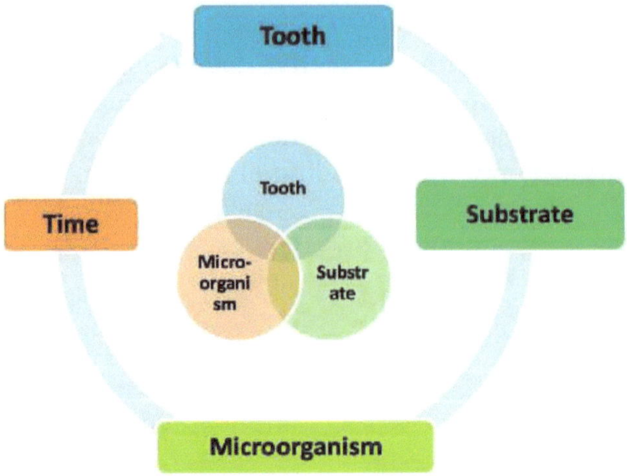

Fig. (2). Etiology of dental caries.

As depicted in Fig. (**3**), the components of a cariogram model are as follows:

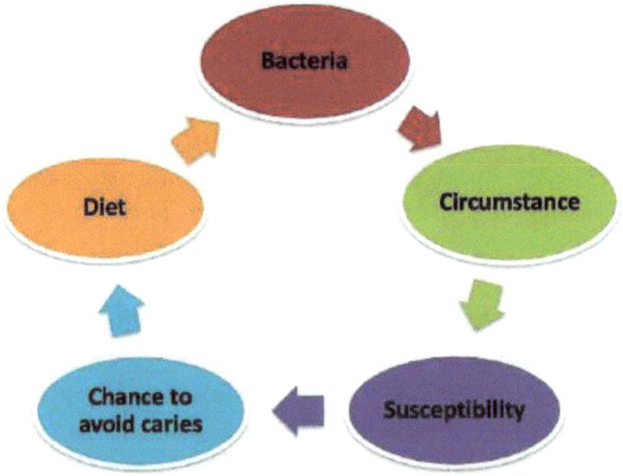

Fig. (3). Cariogram model [4].

Chance: Chance to prevent new cavities in the future

Diet: Consumption of food types and their sources

Bacteria: Numbers and types of bacteria in plaque

Susceptibility: Tooth defense (fluorides) and saliva characteristics

Circumstances: History of caries and systemic diseases

The main microorganism involved in the initial phase of dental caries is *S. mutans,* which colonizes smooth surfaces, pits, and fissures. Colonization by *S. mutans* is abided by the production of glucans and dextrans, insoluble sticky extracellular polysaccharides that increase adhesion to the tooth surface, resulting in demineralization and cavity formation [4]. Thus, dental caries is a dynamic process, which involves demineralization and remineralization (Figs. **4** & **5**).

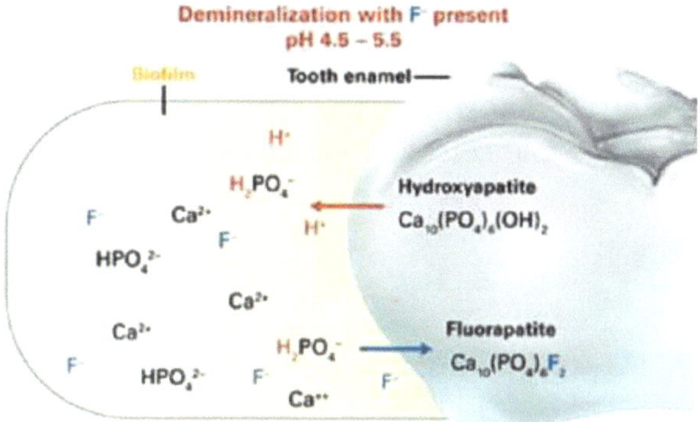

Fig. (4). Demineralization process [5].

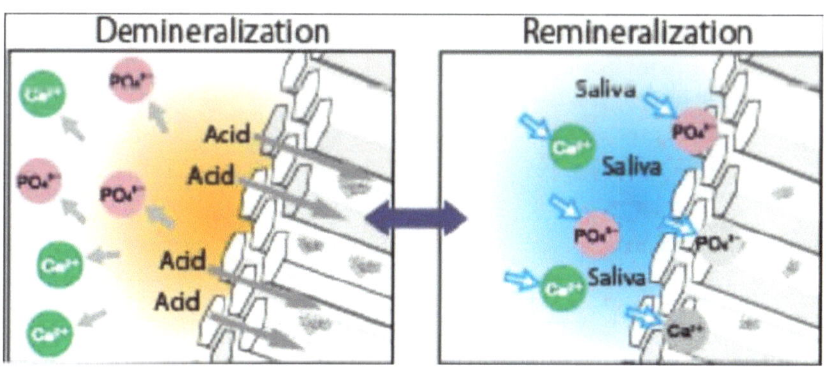

Fig. (5). Demineralization and remineralization processes [6].

The carious process is initiated by bacterial fermentation of carbohydrates, leading to the formation of a variety of organic acids and a reduction in pH. In the early stages of caries formation, hydrogen (H^+) ions are taken up by buffers in plaque and saliva. However, when the pH decreases due to an increase in H^+ ions, the fluid medium is depleted of hydroxide (OH^-) and phosphate ions, which react with H^+ to form H_2O and hydrogen phosphate $(HPO)_4^{2-}$. Upon total depletion of these compounds, the pH can fall below a critical value (*i.e.*, 5.5) [5]. The saliva then becomes undersaturated with respect to hydroxyapatite [5].

A buffer system exists in saliva comprising bicarbonate and ammonia ions. Due to the presence of this system, H^+ ion transfer within the buffer system can raise the pH of saliva within 30–40 minutes. The pH value then becomes neutral, and calcium and phosphate ions are deposited into hard tissue of the teeth. This process is called remineralization, and the remineralization process is faster in the presence of fluoride in the plaque or saliva [6]. Fluorides, sodium-calcium phosphosilicate (bioactive glass), functionalized tricalcium phosphate, casein phosphopeptide-amorphous calcium phosphate, and casein phosphopeptide-amorphous calcium fluoride phosphate are remineralizing agents, as they can be applied to the tooth surface and release ions required for remineralization (Fig. **6**) [7].

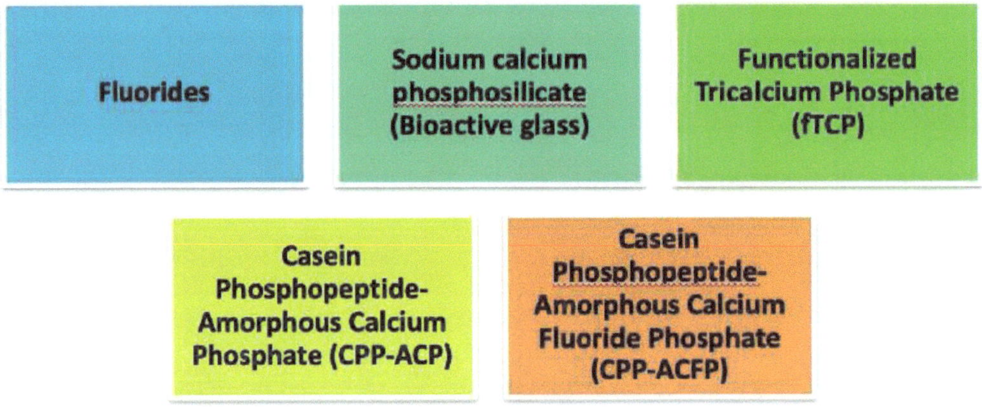

Fig. (6). Remineralization agents [7].

From the diet aspect of caries formation, refined sugars, such as the lactose in milk and fructose in fruit juice, contribute to tooth decay. In terms of tooth decay, starchy foods (*e.g.*, potato chips and popcorn) are worse than sugary foods, as they tend to stick to the tooth surface. Caries prevention depends on the knowledge of balancing between protective and pathogenic factors. Over consumption of refined sugars, along with lack of oral health maintenance can disrupt the balance and arching towards growth of pathogenic factors. Tooth mineral loss is part of the demineralization process, leading to cavity formation and eventual invasion of pulpo-dentinal structures.

Dental Caries Classification

The severity and incidence of dental caries are measured using the Decayed, Missing and Filled (DMF) index of Klein *et al.* or Decayed, Extraction, and Filled index of Gruebbel [8, 9]. Both indexes classify only cavitary carious lesions. Other indexes are used to classify additional phases of carious lesion formation. These include the International Caries Detection and Assessment System (ICDAS), which assesses changes in the tooth surface and histological depth of carious lesions, and Pulp, Ulcer, Fistula, and Abscess (PUFA), which assesses the level of pulpal involvement (*i.e.*, carious lesion severity). Another index known as the Caries Assessment Spectrum and Treatment (CAST) is used to evaluate carious lesion progression [2].

In 2008, the American Dental Association (ADA) and other experts began to develop a caries classification system (CCS) to aid pulpal and periapical disease diagnosis and dental treatment planning. The current version of the ADA CCS is presented in this report. The ADA CCS is intended to be easily applied in clinical practice. As compared with other caries classification methods used for caries diagnosis and treatment, the ADA CCS has some similarities and differences, which are presented in the later section.

Carious lesions can be classified as active or inactive based on their activity. Remineralized carious lesions can be used with caution to show inactive lesions, based on their development. An inactive lesion is defined as a lesion less likely to progress into caries. It depends on the balance between biofilms and environmental factors [4]. Clinicians must be able to determine whether a carious lesion is active or inactive. Inactive lesions require no treatment, as they will not progress and become dental caries. On the other hand, active lesions require treatment to impede demineralization and maintain the ecological balance in the oral cavity. The initial stage of a carious lesion on enamel is called a white spot lesion, which can be seen with the naked eye. A white spot lesion may remain inactive for several years before becoming active [7]. Thus, the initial classification of the lesion as inactive may change over time [7].

Dental Caries Classification

Dental caries classifications based on different factors are outlined below [4, 7]. These factors include lesion location (Figs. **7** and **8**), tissue involvement (Fig. **9**), carious stage (Fig. **10**), lesion severity (Fig. **11**), tooth surface involvement (Fig. **12**), and age (Fig. **13**). There are also dental caries classifications created by WHO (Fig. **14**) and others described further below.

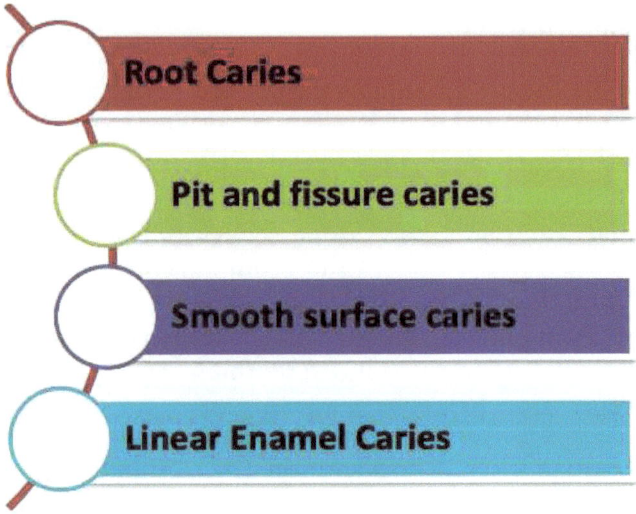

Fig. (7). Classification of dental caries based on their location.

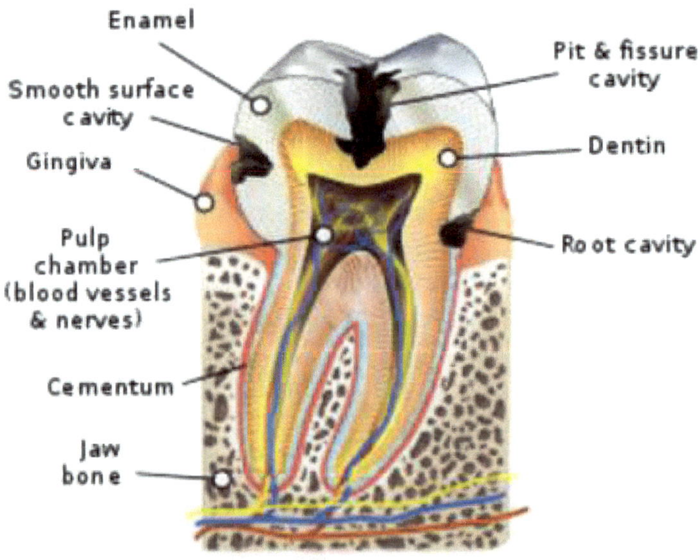

Fig. (8). Illustration of dental caries within the tooth.

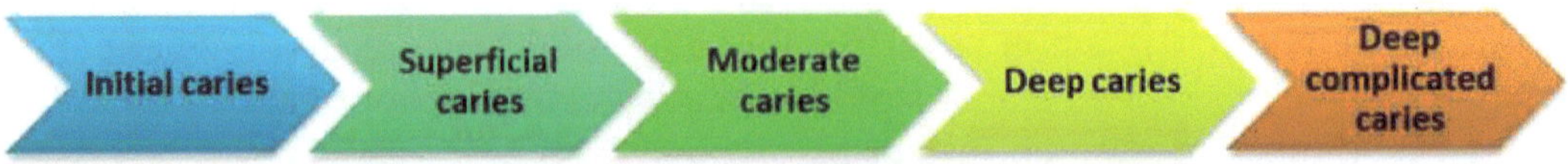
Initial caries
Superficial caries
Moderate caries
Deep caries
Deep complicated caries

Fig. (9). Dental caries classification based on tissue involvement.

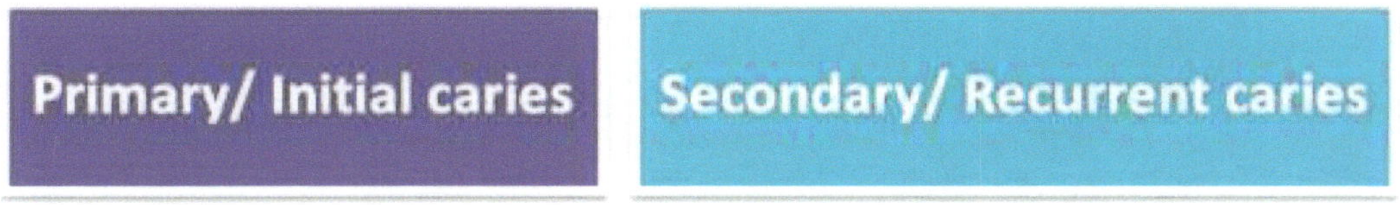
Primary/ Initial caries
Secondary/ Recurrent caries

Fig. (10). Dental caries classification based on the stage of caries growth.

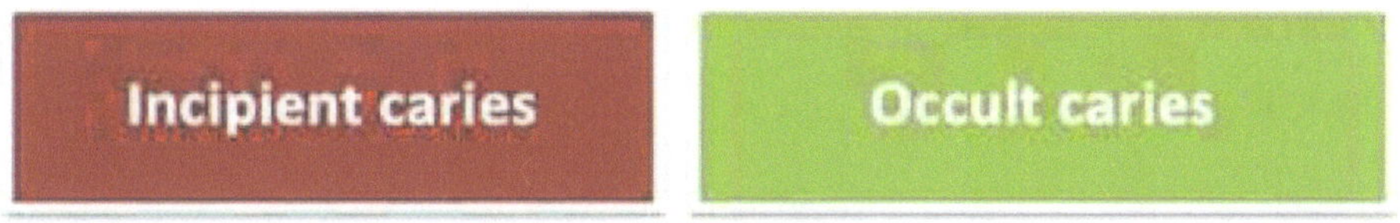
Incipient caries
Occult caries

Fig. (11). Dental caries classification based on lesion severity.

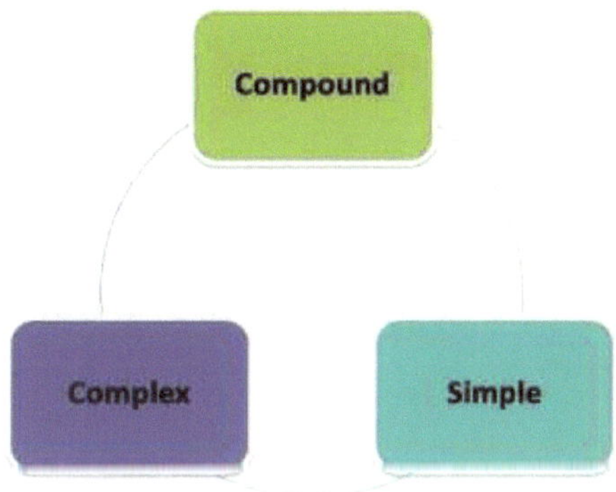

Fig. (12). Dental caries classification based on tooth surface involvement.

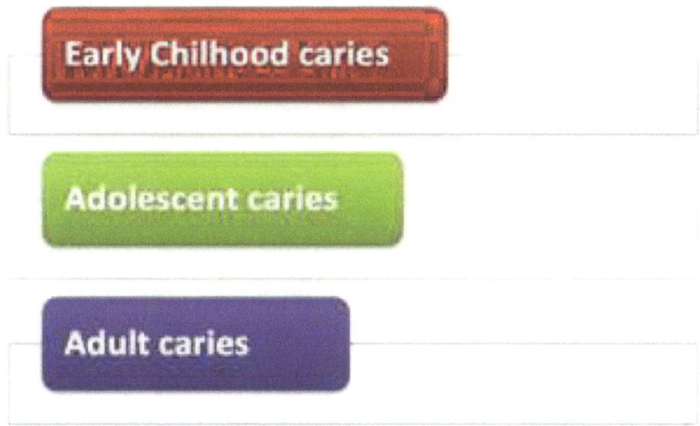
Early Chilhood caries
Adolescent caries
Adult caries

Fig. (13). Dental caries classification based on age.

WHO Classification (1995)

- K02.0 – Caries limited to enamel
  - White spot lesion (Initial caries)
- K02.1 – Caries extending into dentin
- K02.2 – Caries of cementum
- K02.3 – Arrested caries
- K02.4 – Odontoclasia
  - Infantile melanodontia
  - Melanodontoclasia
  - Excludes: internal & external resorption of teeth (K03.3)
- K02.8 – Other specified dental caries
- K02.9 – Dental caries, unspecified

Fig. (14). Dental caries classification according to WHO.

Aside from the previously mentioned classification of caries, Mount and Hume (1997) classified carious lesions according to their location and size, as below:

A). Location

Location 1:	Lesions on pits and fissures of occlusal surfaces of the posterior teeth. These include buccal grooves of lower molars and palatal grooves of upper molars.
Location 2:	Lesions on contact areas of posterior and anterior teeth
Location 3:	Lesions of the gingival third of all teeth

B). Size

Size 1 (mild):	Lesions that have progressed just beyond remineralization
Size 2 (moderate):	Larger lesions, with adequate tooth structure to support restoration
Size 3 (enlarged):	Lesions in which the tooth structure and the restoration are susceptible to fracture
Size 4 (severe):	Lesions that have destroyed most of the tooth structure

Another dental caries classification is called Black's classification (Fig. **15**), which is based on the location of carious lesions on the tooth and the site of the tooth [10]. The classification system is as follows:

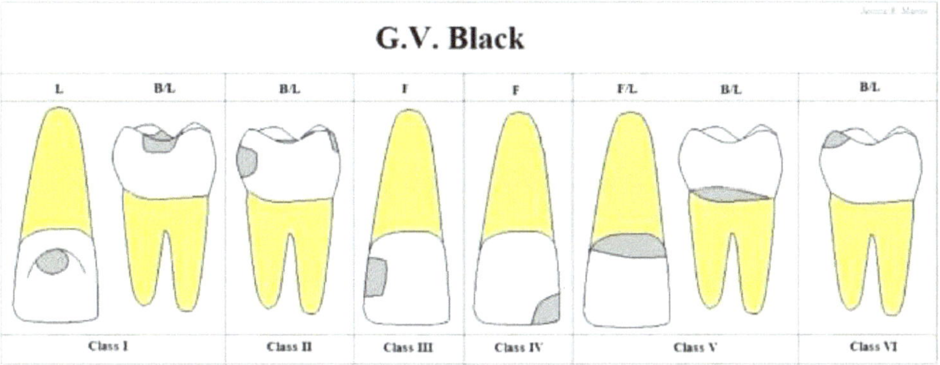

Fig. (15). Black's classification of carious lesions [8].

Class I: Caries on pits and fissures of facial, lingual, and occlusal surfaces on premolars and molars

Class II: Caries on proximal surfaces of posterior teeth

Class III: Caries on proximal surfaces of anterior teeth

Class IV: Caries on proximal and incisal surfaces of anterior teeth

Class V: Caries on facial and lingual surfaces in the cervical third of teeth

Class VI: Lesions on incisal edges of anterior teeth and cusp tips of posterior teeth

International Caries Detection and Assessment System (ICDAS) is a system developed by proven clinicians, epidemiologists, and researchers to provide better quality data of dental caries and to allow customized management of total caries in accordance with the condition of the patient [2]. American Dental Association Caries Classification System (ADA CCS) classifies caries as a disease that progresses with time, in which implications for patient treatment are affected. This classification attempts to maintain a balance between data collection and constraints imposed by time constraints (Tables **1** and **2**).

Table 1. ADA classification system.

No caries	No lesion on the tooth surface
Initial enamel caries	Visible, no cavity lesion and limited to enamel
Moderate dentin caries	Destruction of enamel or loss of root cementum, with no cavity on dentin
Severe dentin caries	Extensive cavity on enamel and dentin

Table 2. ADA chart entry coding [8].

-	Class 1 (Sound teeth)	Class 2 (initial lesion)	Class 4 (moderate lesion)	Class 6 (extensive lesion)
Pit and fissure (P)	P.0	P.2	P.4	P.6
Approximal (A)	A.0	A.2	A.4	A.6
Cervical and smooth surfaces (C)	C.0	C.2	C.4	C.6
Root surfaces (R)	R.0	R.2	R.4	R.6

Another classification is called site-stage (Si/STA) classification, which is the same as the Mount–Hume system [11]. Both systems classify carious lesions according to the lesion site and stage [4].

The Caries Assessment Spectrum and Treatment (CAST) index shows the different stages of caries is shown in Table **3**.

Table 3. CAST index codes and criteria [12].

Characteristics	Code	Description
-	0	Healthy – no carious lesions seen
Sealed	1	Sealed pits and fissures partially or completely sealed with sealant filling
Restored	2	Cavity restored with direct restorative filling, without dentine involvement and no fistula/abscess seen
Enamel	3	Alteration of enamel, such as visible spots on enamel (whitish or brownish spots) and destruction of localized enamel but no visible dentinal involvement
Dentine	4	Dentinal changes, including discoloration of dentine visible through the enamel and sometimes localized damage
Pulp	5	Distinct cavitation into dentine and no (expected) pulpal involvement present
	6	Carious lesion extending into the pulp chamber, with a cavity in the pulp chamber and only the tooth root visible
	7	Abscess/fistula: dental abscess due to a carious lesion in the pulp chamber, with the abscess containing pus and reaching the sinus area
Lost	8	Tooth extraction due to a carious lesion
Other	9	Unclassified carious lesion

While dental classifications have been made thus far, a special case of caries, which is called rampant caries, may emerge. Rampant caries refers to the sudden appearance of widespread, rapidly burrowing types of caries, which damage enamel and result in early pulpal involvement [13]. Such caries affects erupted teeth, usually regarded as immune to ordinary decay. Patients with rampant caries have five or more new carious lesions on tooth surfaces each year. This dental condition is one of the most difficult cases for dentists due to the complexity in determining dental treatment and a future preventive plan. Based on the severity of rampant caries, they can be classified as bottle or nursing caries, early childhood caries, radiation caries, or drug-induced caries [13].

Transmission of Microorganisms from Mother to Child

Li and Caufield [14] showed that microorganisms can be transmitted vertically from mother to infant. They collected saliva samples from mothers and new-borns every 3 months for 3 years and identified oral microorganisms using 16s metagenomics. In 71% of cases, the microorganisms identified in the mothers' samples were the same as those in the infants' samples. It is important to note that female infants inherit oral microbiome profile that are substantially more like their mothers than male infants (88% and 53%). The results of the study by Li and Caufield [14] show that several strains of microorganisms can be transmitted from mother to infants and that sex determines the likelihood of similarity of microorganisms [14].

Intrafamily Transmission of Microorganisms to Children

Kulkarni *et al*. [15]. conducted restriction endonuclease analysis (REA) of cellular DNA of 396 clinical strains of *S. mutans* and conveyed that the study of microorganism transmission can be conducted using REA and documented types of microorganism strains. *Eco*RI and *Hind*III enzymes were used to digest DNA, then electrophoresed on agarose gel, and the visualized bands were compared. The study used fresh isolates from 58 participants and included 19 strains from each member of five families. The pattern of these microorganisms is different from each other, excluding from the same family. The band profiles reveal similar results intrafamily-wise. The study also revealed different patterns of *S. mutans* in the different families. The participants had a high level of multiple REA forms (up to five). This study provides evidence of intrafamily transmission of microorganisms to children within the same family. However, interestingly, evidence from Kulkarni *et al*. [15] also discerned the possibility of transmission from different families into children.

Diagnosis

Untreated carious lesions can lead to pulpal and periapical diseases. Pulpal and periapical diagnoses have been developed to provide the proper treatment plan options. Establishing a diagnosis requires knowledge, skills, and the ability to interpret and interact with the patient. Both subjective (based on the clinician's deduction) and objective (based on the patient's medical record) examinations are required to ensure the correct diagnosis and a successful treatment plan.

The depth and area of caries cannot be used as a benchmark for establishing the diagnosis of pulpal and periapical diseases. Clinical signs, symptoms, and histopathology are more suitable than caries depth/area in the differential diagnosis of pulpal diseases. Pulpal and periapical disease terminologies and classifications used by the American Association of Endodontists (AAE) are shown in Table **4**.

Table 4. Recommended diagnostic terminology based on AAE consensus conference [16].

Pulpal	-
Normal pulp	Clinical diagnostic category in which pulp is symptom free and normally responsive to pulp testing
Reversible pulpitis	Clinical diagnosis based on subjective and objective findings pointing to resolution of pulpal inflammation
Symptomatic irreversible pulpitis	Clinical diagnosis based on subjective and objective findings pointing to nonhealing of vital inflamed pulp, accompanied by lingering thermal pain, spontaneous pain, and referred pain
Asymptomatic irreversible pulpitis	Clinical diagnosis based on subjective and objective findings pointing to nonhealing of vital inflamed pulp, with no clinical symptoms but inflammation related to caries, caries excavation, and trauma
Pulp necrosis	Clinical diagnostic category indicating death of dental pulp, where pulp is usually nonresponsive to pulpal testing
Previously treated	Clinical diagnostic category indicating that the tooth has been endodontically treated and that canals have been obturated with various filling materials other than intracanal medicaments
Previously initiated therapy	Clinical diagnostic category indicating that the tooth has been previously treated by partial endodontic therapy (*e.g.*, pulpotomy, pulpectomy)

Apical	-
Normal apical tissues	Teeth with normal periradicular tissues that are not sensitive to percussion or palpation testing; intact lamina dura surrounding the root and uniform periodontal ligament space
Symptomatic apical periodontitis	Inflammation, usually of the apical periodontium, producing clinical symptoms, including a painful response to biting and/or percussion or palpation, which may or may not be associated with an apical radiolucent area
Asymptomatic apical periodontitis	Inflammation and destruction of apical periodontium of pulpal origin, appears as an apical radiolucent area, and does not produce clinical symptoms

(Table 4) cont.....

Apical	-
Acute apical abscess	An inflammatory reaction to pulpal infection and necrosis characterized by rapid onset, spontaneous pain, tenderness of the tooth to pressure, pus formation, and swelling of associated tissues
Chronic apical abscess	An inflammatory reaction to pulpal infection and necrosis characterized by gradual onset, little or no discomfort, and intermittent discharge of pus through an associated sinus tract
Condensing osteitis	Diffuse radiopaque lesion representing a localized bony reaction to a low-grade inflammatory stimulus, usually seen at the apex of the tooth

CONCLUSION

Several new classifications of dental caries have been proposed in the last decade. Of these, Black's classification remains the most widely accepted. We should identify the carious lesion from the early stage of remineralizable before dental restorative treatment is required. Caries progression affects the dental pulp, leading to pulpal and periapical diseases. The diagnosis of pulpal and periapical diseases is crucial to determine treatment planning.

CONSENT FOR PUBLICATION

Not applicable.

CONFLICT OF INTEREST

The author(s) declare no conflict of interest, financial or otherwise.

ACKNOWLEDGEMENT

Declared none.

REFERENCE

[1] Rathee M, Sapra A. Dental Caries.StatPearls. Treasure Island, FL: StatPearls Publishing 2021.https://www.ncbi.nlm.nih.gov/books/NBK551699/ Updated 2021 Mar 12 Internet.

[2] 2021.https://www.dentalhealth.ie/your-oral-health/terms/dental-caries-tooth-decay/

[3] Pitts NB, Zero DT, Marsh PD, *et al.* Dental caries. Nat Rev Dis Primers 2017; 3(1): 17030. [http://dx.doi.org/10.1038/nrdp.2017.30] [PMID: 28540937]

[4] Bratthall D, Hänsel Petersson G. Cariogram - a multifactorial risk assessment model for a multifactorial disease. Community Dent Oral Epidemiol 2005; 33(4): 256-64. [http://dx.doi.org/10.1111/j.1600-0528.2005.00233.x] [PMID: 16008632]

[5] Nakano K, Nomura R, Nakagawa I, Hamada S, Ooshima T. Role of glucose side chains with serotype-specific polysaccharide in the cariogenicity of *Streptococcus mutans.* Caries Res 2005; 39(4): 262-8. [http://dx.doi.org/10.1159/000084831] [PMID: 15942184]

[6] Featherstone JD. The continuum of dental caries: evidence for a dynamic disease process. J Dent Res

2004; 83: C39-42.

[7] Mittal R, Relhan N, Tangri T. Remineralizing Agents: A Comprehensive Review. International Journal of Clinical Preventive Dentistry 2017; 13(1): 1-4. [http://dx.doi.org/10.15236/ijcpd.2017.13.1.1]

[8] Klein H, Palmer CE, Knutson JW. Studies on dental caries: I. Dental status and dental needs of elementary school children. Public Health Reports (1896-1970) 1938; 751-65.

[9] Gruebbel AO. A measurement of dental caries prevalence and treatment service for deciduous teeth. J Dent Res 1944; 23(3): 163-8. [http://dx.doi.org/10.1177/00220345440230030201]

[10] Young DA, Nový BB, Zeller GG, *et al.* The American Dental Association caries classification system for clinical practice: a report of the American Dental Association Council on Scientific Affairs. J Am Dent Assoc 2015; 146(2): 79-86. [http://dx.doi.org/10.1016/j.adaj.2014.11.018] [PMID: 25637205]

[11] Mount GJ, Tyas MJ, Duke ES, Lasfargues JJ, Kaleka R, Hume WR. A proposal for a new classification of lesions of exposed tooth surfaces. Int Dent J 2006; 56(2): 82-91. [http://dx.doi.org/10.1111/j.1875-595X.2006.tb00078.x] [PMID: 16620036]

[12] Leal SC, Ribeiro APD, Frencken JE. Caries Assessment Spectrum and Treatment (CAST): a novel epidemiological instrument. Caries Res 2017; 51(5): 500-6. [http://dx.doi.org/10.1159/000479042] [PMID: 28968606]

[13] Yusuf TN, Jeffrey J. Comprehensive Treatment for Eight Years Old Child with Rampant Caries. Journal of Medicine and Health 2020; 2(5) [http://dx.doi.org/10.28932/jmh.v2i5.1843]

[14] Li Y, Caufield PW, Dasanayake AP, Wiener HW, Vermund SH. Mode of delivery and other maternal factors influence the acquisition of *Streptococcus mutans* in infants. J Dent Res 2005; 84(9): 806-11. [http://dx.doi.org/10.1177/154405910508400905] [PMID: 16109988]

[15] Kulkarni GV, Chan KH, Sandham HJ. An investigation into the use of restriction endonuclease analysis for the study of transmission of mutans streptococci. J Dent Res 1989; 68(7): 1155-61. [http://dx.doi.org/10.1177/00220345890680070401] [PMID: 2632600]

[16] Glickman GN. AAE Consensus Conference on Diagnostic Terminology: Background and Perspectives. 1619-20.

CHAPTER 7

Role of Diet in Dental Caries

Satyawan Damle[1,*], **Prachi Goyal**[2] and **Dhanashree Sakhare**[3]

[1] *Nair Hospital Dental College, Mumbai, and Former Vice-Chancellor M. University Mullana Ambala, Haryana, India*

[2] *Maharishi Markandeshwar College of Dental Sciences and Research, Ambala, India*

[3] *Founder Lavanika Dental Academy, Melbourne, Australia*

Abstract: The importance of sugars as a cause of dental caries is underemphasized and not prominent in preventive strategies. Quantitative analysis shows a log-linear dose-response relationship between sucrose or its monosaccharide intakes and the progressive lifelong development of caries. This results in a substantial dental health burden throughout life. Processed starches have cariogenic potential when accompanying sucrose. Dental diseases impair quality of life and hurt self-esteem, eating ability and health, causing pain, anxiety, and impaired social functioning. So, it was also thought that diet could be controlled or modified, to exert an anti-caries effect. Several experiments, studies and research have been carried out to assess the effect of diet on dental caries.

Keywords: Dental Caries, Diet counselling, Sugar studies, Sugar Substitutes.

INTRODUCTION

Dental caries is the most prevalent Non-Communicable Disease (NCD) globally and affects all age groups across the life course. Despite the accepted scientific evidence that caries creates incredibly significant personal, societal, and economic burdens across the world and that caries presents the largest numerical impact on oral health, the disease has typically been invisible in health policies. This situation appears to be paradoxical, as the burdens and pain caused by caries and cavities are preventable and addressing the risk factors for cavities can also reduce other non-communicable diseases and improve general health. The main cause of tooth loss is dental caries (Fig. **1**), in which diet plays an important role.

* **Corresponding author Satyawan Damle:** Nair Hospital Dental College Mumbai, and Former Vice-Chancellor M University Mullana Ambala, Haryana, India; Tel: +91 9729062515; E-mail: sgdamble@gmail.com

Satyawan Damle, Ritesh Kalaskar, Dhanashree Sakhare & Abdulkadeer Jetpurwala (Eds.)

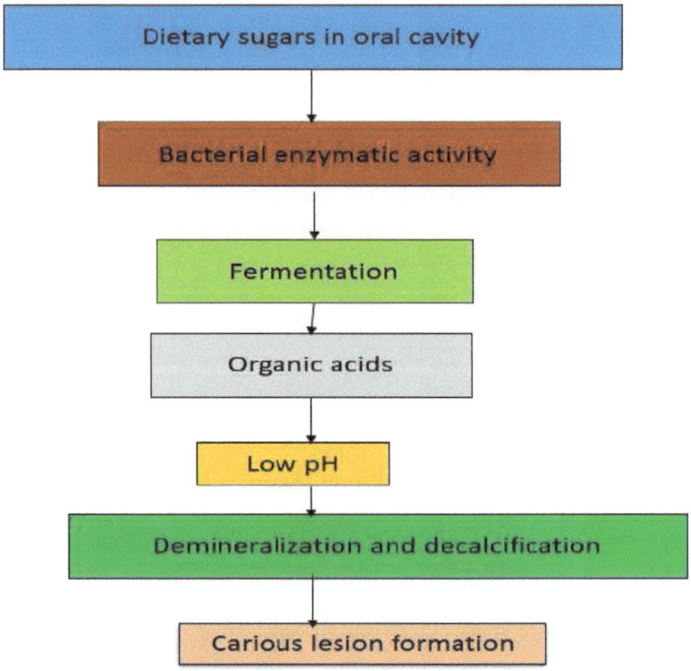

Fig. (1). Factors and sub-factors that influence caries development.

Oral health is related to diet in many ways; for example, nutrition influences craniofacial development and oral mucosal and dental diseases, including dental caries, enamel defects and periodontal disease. Dental diseases impair quality of life and hurt self-esteem, eating ability and health, causing pain, anxiety, and impaired social functioning. Tooth loss reduces the ability to eat a nutritious diet, the enjoyment of food and confidence to socialize. It was also thought that diet could be controlled or modified, to exert an anti-caries effect. A few experiments, studies and research have been carried out to assess the effect of diet on dental caries. After the Second World War, advice about a nutritious diet often encouraged mothers to give their young children a diet rich in calcium and vitamin D, so that they would develop strong bones and teeth, which would be less susceptible to decay. Although this was sound advice as far as the bones are concerned, there has always been little evidence to substantiate the view that good nutrition in early life helps to prevent dental decay by a systemic effect. This certainly does not mean that good nutrition should be discouraged; it merely reflects the current view, that diet has a much greater effect locally in the mouth than it does pre-eruptively, while the teeth are still forming.

Definition

Dental Caries is a biofilm-mediated, diet modulated, multifactorial, non-communicable, dynamic disease resulting in a net mineral loss of dental hard tissues. It is determined by biological, behavioural, psychosocial, and environmental factors. Owing to this process, a caries lesion develops [1].

"In dentine, when no cavities are detected, it is termed as cavity-free. In enamel, when no cavities are detected, it is termed caries-free." However, thorough clinical examination may reveal the presence of non-cavitated and/or micro-cavitated carious lesions. Occult caries is known as PEIR (pre-eruptive intracoronal resorption).

Caries Prevention refers to the inhibition of the initiation of caries lesions. Effective primary prevention interventions allow this to be successful. However, once the caries process has been initiated, movement to an appropriate caries care/management program is desirable to ensure that the lesions do not progress and that caries is arrested.

Dental caries is the result of complex interactions involving the individual (nutrition, genetics, behaviour, race, and age), plaque bacteria, saliva flow and composition and the environment. Diet is one very important element of the environment that can be at risk and so contribute to dental caries. Diet exerts a profound effect on dental caries locally in the mouth by reacting with the enamel surface and serving as a *substrate for cariogenic* microorganisms, which produce acid thereby reducing the pH and causing dissolution of the tooth surface [2].

Cariogenicity of Diet

Cariogenic Potential – "A food's ability to foster caries in humans under conditions conducive to carious lesion formation".

Cariogenicity – "The true cariogenicity of a food can only be established by experimentally determining in humans the extent of tooth decay associated with a given food." **(Stamm JW *et al.*, 1986)**

• When a tooth enters the 'restorative spiral', it becomes more and more complex and expensive, often resulting in multiple replaced restorations of increasing.

• The severity of the affected tooth at each stage of the cycle reaches a significantly higher risk of eventual extraction.

• Despite this knowledge, and some notable attempts to change, in many countries, the balance of dental education remains largely focused on a surgical approach to dentistry, resulting in a workforce who are still often biased towards restorative rather than preventive intervention. The effective use of established methods of primary, secondary, and tertiary caries prevention allows for the arresting of early-stage disease and prevents the initiation of new lesions before the tooth requiring (Figs. **2** & **3**).

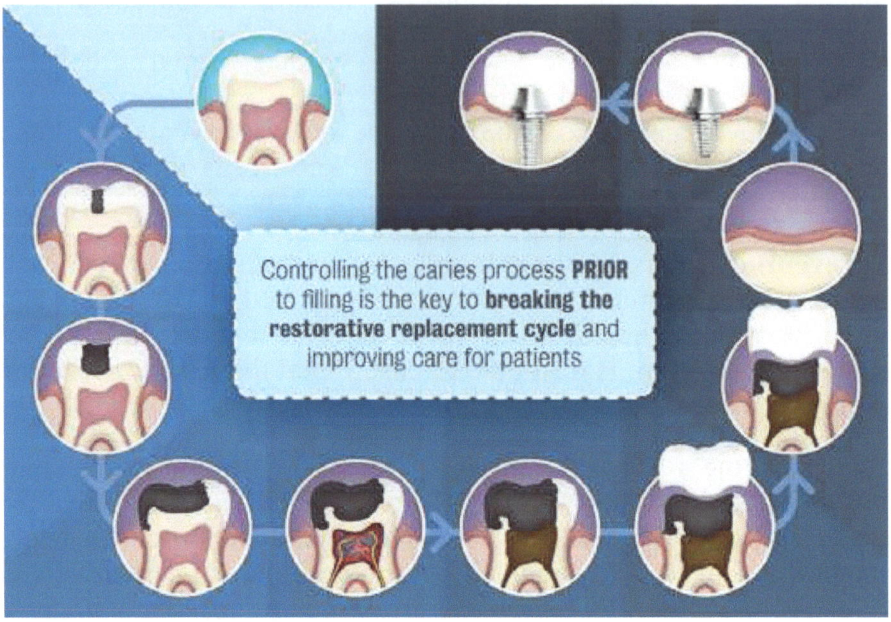

Fig. (2). Diagrammatic representation of the caries process leading to loss of tooth.

• In children from conception to approximately 11 years, if nutrition is inadequate, the formation of enamel can be affected; this causes pits and areas of roughness, which can be more susceptible to dental caries.

• Infants and toddlers are put to bed with dummies dipped in syrup or with bottles containing fluids other than water.

• Persons who suffer from eating disorders, such as anorexia and bulimia, where vomiting is induced so causing the abnormal oral acid environment [2] for decay.

• Elderly people are at risk due to a higher incidence of chronic diseases and multiple drug (usually prescribed) use, inadequate oral hygiene, and lack of food variety, all of which led to poor dental health.

• Persons with diabetes are at a higher risk; potential causes include increased salivary glucose levels in inadequately controlled diabetes, decreased salivary flow and dry mouth.

• Persons living in a community without a fluoridated water supply.

• Fluoride decreases the caries rate due to its effect on the tooth surface; it reverses the demineralising effect of acids produced by plaque.

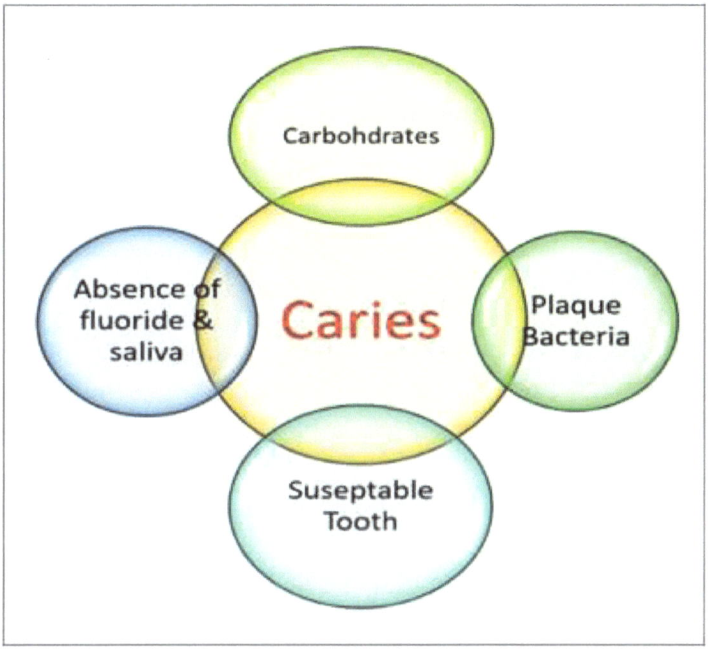

Fig. (3). Diagrammatic representation of the Caries development process based on the stage of carious lesion.

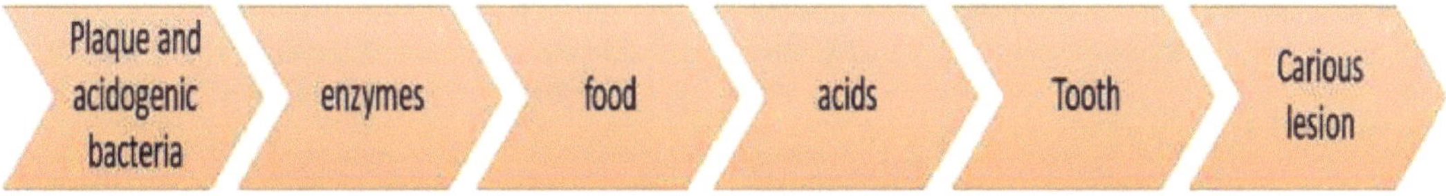
Plaque and acidogenic bacteria
enzymes
food
acids
Tooth
Carious lesion

Fig. (4). Etiology of dental caries

To evaluate the cariogenicity of diet, the balance between the other causative as well as protective factors should be taken into consideration (Fig **4**):

1. Nature of the diet
2. Retention and oral clearance time of dietary components
3. Intake frequency
4. Chemical composition
5. Protective components in the diet

When the causative factors overpower the protective factors in the diet, it is termed **'Cariogenic'** (Fig. **5**).

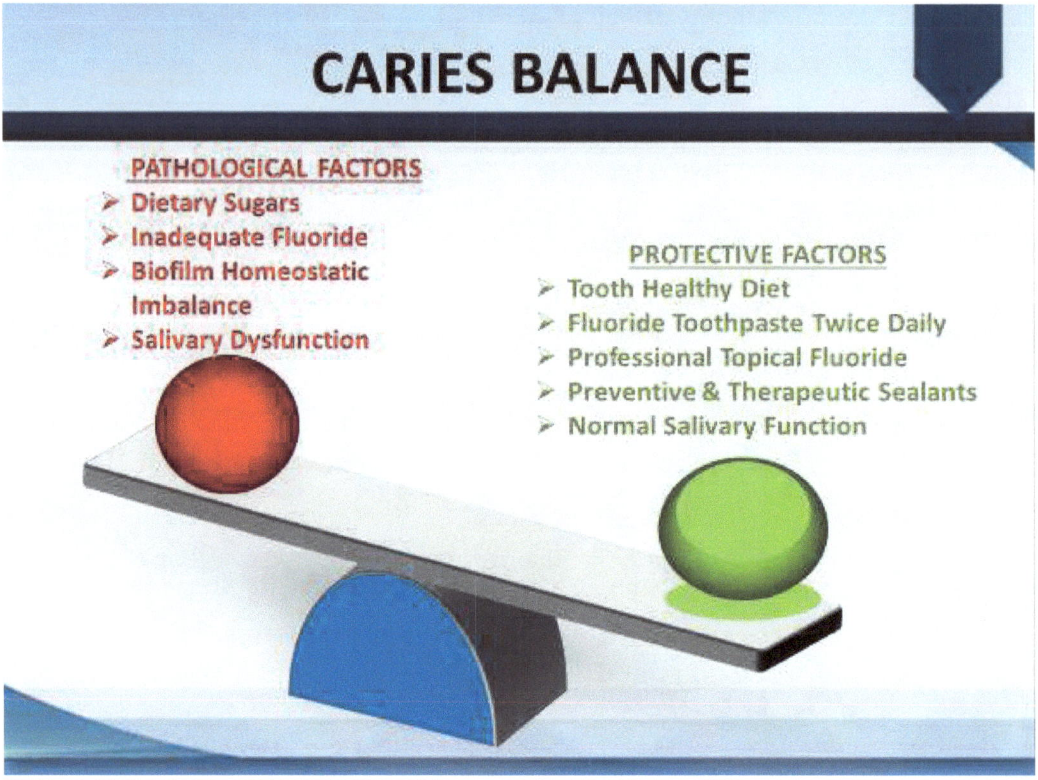

Fig. (5). Diagrammatic representation of Oral health Caries balance based on lesion severity.

Nature of the Diet

The form of the fermentable carbohydrate directly influences the duration of exposure and retention of the food on the teeth. Prolonged oral retention of cariogenic components of food may lead to extended periods of acid production and demineralization and shortened periods of remineralization. The duration may also be influenced by the frequency and amount of fermentable carbohydrates consumed. Liquid sugars, such as those found in beverages and milk drinks, pass through the oral cavity quickly with limited contact time or adherence to tooth surfaces. However, fluid intake patterns can influence the caries risk of the beverages. Holding sugar-containing beverages in the oral cavity for a prolonged time or constant sipping of a sugared beverage increases the risk of caries. Long-lasting sources of sugars, such as hard candies, breath mints, and lollipops, have extended exposure time in the oral cavity because the sugars are gradually released during consumption. Dental erosion is the chemical dissolution of tooth structure in the absence of bacteria when the environment is acidic (pH<4).

Retention and Oral Clearance Time of Dietary Components

Oral clearance properties vary in person and depend on metabolism by microorganisms, adsorption onto oral surfaces, degradation by plaque and salivary enzymes, saliva flow, and swallowing. Most carbohydrates will be cleared by these simultaneous mechanisms. Retentiveness of foods is not the same as stickiness. A caramel or jellybean may be sticky, but its retentive properties are low, and they are cleared from the oral cavity faster than are retentive foods such as cookies or chips.

The study showed that the longer that food is retained in the oral cavity, the greater the potential the starch must break down into sugars and contribute to the caries process. The initial content of sugars was not the culprit; rather, it was the type of starch and extent of starch retention time in the oral cavity that determined the relative cariogenic risk of the food (Fig. **5**).

Intake Frequency

The frequency of consumption seems to be a significant contributor to the cariogenicity of the diet, although **Bowen *et al.* (1983)** concluded that it is not the frequency of ingestion per se that is related to the development of caries but the time that sugars are available to microorganisms in the mouth. The importance of frequency is clear when caries is regarded as the outcome of the alternation of demineralization and remineralization. Higher frequency means more demineralization and less remineralization. The duration of the decrease in pH after intake of a cariogenic food is an important confounder in this relation.

Chemical Composition

Carbohydrates are classified as monosaccharides, disaccharides, and polysaccharides. Sucrose, which is a disaccharide consisting of fructose and glucose, is more easily fermentable than polysaccharides like starch. Earlier it was thought that the consumption of sugars, mainly sucrose was the key factor in the development of tooth decay. However, processed, cooked, starchy foods, especially when combined with refined sugars (doughnut, pastry, potato chips), also contribute to dental caries.

Diet and nutrition may favour remineralization when their content is high in calcium, phosphate, and protein. In experiments using processed cheese and sucrose solutions, **Jensen, and Wefel (1990)** showed that processed cheese was anti-cariogenic. Cheese consumption followed by a 10% sucrose solution resulted in a pH of 6.5 compared with a pH of 6.3 for cheese alone and a pH of 4.3 for sucrose alone.

Mechanisms proposed to explain the anti-cariogenic effects of cheeses are as follows:

1. Increased salivary flow and the subsequent buffering effect, which can neutralize plaque acids.
2. Inhibition of plaque bacteria and the effect of that inhibition on reducing the number of bacteria, thereby reducing acid production; and
3. Intake of increased alkaline substances, calcium, inorganic phosphate, and casein, which decrease demineralization and enhance remineralization.

***Acid Content*:** The acidity of individual foods can precipitate erosion. The erosive potential, however, depends also on whether the oral buffer systems can neutralize the food. Because the critical pH for enamel dissolution is 5.5, any food with a pH lower than 5.5 may contribute to or stimulate erosion. In persons with adequate saliva and good oral hygiene habits, these fluids and foods pose a minimal risk when consumed as part of a balanced diet. Large doses of chewable vitamin C may also cause a decrease in pH because of its citric acid content, which contributes to tooth erosion.

Protective Component in the Diet (Fig. 6)

Some components of food are somewhat caries inhibiting (Cariostatic) and have been called protective, especially products that are rich in calcium and phosphates.

They act by

1. Reducing the rate of dissolution of hydroxyapatite.
2. Reducing the fall in plaque pH by buffering acids produced by fermentation
3. Enhancing remineralisation
4. Modifying formation and composition of pellicle and plaque

Components of diet that inhibit caries up to a certain extent are calcium, peanuts, cocoa, lectin, cheese *etc* [3].

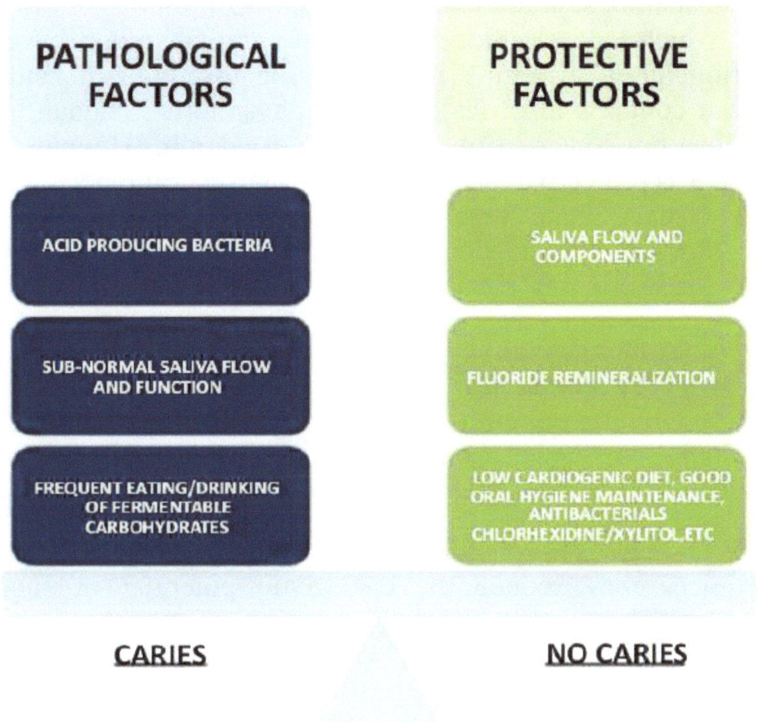

Fig. (6). Protective component in the diet.

Reports from the past 2 decades of the 20th century have shown that a small percentage of the variance in caries increase may be explained by dietary components since the introduction and use of fluoridated toothpaste. The relation between sugars and dental caries is difficult to quantify because of inherent limitations. It is well known that

1. Variability in patterns of sugars consumption affects the duration of exposure of the teeth to sugars,
2. Dietary recalls or food diaries only provide an approximation of actual sugars consumption and food consumption patterns,
3. Patterns of sugars consumption are reported on an annual basis, but caries formation can take several years, and
4. Caries prevalence is influenced by several factors that are difficult to control, including the dietary mineral content (fluoride, calcium, and phosphorus), health care, oral hygiene habits, and education level. The following studies must be considered in light of these concerns [4].

Milk**:** It is a substantial source of sugars in the diet of young children. It is rich in lactose sugar, which is less acidogenic. Various animal studies have shown milk to be anti-cariogenic. Cow's milk contains 5% lactose but is considered safe for teeth because it contains much calcium and phosphorus. Human breast milk is higher in lactose but lower in phosphorus and calcium. Human milk contains more sugar but less protective factors and there are several reports of dental caries in infants who have been breastfed on demand for many years. Normal breastfeeding does not cause dental caries whereas prolonged and nocturnal suckling can increase caries risk.

Cheese**:** Numerous animal and experimental studies indicated that cheese is anti-cariogenic. Cheese consumption following sugary snacks abolishes the fall in pH as it stimulates salivary secretion and increases plaque calcium concentration. Various Enamel slab experiments have shown that cheese promotes the remineralization of previously demineralized enamel.

Cocoa, Coffee & Tea: Polyphenols such as tannins in cocoa, coffee, tea, and many fruit juices may reduce the cariogenic potential of foods. *In vitro* experiments have shown that these polyphenolic compounds, in addition to fluoride & flavonoids may interfere with the glucosyltransferase activity of mutans streptococci, which may reduce plaque formation. In rat experiments, tea polyphenols reduced caries. Black tea extract inhibits salivary amylase activity thus reducing dental caries [5].

Sugar Studies

Sugar is added to food for a multitude of functions: fermentation, preservation, physical and chemical, and to satisfy the consumer's preference for sweetness. Unfortunately, sugar consumption is also a main etiological factor for dental caries (Fig. 7). The relationship between sugar and caries was established in the latter half of the 19th century. Many factors influence this relationship: the availability of sugar for bacterial digestion, the presence of acidogenic bacteria in the plaque on teeth, and the ability of fluoride and saliva to counteract bacteria and acids. The importance of the frequency of administering sugars over the amount has been demonstrated in various studies on humans. Through guidelines, world and national health organizations advocate the reduction of sugar consumption to below 10E% (daily dietary energy percentage consumption per capita), but voluntary implementation on an individual basis is difficult for many, and maybe more compulsory strategies that aim to reduce both the amount and frequency of sugar intake are needed. The influence of dietary sugars on dental caries has been a very dominant feature. A very strong relationship between sucrose consumption with caries experience can be observed in a variety of epidemiological, clinical and laboratory studies [6, 7].

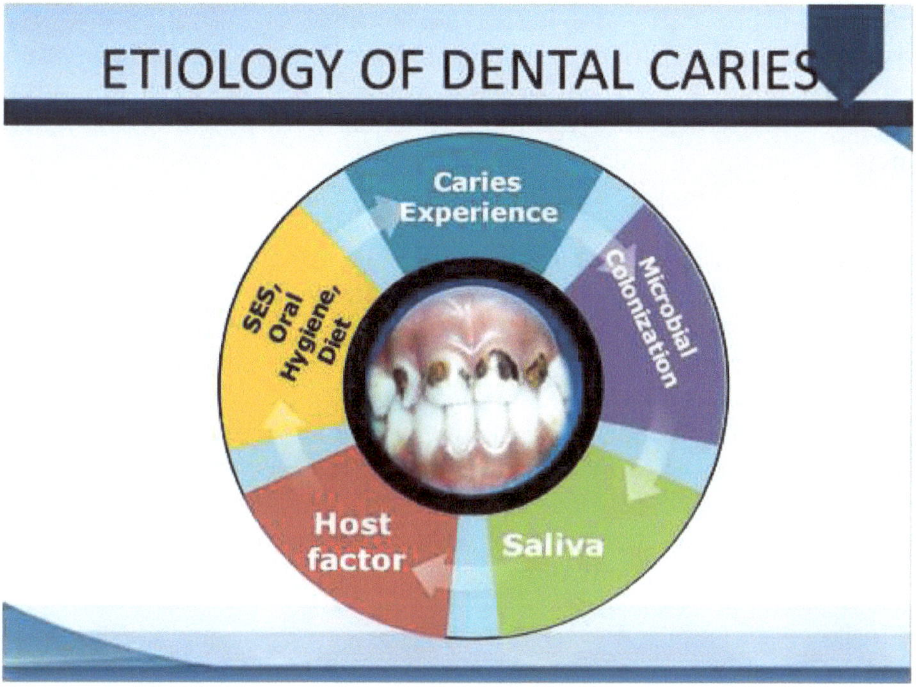

Fig. (7). Etiology of Dental caries.

Sucrose – The Arch Criminal

'Sucrose is the Arch Criminal of Dental Caries' has been softened over the years, it continues to be the most common form of added sugar in the diet, even with the continuation of the trend toward increased use of high fructose corn syrup in many industrialized countries. There does not appear to be any difference in the acidogenic potential or the ability to directly induce *in situ* enamel demineralization among the common sugars, sucrose, maltose, glucose, and fructose. Lactose has less acidogenic potential than the other sugars and, as a constituent of milk is not considered cariogenic mainly due to the protective factors in milk. Dental caries is a bacterial disease that affects the hard tissue of the tooth, which is formed through complex reactions over time between acid-producing microorganisms and fermentable carbohydrates, proceeding to the formation of a cavity [8].

Dental caries is a global public health issue worldwide and the most common non-communicable disease. And the most popular condition is enclosed in the 2015 Global Burden of Disease study, ranking the 1st for caries of permanent teeth affecting 2.3 billion people and 12th for deciduous teeth affecting 560 million children. The problem is more expensive to treat, consuming 5–10% of healthcare budgets in developed countries and is a common reason for hospitalization. The occurrences of dental caries are increasing because of unlimited use of sugary foods, poor oral care practices, and inadequate health service utilization. The burden of caries was higher in economically disadvantageous communities. Across all age groups, dental caries affects the quality of life, affecting individuals and society's economy and leading tonto treatment problems, tooth loss and pain, and slow language development in children.

Sucrose has been given special importance due to its involvement as the sole substrate in the synthesis of extracellular (water-soluble and water-insoluble) glucans meditated by microbial glycosyltransferases, which have been the subject of intense study for many years. Glucans can form a major component of the structural intermicrobial matrix of dental plaque (Fig. **8**). It has been proposed that water-insoluble glucans enhance the ability of mutans streptococci to accumulate on the smooth surfaces of teeth. When compared to other dietary sugars (glucose, fructose, and lactose) in the rat caries model, sucrose is more cariogenic in some studies. However, the effect appears to be strain-specific and is also influenced by the type of animal model and the effect is generally associated with smooth surfaces [9].

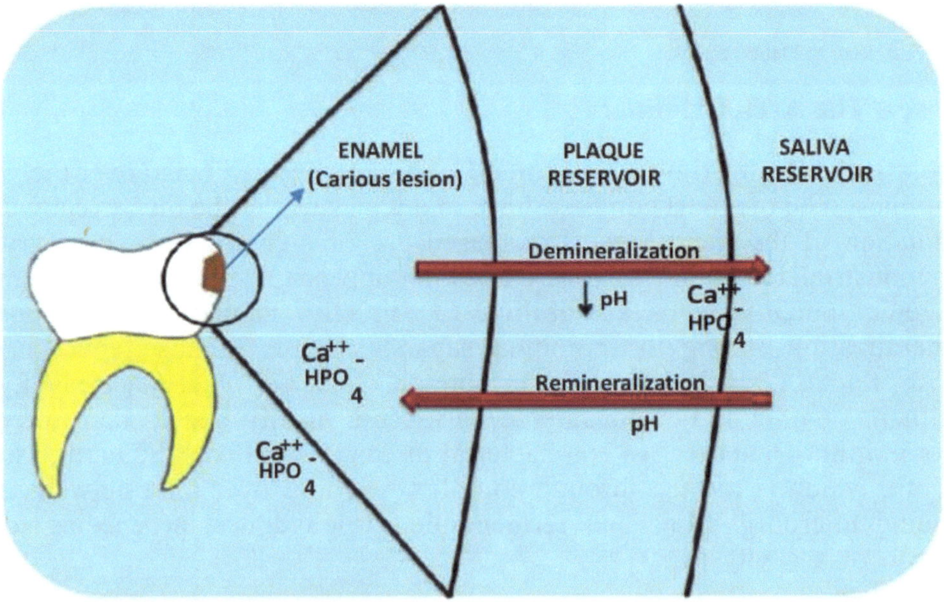

Fig. (8). Remineralization and demineralization.

The authors have suggested that the replacement of sucrose with monosaccharides may reduce proximal- and smooth-surface caries. Several studies have indicated that the caries-associated virulence of glucan may have more to do with an alteration in plaque ecology than effects on the accumulation of specific bacteria in plaque. The same happened when whereby sucrose-mediated synthesis of glucans increases the porosity of plaque, permitting deeper penetration of dictary sugar into the biofilm and greater acid production immediately adjacent to the tooth surface. In studies using an intraoral caries model, *Mutans streptococcus* plaque prepared from sucrose-containing cultures was found to have markedly enhanced demineralization potential compared with glucose-grown plaque. The rate decreased from 1-3 years. The effect has been attributed to an alteration of the diffusion properties of plaque due to the presence of water-insoluble glucan synthesized from sucrose. Recent studies have found a relationship between water-insoluble glucan synthesis by mutans streptococcal strains and caries incidence in young children and suggested that the capacity of mutans streptococci to synthesize insoluble glucans may be more important than their levels in plaque (Figs. **9** & **10**).

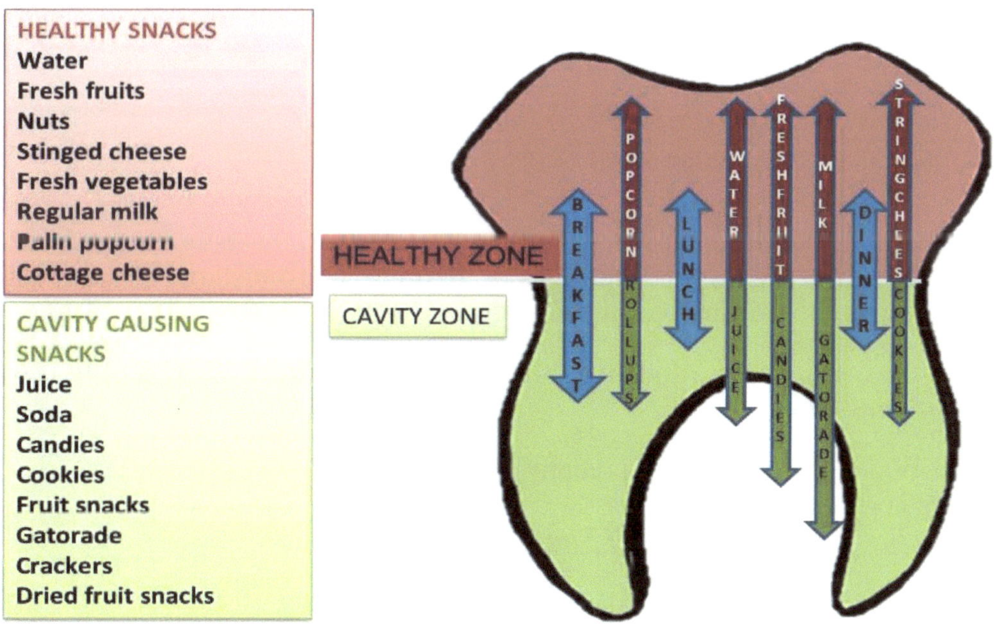

Fig. (9). Diagrammatic representation of healthy zone and cavity zone.

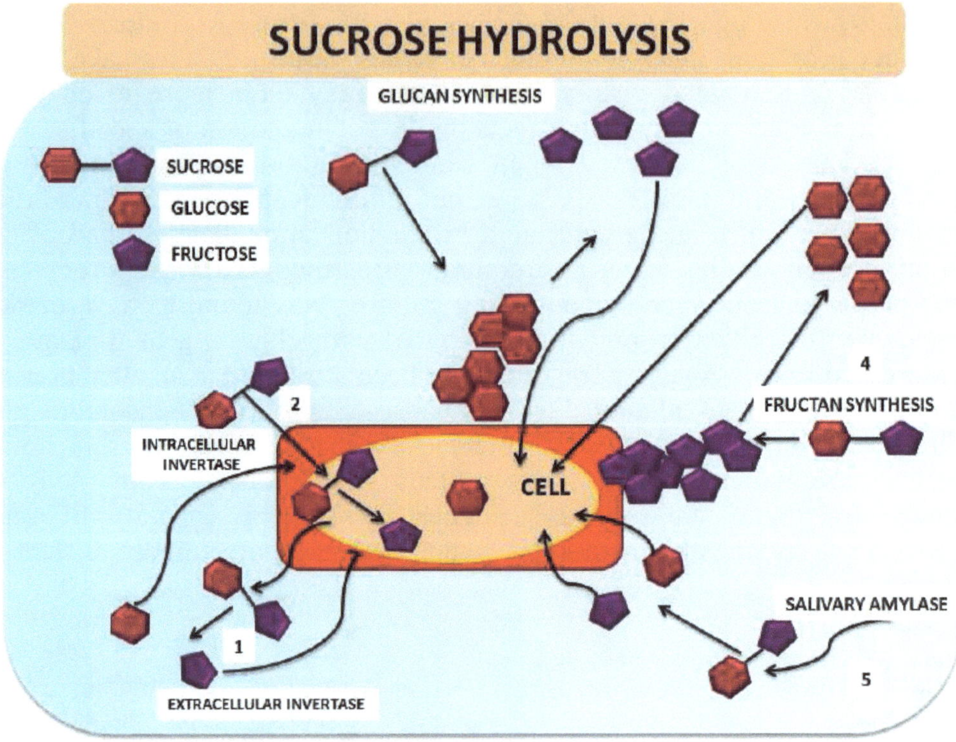

Fig. (10). Mechanisms of sucrose hydrolysis by oral bacteria.

Studies conducted on people consuming sugars and investigation of caries experience have shown that there is a definite relationship between sugar consumed and the occurrence of tooth decay.

Studies Assessing Relationship Between Sugar and Caries [9 - 11], *Observational Human Studies-*

- World-Wide Epidemiology (Screebny 1982)
- Tristan da cunha (Fisher 1986)
- ***Groups Eating Low Amount of Sugar:***
    - Hopewood house (Harris 1963)
    - Hereditary fructose intolerance (Newbrun 1989)
    - Dentist children (BRADFORD & Crabb 1961)
    - Wartime Diets (Takahashi 1961)
- ***Groups Eating High Amounts of Sugar:***
  -Sugar-cane chewers (Frencken 1989)
  -Workers in confectionary factories (Anaise 1978)
  -children taking sugar-based medicines (Roberts & Roberts 1979)

Inventional Human Studies-

-Vipeholm study (Gustaffson *et al.* 1954)
- Turku study (Scheinin & Makinen)

Animal Experiments-

- Frequency of feeding (Konig *et al.* 1968)
- Concentration of sugar (Shawm, 1979)
- Type of sugar (Grenby *et al* 1973)

Enamel Slab Experiments -

- Lesion formation (Koulourides *et al* 1976)

Plaque pH Experiments

- Acidogenicity tests (*Imfeld* 1977)

Incubation Experiments -

- Test tube experiments (Grenby *et al.* 1989)

Modern Diet *Versus* Primitive Diet

Epidemiological studies have shown that the incidence of dental caries differs immensely among population groups. Although part of the variance can be attributed to genetic factors, the diets of different ethnic groups probably account for the major differences. Skeletal remains from sucrose cultures showed that dental caries incidence was much lower. For example, the caries prevalence among ancient Hawaiians was extremely low, especially throughout childhood and early adulthood. In older members (40 years and older), it usually increased due to cervical root caries complicated by concurrent periodontal disease. By contrast, the children in Hawaii today have one of the highest dental caries incidences.

Dental caries incidence in native populations (Australian Aborigines, Bantu tribes of South Africa, the New Zealand Maoris, the Eskimos) was very low before the introduction of the modern diet but increased dramatically after the introduction of the North American/ European culture. The children of Tristan da Cunha were remarkably free of caries in 1937. They became progressively affected with severe dental caries, as they grew more sophisticated in terms of lifestyle and the adoption of a modern diet.

Human Observational Studies

Hopewood House Study, Sullivan & Harris, 1958 (Fig. **11**).

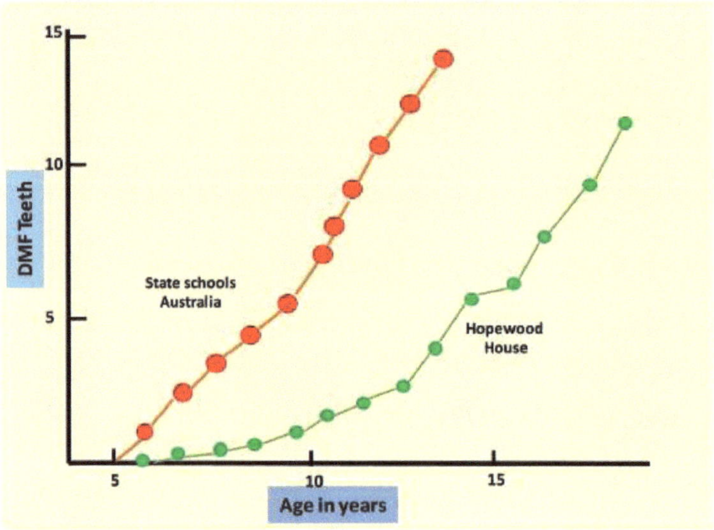

Fig. (11). The number of decayed, missing or filled (DMF) teeth with caries in the general population compared to children in Hopewood House.

- In 1942, an eccentric businessman transformed a spacious mansion into a motherhouse at Bowral, Australia. 80 children who were in their early infancy were given a vegetarian diet that was adequate but Spartan regarding sugars.
- Wholemeal bread, porridge, biscuits, wheat germ, fruits and vegetables, cheese, milk, and butter were given to the children.
- Uncooked food and meals supplemented by vitamin concentrates were given to retaining their natural state.
- Most striking feature was the notable absence of white or brown sugar & sugar-flour confections.
- F content of water & food was insignificant & no tea was consumed.

Results

- At the end of the 10 years, they ranged from 7 to 14 years.
- At the end of a 10-years, 13 years old children of the house had a mean DMF per child of 1.6, and the corresponding Fig for the general child population of the state of Bowral was 10.7.

- Only 0.4% of 13 years old of state were free from caries, while 53% of Hopewood children – had caries-free as well House children's oral hygiene was poor, calculus was uncommon, but gingivitis was prevalent in about 75% of children.

CONCLUSION

- In institutionalized children, caries can be reduced to insignificant levels by a Spartan diet, without beneficial effects of F & in the presence of unfavourable oral hygiene.
- Children in communal homes have lower caries rates as compared to children living with parents, as sugar-containing foods are not available between meals.

Low Sugar Diet Has Low Levels of Dental Caries

• Low caries experience has been reported in groups of people who have a habitually low intake of dietary sugars, *e.g.*

• Children of dentists **(Barford & Crabb 1961)**.

• Children in institutions where strict dietary regimes are followed.

• Children with hereditary fructose intolerance.

High Sugar Diet Has High Levels of Dental Caries

Evidence shows - many groups of people with habitually high consumption of sugars also have a high level of caries.

Examples include-

1. Confectionery industry workers & children with chronic diseases require long-term sugar-containing medicines (Roberts & Roberts, 1979).
2. Studies have shown up to 71% higher caries in the confectionery industry than factory workers from other industries (Anaise 1978).
3. Some medical conditions such as phenylketonuria require diets that are high in refined sugars.

Nikiforuk and Fraser in 1981

Nutrition may cause enamel hypoplasia was presented by Nikiforuk and Fraser in 1981. Their study involved the thorough examination of 56 patients in Toronto, Canada, for 25 years. Ten patients had hereditary vitamin D dependency rickets, 25 patients had X-linked hypophosphatemia, and 21 patients had hypo parathyroid/pseudohypoparathyroidism conditions. Enamel hypoplasia only occurred in children with hypocalcaemia, and no relation was found between enamel hypoplasia and plasma phosphorus levels.

Worldwide Epidemiological Observational Studies, Sreebny Lm 1982

• He found a relationship between sucrose consumption & dental caries. He correlated the dental caries experience of primary dentition (dmft) of 5-6yr old with sugar supplies data of 23 countries: & the dental caries experience of 12yr olds to sugar supply of 47 countries. He reported that in populations with the availability of sucrose (57-115g/person/day), 12yr old children had dmft ranging from 3.2 to 4.8 compared with 0.1-2.7 in paired children in populations having average sucrose intake <50g/person/day.

• He observed a significant correlation.

+0.31 for primary dentition.

+0.7 for permanent dentition.

Reports suggested that ~ 50% of the variability in caries could be explained by the sucrose available [10, 11].

***Conclusion*:** Communities or groups of people who had very low intakes of sugar showed very low caries scores, & those that had very high availability of sugars in their diets at that time developed high numbers of carious lesions

- A later analysis conducted in 1994, did not find such a strong association between per capita sugar availability & mean DMFT of 12yr old in developed countries, whereas the association continued to be noted in developing countries.
- Sugars are consumed in different physical forms with different foods & dietary patterns that affect the clearance rate of dietary sugars.
- The data, whether obtained from food balance sheets or dietary surveys, represent an approximation of actual sugar consumption.
- Caries prevalence is influenced by other factors, including fluorides availability, health services, education, oral hygiene practices, & other habits.

Tristan Da Cunha, (Fisher 1986)

During Volcanic eruptions on the island, the population was made to move to England in 1962. A dental examination was carried out in 1962 and on return to the island in 1966. Before emigration, the population was on a simple diet and caries in the first molars in 6-19 years was=0, and it increased to 50% after emigration. Change in the diet influenced to the development of caries to levels that were equal to those in England at that time.

Hereditary Fructose Intolerance (Hfi) (Newbrun 1909)

He tabulated the caries Prevalence of 31 persons with HFI & found that the dental caries prevalence was extremely low. Hereditary Fructose Intolerance is caused by the remarkably reduced levels of hepatic fructose 1- phosphate aldolase. Persons affected with this rare metabolic disorder tend to avoid any food that contains fructose or sucrose because it causes symptoms of nausea, vomiting, malaise, tremor, excessive sweating & even coma due to fructosemia.

World War II Rationing

In countries with a level of sugar consumption of less than 18 kg/person/year, caries experience is consistently low. The reduced availability of sugar during the Second World War was mirrored by a reduction in dental caries, which subsequently increased when the restriction was lifted. During Wartime dietary restrictions, the same happened when there was an increase in potatoes, fish, vegetables & unrefined flour & a decrease in sugar & fat consumption. Analysis of caries rates in Scandinavian countries by Toverud 1957; found caries rates in permanent molars decreased 1-3 years after a reduction in sugar intake in 7-8 year-olds. Caries rates increase sharply 1-2 years after the rise of sucrose in post-war diets of children. Similar findings were reported in Japan & Switzerland (Marthaler 1967); the rate decreased from 1-to 3 years.

Interventional Studies

Vipeholm Study (Gustaffson et al. 1954) (Fig. 12)

Davies summarized this in 1955. *In 1939, the Swedish Govt. requested the Royal Medical Board to investigate*- 'what measures should be taken to reduce the frequency of most common dental disease in Sweden'.

This request led to a study at the VIPEHOLM HOSPITAL, LUND. A longitudinal study under well-controlled conditions was carried out with the aim of:

- To determine the effects of frequency and quality of sugar intake on the formation of carious lesions.
- To find out -
    - Does an increase in carbohydrates (mostly sugar) intake cause an increase in dental caries?

- Does a decrease in carbohydrates (mostly sugar) intake produce an increase in dental caries?
- Can caries formation be reduced?

Method: 436 Adults inmates from the mental institution were included for 5 years with a diet that contained little sugar with no provision for in-between meal snacks, which was divided into 7 groups:

Seven GROUPS-

- Control group
- Sucrose group
- Bread group
- Chocolate group
- Caramel group
- 8 toffee group
- 24 toffee group

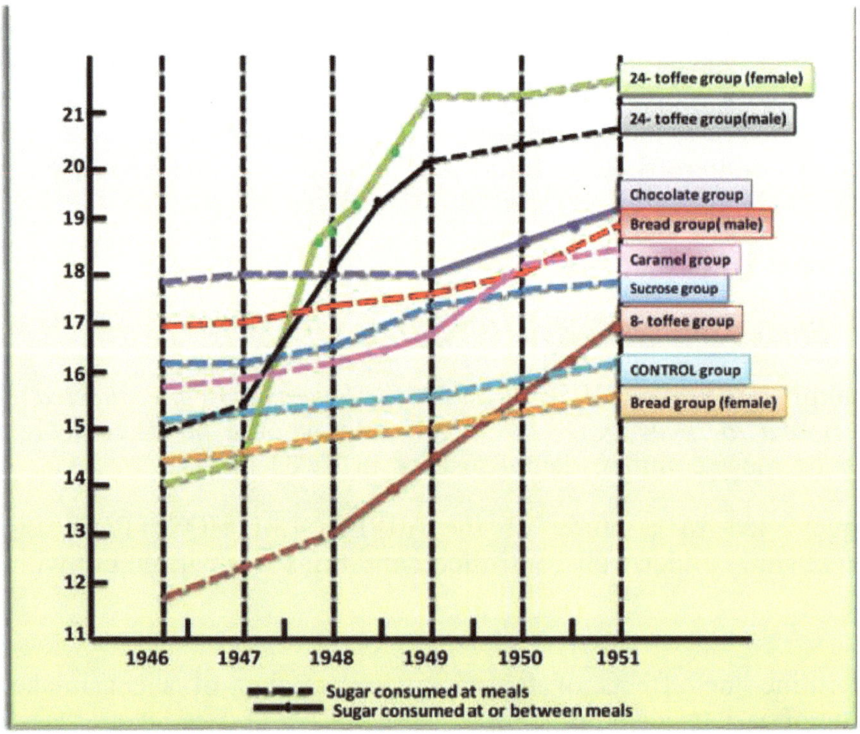

Fig. (12). Vipeholm study: the incidence of caries caused by different amounts and types of dietary carbohydrates.

CONCLUSION

- ↑ Carbohydrates mainly sugar ↑ caries activity.
- Caries risk greater - sugar consumed -retained on the tooth surface.
- Caries activity greatest – sugar consumed between meals.
- Varies widely between individuals.
- Withdrawal of the sugar-rich foods ↓ caries activity rapidly.
- High concentration -prolonged retention - caries activity ↑.
- Clearance time of sugar correlates closely with caries activity.

Turku Sugar Study (Scheinin & Makinen, 1975)

This study was carried out in Turku, Finland. This is the 2nd important intervention study which is a controlled longitudinal study carried out for 2yr as a feeding study on 125 young adults. The study aimed to compare the cariogenicity of sucrose, fructose & Xylitol. 125 subjects (15-45 years) divided into 3 groups (Fig. **13**):

- Sucrose Group- 35 People
- Fructose Group- 38 People
- Xylitol Group- 52 People

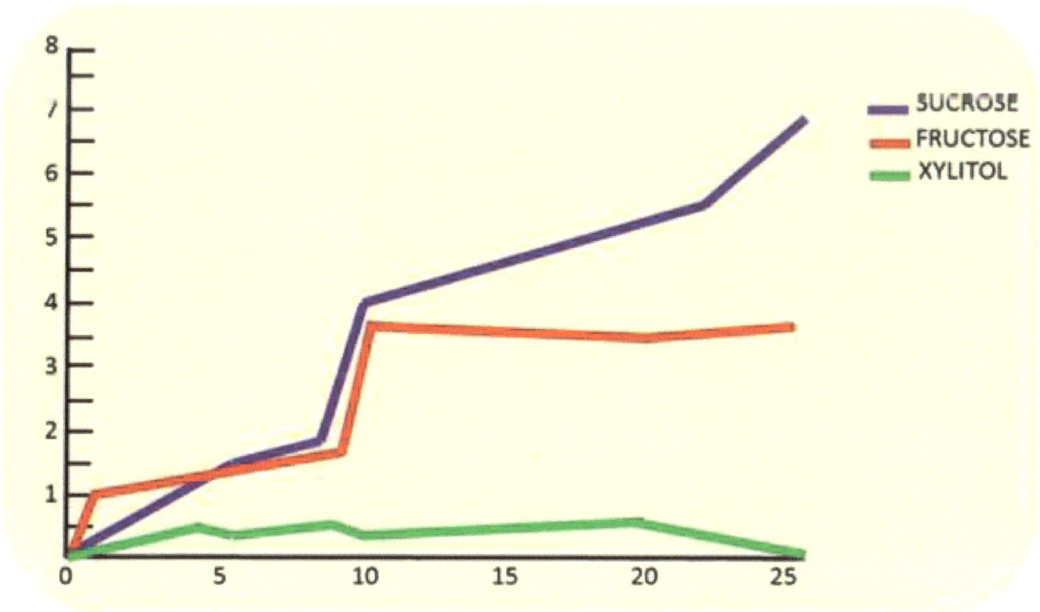

Fig. (13). Comparison of caries increment.

RESULTS

- After 1 year: - sucrose & fructose showed equal cariogenicity while xylitol showed no caries
- At the end of the 2nd year: - caries increased in the sucrose group, remained unchanged in the fructose group & DMFS in the xylitol group fell to = 0.

***Conclusion*:** Fructose was less cariogenic than sucrose. Xylitol was non-cariogenic or even anticariogenic.

Enamel Slab Experiments

Ostram and Koulorides 1976 first measured hardness changes of enamel using an intraoral appliance that was placed inside the mouth for 1 week.

There is a use of oral appliances that hold slabs of bovine or human enamel. The slabs were exposed to the dietary factors being tested by consumption, with slabs *in situ* or by removal of appliances several times a day to dip into vessels containing dietary test substances. Plaque forms on the enamel slabs that remain in the mouth for 1 to 6 weeks. Changes in enamel hardness or degree of demineralization were measured.

The research workers then showed:

- Sugars cause demineralization.
- Non-fermentable non-sugar sweeteners aid remineralization.
- Increasing frequency and concentration of sugars increase demineralization.

Advantages of enamel slab experiments.

- Measure demineralization and not just acidogenic potential.
- Account for the protective role of saliva.

Plaque pH Studies - Acidogenicity Tests (Imfeld 1977)

These studies measure changes in pH of plaque following consumption of carbohydrates. This measures acidogenic potential, which is taken as an indirect measure of cariogenic potential.

1. Metal probes are used (antimony, iridium, palladium), which can be inserted inside the situ into the plaque.

2. Glass probes.
3. Miniature glass electrodes built into the partial denture.
4. Harvesting method: involves removing small samples of plaque from representative teeth and measurement of plaque pH on an electrode outside the mouth.

Stephan curve: Stephan (1940, 1944) demonstrated the relationship between sugar exposure resulting in the acidification of dental plaque and caries experience (Fig. **14**).

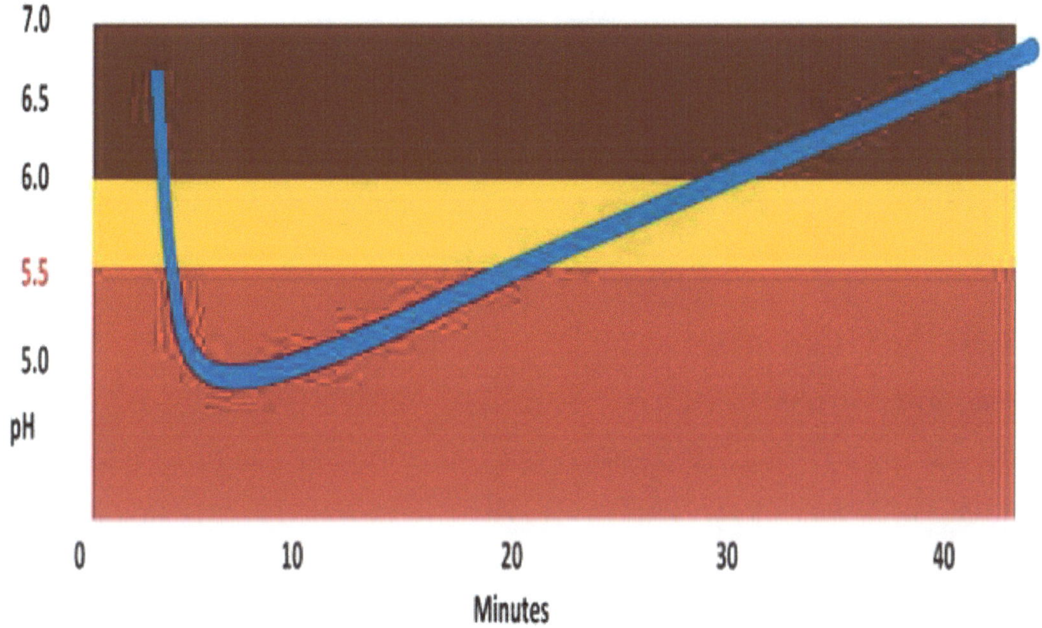

Fig. (14). The Stephan curves.

Plaque pH studies measure plaque acid production following consumption of a substance but not caries development. Therefore, they do not consider protective factors in foods and the effects of other components of the diet. Many of the plaque pH studies that show falls in pH below the critical pH of 5.5 with cooked starchy foods have been conducted using the indwelling electrode technique in order not to disturb the plaque. However, the indwelling electrode is recognised as being hypersensitive and non-discriminating.

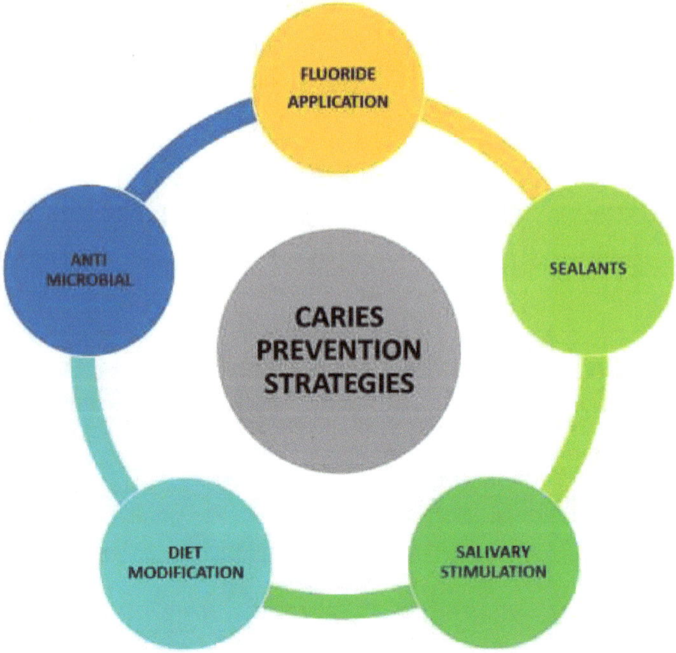
FLUORIDE APPLICATION
SEALANTS
SALIVARY STIMULATION
DIET MODIFICATION
ANTI MICROBIAL
CARIES PREVENTION STRATEGIES

Fig. (15). Caries Prevention Strategies.

Author(s) Main Conclusion (Fig. 15).

Marthaler (1967)	foodstuffs containing simple sugars are far more cariogenic than common starchy foods
Newbrun (1969)	called for the specific elimination of sucrose or sucrose-containing foods rather than restricting total carbohydrate consumption
Bibby (1975)	snack foods share importance with sucrose in caries causation
Sreebny (1982a)	total consumption and frequency of intake contribute to dental caries; lacking evidence about the precise definition of the relationship
Newbrun (1982a)	compelling evidence that the proportion of sucrose in food is one important determinant of its cariogenicity
Sheiham (1983)	sugar is the principal cause of caries in industrialized countries; recommended that sugar consumption be reduced to 15 kg/person/year or below
Shaw (1983)	studies in animals consistent with the clinical evidence on the relationship between sugar and caries
Rugg-Gunn (1986)	cariogenicity of staple starchy foods is low; the addition of sucrose to cooked starch is comparable to similar quantities of sucrose; fresh fruits appear to have low cariogenicity
Bowen and Birkhed (1986)	frequency of eating sugars is of greater importance than total sugar consumption

Marthaler (1967)	**foodstuffs containing simple sugars are far more cariogenic than common starchy foods**
Walker and Cleaton-Jones (1989)	degree of incrimination of sugar as a cause of caries is grossly exaggerated; questioned predictions of reductions in caries from decreases in sugar and snack intakes
Marthaler (1990)	despite dramatic reductions in caries due primarily to the widespread use of fluoride, sugars continue to be the main threat to dental health
Rugg-Gunn (1990)	dietary modification involving restriction on the frequency and amount of extrinsic sugars can be more effective than other control measures
Konig and Navia (1995)	acknowledged the relationship between frequency and sugar intake and caries; recommended removing the focus away from elimination of sugar and towards improved oral hygiene and use of fluoride toothpaste
Ruxton *et al.* (1999)	evidence strongly supports the formulation of advice on frequency of consumption, not amount
Konig (2000)	dental health problems do not require any dietary recommendations other than those required for the maintenance of general health
van Loveren (2000)	if good oral hygiene is maintained and fluoride is supplied frequently, teeth will remain intact even if carbohydrate-containing food is frequently eaten
Sheiham (2001)	sugars, particularly sucrose, are the most important dietary cause of caries; the intake of extrinsic sugars greater than 4 times a day increases caries risk; sugar consumption should not exceed 60 g/day for teenagers and adults and proportionally less for younger children

Data From National Surveys.

Sreebny (1982b)	DMFT in 6-year-olds from 23 nations and DMFT in 12-year-olds from 47 nations; sugar supply (g/person/day) significant positive correlation (r = 0.72; p! 0.005) between caries prevalence and national sugar supplies for 12-year-olds only; ingestion of 50 g of sugar/day may be the upper limit of 'safe' or 'acceptable' sugar consumption
Woodward and Walker (1994)	DMFT in 12-year-olds from 90 nations; sugar supply (kg/person/year) linear relationship between DMFT and sugar consumption when all 90 nations were included; no evidence of a relationship with a separate analysis of 29 industrialized nations
Miyazaki and Morimoto (1996)	DMFT in 12-year-olds (kg sugar/year); 1957–1987; low fluoride exposure excellent correlation (r = 0.91; p! 0.01) between DMFT and per capita sugar consumption in Japan
van Palenstein Helderman *et al.* (1996)	Caries experience in Africa, Europe, and North America; salivary mutans streptococci caries experience on three continents is attributable to dietary differences and not prevailing mutans streptococci species
Downer (1999)	DMFT in 5-year-olds and DMFT in 12-year-olds; available sugar (kg/person/year) strong positive correlation over time (50 years) between caries experience and national sucrose availability in the UK

Sugar Clock (Fig. 16)

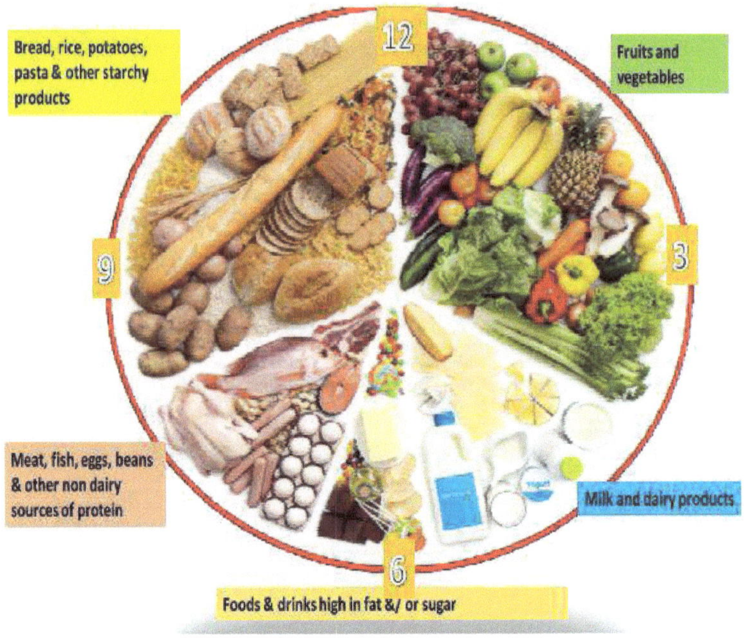

Fig. (16). Sugar Clock.

The concept of a "sugar clock" must be stressed. This means that we must explain to the parents/caretaker, the importance of abstaining from frequent snacking throughout the day. This will decrease the amount of time the pH of oral fluids remains below the critical pH (5.2 to 5.5) and thus fewer demineralization attacks on the tooth (Fig. **17**).

Sugar Substitutes: Consumption of a diet rich in sucrose often results in high caries activity. Replacing sucrose with the alternatives called sugar substitutes can help in reducing the caries activity. They are commonly classified as:

Non-caloric Sweeteners	Caloric Sweeteners
Aspartame	Palatinit, Lycasin
Cyclamate	Sorbitol, Xylitol
Saccharine	Lactitol
Acesulfame K	Maltitol
Sucralose	Mannitol

Non-caloric sweeteners: They are also referred to as intense sweeteners as they are much sweeter than sugars, weight by weight. They yield little or no energy, provide no bulk, and are used in very small quantities, especially in drinks or are blended with sugar substitutes in foods and snacks.

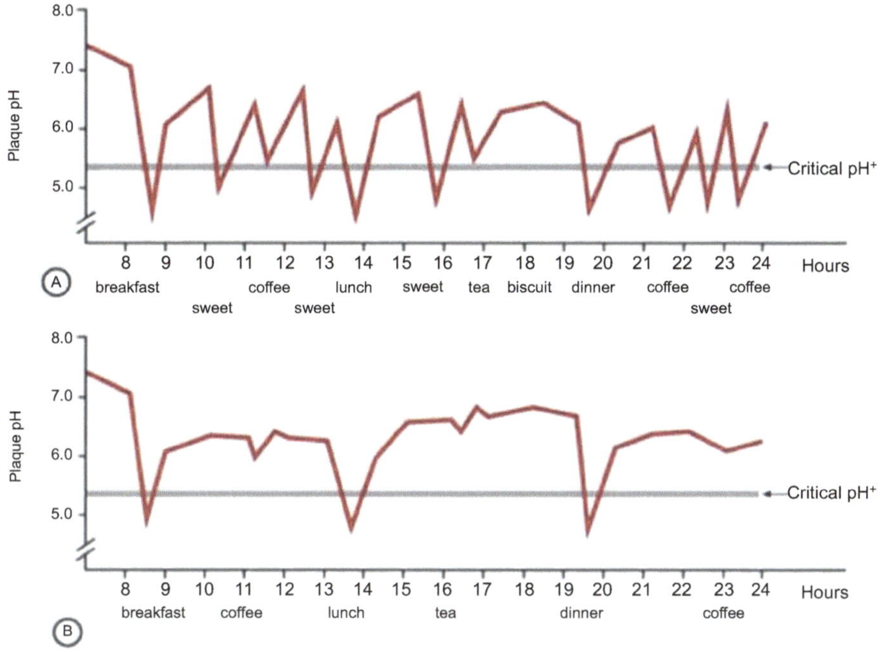

Fig. (17). Frequent snacking leads to repeated acid attacks and rapid demineralization. (M- Meals, S- Snacks).

Xylitol — a 5-carbon sugar, which cannot be metabolized by oral Microflora. These anti-cariogenic effects are attributable to antimicrobial action, stimulation of saliva resulting in increased buffer activity & an increase in pH, and enhanced remineralization. Xylitol is not fermented by cariogenic plaque bacteria and, thus, does not lower the pH of plaque. Because plaque pH does not decrease, enamel demineralization is prevented, and plaque bacteria do not proliferate. Xylitol reduces the accumulation of plaque on the tooth surface. Since plaque pH does not drop when xylitol-sweetened gum is chewed, remineralization is enhanced. Regular chewing of xylitol-sweetened gum has specific inhibiting effects on the growth of mutans streptococci in the mouth. This suggests that there may be permanent reductions in oral mutans streptococci levels from this practice. Chewing any gum stimulates the flow of saliva, which enhances the buffering effect in plaque. This property is not unique to xylitol-sweetened gum; the chewing effect by itself is seen as beneficial.

***Caloric sweeteners*:** These are also referred to as nutritive sugar substitutes or as carbohydrate, sugar substitutes because they are carbohydrates or carbohydrate derivatives. The most important group is the sugar alcohols, also called glycitols, polyols or polyalcohols. They can be metabolized to yield energy and add to the bulk of food products. As they equally or less sweet taste than sucrose, they often need blending with intense sweeteners.

Sorbitol is sweetened gums that simulate saliva without causing a drop in the critical pH and is equal to xylitol gum in terms of caries control. Sorbitol, however, should be considered a low cariogenic sweetener rather than a non-cariogenic one because consumption of larger amounts (more than two sticks of chewing gum per day) increases both the acid production in plaque and the number of sorbitol-fermenting microorganisms. Sorbitol is a solution (such as in a soft drink) that can be fermented, though slowly, by mutans streptococci. Cariogenic microorganisms can “learn” to metabolize sorbitol when their sugar supply is restricted; this form of adaptation to sorbitol has been demonstrated in animals. Firestone and Navia suggested that this adaptation could have occurred owing to selection by sorbitol-fermenting bacteria or induction by sorbitol-specific metabolizing enzymes.

The use of non-sugar sweeteners is growing rapidly, particularly in confectionery and soft drinks. Products that have passed a well-established acidogenicity test can be labelled with the ‘Happy Tooth’ logo – a protected trademark that informs the consumer that these products are dentally safe. Tooth-friendly sweets are available in about 26 countries. A non-profit association called Tooth friendly Sweets International was formed in the 1980s to promote dentally healthy snack food. In Switzerland, about 20% of the confectionery sold carries the ‘Happy Tooth’ logo. There is good evidence that sugarless chewing gums are not only non-cariogenic, but they positively prevent dental caries by stimulating the salivary flow [8 - 12].

Diet Counseling

Points considered in the examination	Measures to reduce caries risk and/or to stop ongoing caries activity
Frequency of meal	The number of meals + snacks should be kept at a low level.
Amount and concentration	Low sugar consumption is desirable from a cariological point of view.
Oral clearance of sugar	Sugar should be eliminated as fast as possible from the oral cavity.
Consistency of food	Food needing active chewing leads to increased salivation, which is desirable.

Points considered in the examination	Measures to reduce caries risk and/or to stop ongoing caries activity
Fermentable carbohydrates	Polysaccharides, disaccharides, and monosaccharides can contribute to the acid formation in the oral cavity, but the capacity differs between products.
Sugar substitute	The use of sugar substitutes results in a lower acid formation.
Protective and favourable element in the diet	Fluoride in food or drinking water has a pronounced caries inhibiting effect. Phosphate, calcium, fat, protein *etc.* have been tested and found to have certain caries inhibiting effects in animals.

Diet is a matter of individual choice influenced by age, ethnic & religious customs, family & peer group, advertisements, and economics. Diet counselling is one of the important aspects of dental caries prevention. The individual's compliance with the dietary advice given is very important. If they fail to follow the instructions given to them, the result is bound to be unproductive.

The following scheme states the course of action,

1. A thorough examination, including the dental and medical history. The treatment plan should then be outlined.
2. Evaluation of the probable causes.
3. Starting patient counselling regarding diet
4. Evaluation of compliance of the patient.
5. Determination of regular eating habits.
6. Continuation of dietary advice.
7. Giving the patient a personalized programme for change.

The record of the dietary intake should be maintained by the patient/parent. Thorough information regarding what food was consumed, how much of it was consumed, when was it consumed, *etc.* should be recorded.

FOOD PYRAMID

A commonly used tool for planning a balanced diet is the Food pyramid. It categorizes foods of common origin and similar nutrients into food groups. In such classification systems, the energy, fat and sugar concentration are extremely variable within food groups. Food processing typically leads to foods with lower nutrients and higher fat, sugar, and energy concentrations. A variety of foodstuffs from all food groups should be consumed to meet the nutrient and energy requirements. Sweet and white carbohydrates (bread, pasta *etc.*) and food with high cholesterol should be eaten sparingly (Fig. **18**).

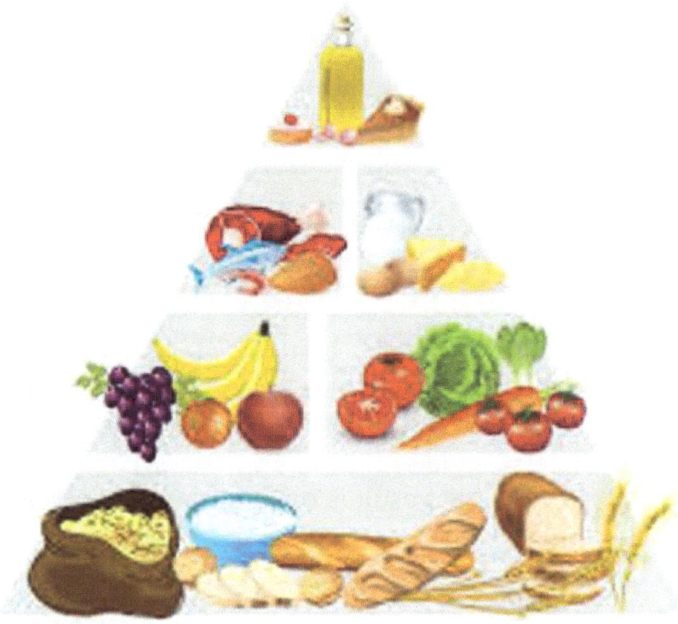

Fig. (18). Food Pyramid.

Dietary Advice for Different Age Groups

Babies: Babies do not need drinks other than breast milk or formula, although water or diluted juices can be offered after the age of 6 months, or in very hot weather. Juices should not be put in a bottle, nor should the baby be put to bed with a bottle of milk or juice to suck. This long-term bathing of teeth in sweet/acid solution causes tooth decay, which can result in loss of teeth. This will affect the growth of healthy permanent or 'second' teeth. Juice should be diluted with 1 to 2 times as much water and served in a baby's cup. Once a baby can sit alone and can make chewing movements it is time to encourage chewing and biting, even if a baby does not have any teeth. This will help with teething and with talking. Food high in sugar can contribute to tooth decay. Sweet foods should not be used as a reward…it is best to use lots of cuddles and attention or a special toy instead. Sugary foods such as honey should NEVER be put on a baby's dummy.

Childhood: This is an important time to develop tooth care habits:

- Use fluoride toothpaste and a soft toothbrush to clean teeth.
- Clean teeth twice daily – after breakfast, before going to school and after the evening meal, before going to bed. Use a soft toothbrush and children's low fluoride toothpaste.

- Visit the dentist regularly.
- For between-meal snacks, choose fruit, raw vegetables, or cheese.
- While at school, swish the mouth out with fresh water after snacking and after having lunch.
- Avoid sugary snacks.
- The Healthy Eating Pyramid is a good guide to food intake and aids in limiting the number of foods high in sugar.

Adolescence: It is normal for young people to supplement their meals with snacks. The frequent intake of foods and drinks high in sugar continually supplies the plaque bacteria with food and increases the amount of decay-causing acid that is produced. It takes up to 40 minutes for the plaque acid to return to a 'healthy' level therefore, it is preferable for the type of snack foods eaten to be fruits, vegetables or cheeses and milk or water.

Regular visits to the dentist and good dental hygiene, including flossing and the use of fluoride toothpaste, will help young people to maintain healthy teeth into adulthood [13, 14].

CONCLUSION

Changing dietary habits to improve health is not easy. It is important to realize that dietary habits do change and that the health professional must encourage them to change in the right direction. This involves much more than merely giving advice; health promotion must ensure that it is as easy as possible for people to change their diet in the right direction. Health professionals should provide expertise at national and community levels so that health promotion is based on the best scientific evidence.

CONSENT FOR PUBLICATION

Not applicable.

CONFLICT OF INTEREST

The author(s) declare no conflict of interest, financial or otherwise.

ACKNOWLEDGEMENT

Declared none.

REFERENCES

[1] Machiulskiene V, Campus G, Carvalho JC, *et al.* Terminology of Dental Caries and Dental Caries Management: Consensus Report of a Workshop Organized by ORCA and Cariology Research Group

of IADR. Caries Res 2020; 54(1): 7-14.
[http://dx.doi.org/10.1159/000503309] [PMID: 31590168]

[2] Pitts N, Mazevet M, Mayne C. Towards a cavity-free future How do we accelerate a policy shift towards increased resource allocation for caries prevention and control? The Alliance for a Cavity-Free Future, King's College, London 2017.
[http://dx.doi.org/10.18742/pub01-024]

[3] The Alliance for a Cavity-Free Future, The Alliance for a Cavity-Free Future. Accessed 18/03/2021 Available from https://www. acffglobal.org https://www. acffglobal.org

[4] World Health Organization, Oral Health. 2021.

[5] World Health Organization, Oral Health: Achieving better oral health as part of the universal health coverage and non-communicable disease agendas towards 2030. 2020.

[6] Glick M, *et al.* Vision 2030: Delivering Optimal Oral Health for All. 2021, FDI World Dental Federation: Geneva. Int Dent J. 2021; 71: pp. (1)3-4.

[7] Varenne B, Fox CH. The Role of Research in the WHO Oral Health Resolution. JDR Clin Trans Res 2021; 6(2): 112-4.
[http://dx.doi.org/10.1177/2380084421997095] [PMID: 33719671]

[8] Pitts NB, Zero DT, Marsh PD, *et al.* Dental caries. Nat Rev Dis Primers 2017; 3(1): 17030.
[http://dx.doi.org/10.1038/nrdp.2017.30] [PMID: 28540937]

[9] Selwitz RH, Ismail AI, Pitts NB. Dental caries. Lancet 2007; 369(9555): 51-9.
[http://dx.doi.org/10.1016/S0140-6736(07)60031-2] [PMID: 17208642]

[10] Phantumvanit P, Makino Y, Ogawa H. WHO Global Consultation on Public Health Intervention against Early Childhood Caries. Community Dent Oral Epidemiol 2018; 46(3): 280-7.
[http://dx.doi.org/10.1111/cdoe.12362]

[11] Pitts N, Zero D. White Paper on Dental Caries Prevention and Management A summary of the current evidence and the key issues in controlling this preventable disease. FDI World Dental Federation 2016.

[12] FDI World Dental Federation, FDI Policy Statement– Carious Lesions and First Restorative Treatment, in FDI General Assemb 2019.

[13] Peres MA, Macpherson LMD, Weyant RJ, *et al.* Oral diseases: a global public health challenge. Lancet 2019; 394(10194): 249-60.
[http://dx.doi.org/10.1016/S0140-6736(19)31146-8] [PMID: 31327369]

[14] Glick M, Williams DM, Kleinman DV, Vujicic M, Watt RG, Weyant RJ. A new definition for oral health developed by the FDI World Dental Federation opens the door to a universal definition of oral health. Int Dent J 2016; 66(6): 322-4.
[http://dx.doi.org/10.1111/idj.12294] [PMID: 27885673]

CHAPTER 8

Early Childhood Caries

Neerja Singh[1,*] and **Monika Rathore**[1]

[1] *Department of Pedodontics and Preventive Dentistry, BBD College of Dental Sciences, BBD University, Lucknow, U.P., India*

Abstract: Early childhood caries (ECC) is a serious and common public health problem affecting young children across the globe. It is prevalent in both developing and developed countries. ECC starts and progresses rapidly in high-risk children. It can lead to various physical, psychosocial and financial consequences for the child and their family, leading to compromised quality of life. There are some factors unique to this type of caries due to the developmental stage and dependence of the child on the mother or caretaker for feeding and oral hygiene practices. The faulty feeding practices can affect the primary dentition severely. ECC also indicates higher risk of caries development in later stages of life.

The disease can be challenging to manage in advanced stages due to limited specialized personnel and resources and behavioral management problems in young children. An effective prevention protocol is our best tool to manage this disease, reducing the burden the healthcare system and society.

Keywords: Early childhood caries (ECC), Etiology, Clinical features, Prevention and management.

INTRODUCTION

Early childhood caries is one of the most debilitating and common diseases of preschool-aged children leading to the destruction of tooth tissues by combined effects of acids generated from the fermentation of dietary carbohydrates by bacteria, interplay host factors, such as teeth and saliva and the effect of home oral hygiene measures including the use of fluoride.

Decay of primary teeth in children under 6 years of age is referred to as early childhood caries (ECC). The consequences of ECC and poor oral health can influence the overall general health of children and the quality of life of children as well as their parents.

* **Corresponding author Neerja Singh:** Department of Pedodontics and Preventive Dentistry, BBD College of Dental Sciences, BBD University, Lucknow, U.P., India; Tel: +91 98393472271; E-mail: neerjaped@gmail.com

Dental caries is a preventable disease, yet it is the most prevalent childhood disease in the world. In India, this is one of the most common conditions with unattended health needs in children.

Definitions

Early Childhood Caries (ECC) is defined as the presence of one or more decayed (non-cavitated or cavitated lesions), missing (due to caries), or filled tooth surfaces in any primary tooth in a child under the age of six (AAPD 2020).

Severe early childhood caries (S-ECC) is any sign of smooth-surface caries in a child younger than three years of age, and from ages, three to five, a decayed, missing or filled score of greater than or equal to four (age 3), greater than or equal to five (age 4), greater than or equal to six (age 5) [1].

S-ECC

DMFT score ≥ age in years + 1

Early childhood caries has also been termed as Nursing Bottle Caries, Nursing caries, Baby bottle tooth decay, Bottle rot and Maternally Derived *Streptococcus mutans* Disease.

While a child is said to have early childhood caries when even a single tooth shows signs of decay, restoration or is missing, nursing caries is associated with patterns of decay wherein the mandibular anterior teeth are spared from caries.

Rampant Caries

Massler defined rampant caries as ‘suddenly appearing, widespread, rapidly burrowing type of caries, resulting in early involvement of the pulp and affecting those teeth regarded as immune to ordinary decay.

Early childhood caries may also manifest as rampant caries where distinguishingly, the proximal surfaces of mandibular anterior teeth are affected by decay.

ECC, nursing caries and rampant caries can often be considered as a continuum of the same condition when allowed to progress unabated without preventive and therapeutic intervention in the early stage of the disease.

Classification

For the past 20 years, different research groups have attempted to develop classification systems for Early Childhood Caries (ECC) (Fig. **1**). The various classification systems developed include:

1. Based on the severity and the associated etiology (Wyne,1999) [2].

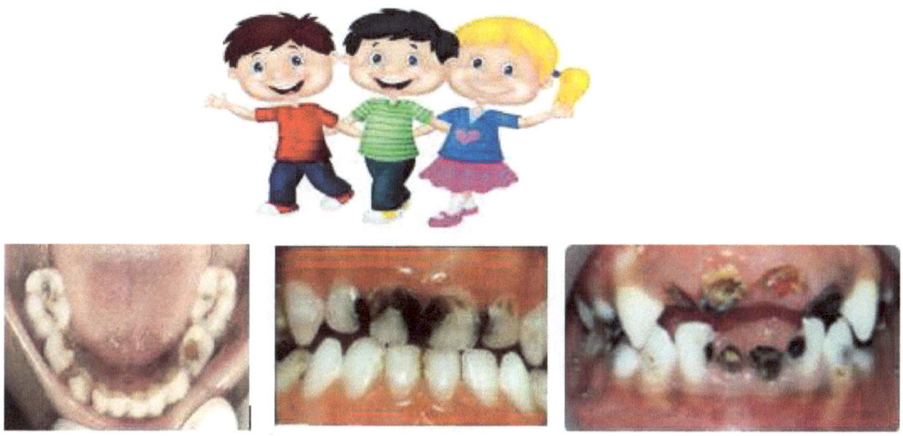

Mild to Moderate ECC	Moderate to Severe ECC	Severe ECC
Isolated carious lesions	'Labiolingual lesions'	Carious lesions affecting almost all surfaces
Incisors and/ or molars are involved	maxillary incisors, with or without molar caries are involved Mandibular incisors are typically unaffected	all teeth including the mandibular incisors are involved
Etiological factors are combination of semi solid/solid food and oral hygiene	Etiological factors are inappropriate use of feeding bottle or at-will breast-feeding or combination of both, with or without poor oral hygiene	Combination of cariogenic food substances and poor oral hygiene

Fig. (1). Classification systems for Early Childhood Caries (ECC).

2. Based on the pattern of tooth involvement (Johnston and Messer, 1994) [3].

- Lesions associated with developmental defects (pit and fissure defects and hypoplasia).
- Smooth surface lesions (labial-lingual lesions, approximal molar lesions).
- Rampant caries- having caries in 14 out of 20 primary teeth, including at least one mandibular incisor.

3. Based on the stage of development of the dentition and severity of dental caries (Verkramp and Wertheim, 1995) (Fig. **2**) [4].

This classification system assumes that dental caries occurs in successive stages, starting late in the first year (10 months) and ending in the fourth year of life (48 months). The four stages were referred to as given in the diagram:

At each stage, a different group of teeth is involved, and dental caries can range from enamel demineralization (opaque white demineralization) to cavitation involving enamel and dentine. Inspite of all the efforts made to classify ECC lesions clinically, there was a great need for a standard system of diagnosis and reporting of ECC for research purposes. Thus, for this purpose, the description of ECC and Severe ECC was formulated by Drury *et al.*, 1999 [1] (Table **1**), (S-ECC) by the participants at the workshop in Bethesda 1999 (Drury *et al*,. 1999)

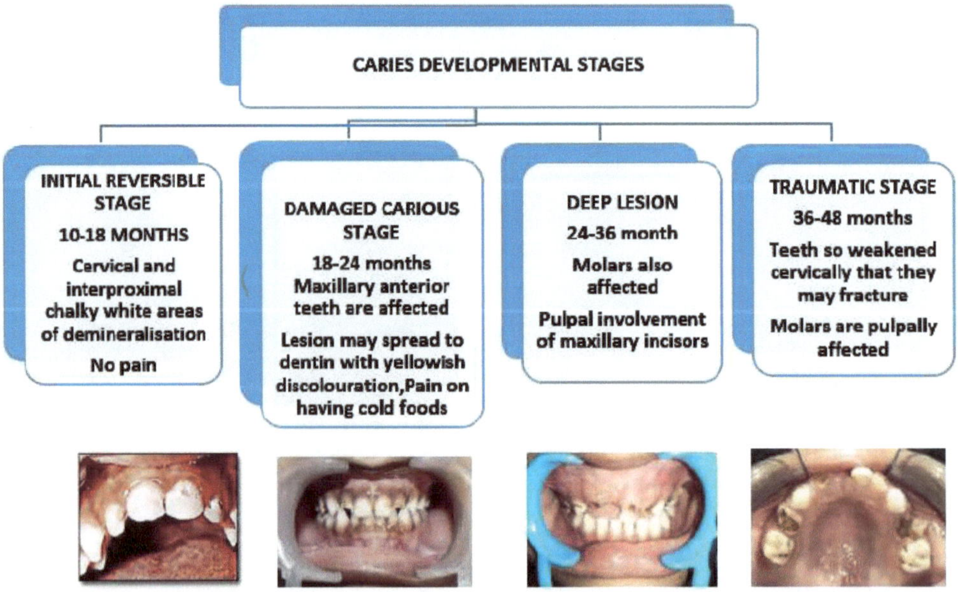

Fig. (2). Developmental stages.

Table 1. Proposed case definitions of Early Childhood Caries (ECC) and Severe Early Childhood Caries.

Age (months)	Early Childhood Caries	Severe Early Childhood Caries
<12	1 or more dmf surfaces	1 or more smooth dmf surfaces
12-23	1 or more dmf surfaces	1 or more smooth dmf surfaces
24-35	1 or more dmf surfaces	1 or more smooth dmf surfaces
36-47	1 or more dmf surfaces	1 or more cavitated, filled, or missing (due to caries) smooth surfaces in primary maxillary anterior teeth or dmfs score >4
48-59	1 or more dmf surfaces	1 or more cavitated, filled, or missing (due to caries) smooth surfaces in primary maxillary anterior teeth or dmfs score >5
60-71	1 or more dmf surfaces	1 or more cavitated, filled, or missing (due to caries) smooth surfaces in primary maxillary anterior teeth or dmfs score >6

Rampant caries is a historic term used to describe multiple caries lesions in the same patient, often used in association with early childhood caries or radiation caries.

Epidemiology

ECC continues to be a pandemic disease worldwide. Prevalence among children aged 3-5 years age varies between continents and countries. The worldwide prevalence of ECC varies significantly depending on many factors. While socioeconomic status plays a very important role, the other factors of significance are race, dietary habits, ethnicity, and oral hygiene status. The high prevalence of ECC is found in underdeveloped countries and less privileged communities. USA has a higher prevalence than European countries, with 40% of children acquiring caries by kindergarten age, while in the United Kingdom, 12% of 3 year-old children had visible caries [4].

In some countries, ECC is localized in specific sectors or population groups. Prevalence is high in many low-income countries, particularly in South-East Asia and Africa and specifically among socioeconomically disadvantaged groups. Most caries is left untreated, which could lead to a lack of physical development and reduced learning ability of children, and the treatment costs could increase. ECC also represents a risk factor for permanent tooth caries. ECC is one of the most prevalent health problems in infants and toddlers. In Japan, the National Oral Health Survey of 2011 showed that 25% of 3-year-olds experienced caries with a rate of decayed and filled primary teeth (dft) of 0.6. A higher prevalence of 36-85% in Asia, 38-45% in Africa and 22-61% in the Middle East is found [5].

Since the late 1940s, most developed countries have experienced significant declines in overall rates of dental caries. The decline in dental caries has been attributed to widespread efforts to improve oral health by increasing access to fluoridated dentifrices (toothpaste) and municipal water supplies. The globalization of food sources and the transition of food habits towards highly processed and sugar-added foods have been key factors in suppressing the rate of improvement in caries experience among at-risk populations.

Etiological Factors

Preschool children represent a unique group who are under continuous changes developmentally and their dental caries progression can be very rapid. Although the caries process is the same for both adults and children, when a young child suffers from ECC the process can happen more quickly. The reasons for rapid progression are related to a combination of the unique behavioral context of a growing child and the susceptible morphology of newly erupting teeth (Fig **3**).

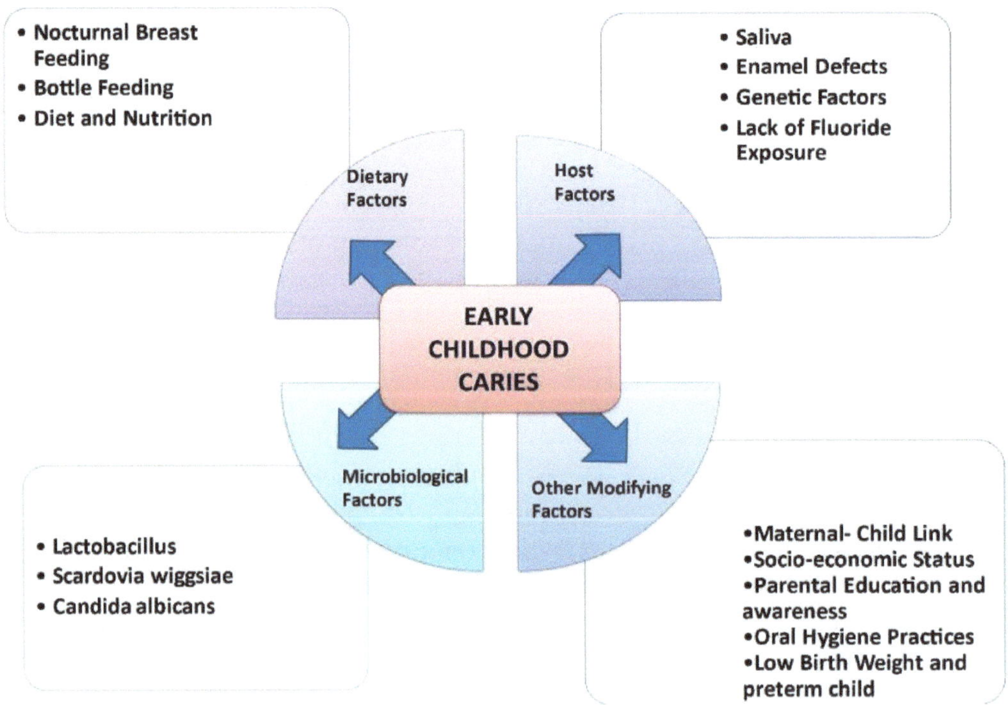

Fig. (3). Etiological Factors.

A. Dietary Factors

1. Breastfeeding
2. Bottle feeding
3. Improper chewing
4. Pouching the food in vestibule
5. Prolonged time taken for completing meals

B. Microbiological Factors

1. Early colonization of Strep. Mutans
2. Poor oral hygiene
    A. Host Factors
        1. Saliva factors
        2. Enamel defects
        3. Genetic factors

C. Other Modifying Factors

1. The maternal-child link to ECC.
2. Socio economic status.
3. Parental education and awareness
4. Oral hygiene practices
5. Low birth weight and preterm babies.
6. Birth order

DIETARY FACTORS

Breastfeeding

The present recommendation from WHO is that children should be exclusively breastfed for the first six months of life. Exclusive breastfeeding during the first six months of life can reduce the risk of gastroenteritis, infections, asthma, atopic disease, and diabetes. The amount of bio-available calcium and phosphate present in human breast milk can prevent the biofilm from reaching a critical pH and thus does not have a cariogenic potential if it is the only source of carbohydrate [6].

The universal availability of refined sugars could modify the relationship between breast milk and the dental caries process. If refined sugars are added to the diet of the young child, the biofilm could become highly cariogenic. When this transformed, cariogenic biofilm is exposed to human breast milk, it may add to caries risk.

While it is accepted that exclusive breastfeeding should continue over the first six months of life, there is currently no consensus on what age breastfeeding should stop. A higher risk of ECC is associated with breastfeeding past 24 months.

Bottle Feeding

Bottle feeding is the main viable alternative to breastfeeding for the delivery of nutrition to the child during infancy. The timing, content, and frequency of drinking are key aspects when describing the risk of bottle-feeding in the ECC process. Children who are offered on-demand bottle feed for a prolonged period, particularly at night time while they are sleeping, have a considerable risk of ECC.

The Diet and ECC

The transition of the child from a liquid diet towards a solid diet is fraught with challenges, and one of those is the addition of free sugars to the diet. This is a significant problem because of the effect that sugar has in transforming the biofilm into a cariogenic biofilm, with a low pH resulting in tooth mineral loss. The *Guideline dietary pattern,* which corresponds most closely to current World Health Organization weaning guidelines, at 6 months, has a protective action against ECC development compared to breastmilk, *Easy-to-prepare foods* and noodles [7]. The *Guidelines dietary pattern* is characterized by high consumption of rice porridge, fish and meat, fresh fruit, and vegetables as core food items throughout the 6 to 12 months period [8].

In terms of sugar, not all sugars are equal in their ability to contribute to disease processes, with free sugars being major contributors to dental caries and chronic disease. Free sugars are all monosaccharides and disaccharides added to foods by the manufacturer, cook or consumer, plus sugars naturally present in honey, syrups, and fruit juices.

One of the most potent vehicles for the delivery of free sugars is sugary liquids which include sweetened medicines, beverages, fruit juices and soft drinks. When a child's mouth is exposed to sugary drinks for a prolonged period, the ability of saliva to neutralize acid gets compromised and the biofilm becomes more acidogenic. The mineral loss that occurs, as a result, is more rapid for immature enamel found in an infant's mouth.

Microbiological Factors

ECC is most caused by Streptococcus mutans *(SM) and* Streptococcus sobrinus. Lactobacilli do not participate in the initiation of a lesion but are actively involved in lesion progression. The levels of mutans streptococci (MS) in the saliva of children increase with age. Children with dental caries show higher levels of mutans streptococci. Based on PCR analysis, a wide range of genetic diversity is seen in cases of children with and without clinically detectable caries [9].

Dental caries is an infectious, transmissible disease. The presence of matching MS genotypes suggests vertical transmission from mothers to children. Feeding habits, gum cleaning, and the number of erupted teeth in children also have a significant effect on MS colonization [10].

Children usually receive S mutans from their mother through vertical transmission and from their siblings and caregivers through horizontal transmission. Infants delivered by caesarean section are more prone to develop S mutans colonization due to their aseptic oral environment.

A further aspect contributing to the complexity of the caries process involves the characteristics of the biofilm and how they will moderate the impact of a cariogenic substrate on the caries balance. Although SM has been established as an etiological factor in the caries process, the presence or absence of SM alone cannot predict caries sensitivity. The predominant model of caries etiology has transitioned from the Specific Plaque Hypothesis to Ecological Plaque Hypotheses, but controversy continues regarding the role played by the MS [11]. The other species associated with ECC are *C. albicans* and *Prevotella* spp. When a biofilm high in cariogenic bacteria is exposed to a cariogenic substrate, then rapid production of acid will occur, but if a healthy biofilm is exposed to the same substrate, then the rate of demineralization will be slower. Also, considering the near-universal presence of S. mutans, when the biofilm is exposed to free sugars with high frequency and oral persistence, then it will transform, and net mineral loss can subsequently occur. This process is independent of the age of the host, or the time of the eruption. If the biofilm is transformed at the time that newly erupted teeth with immature enamel are present, then it is likely that caries will progress more rapidly. If the biofilm is dysbiotic, then more cariogenic bacteria will dominate, and SM will be detectable as a risk indicator.

Scardovia wiggsiae is the pathogen that has been recently proposed as a causative microorganism in severe ECC, even in the absence of mutans streptococci. This pathogen has been isolated from the saliva of children with ECC (Fig **4**) [12].

Host Factors

The expression of dental caries and their clinical signs will be modified by the characteristics of the host. Although biochemical changes occur at the surface of the tooth, it is important to consider the caries process in the context of the individual and the interplay of all the related body systems.

Saliva

Although salivary dysfunction is unusual in young children when saliva has poor quality or is of insufficient quantity, then the antibacterial defenses are reduced, acid and calcium buffering is decreased, and the substrate is cleared less efficiently from the mouth. This places the child at greater risk of caries, particularly if the diet is high in free sugars.

Saliva possesses many innate or acquired defense factors which affect biofilm formation and maturation and inhibit bacterial invasion, growth, and metabolism by different mechanisms. The role of physical properties of saliva (pH, volume, and viscosity) have been well explored, but the role of genetic, proteomic and metabolomic factors remain unexplored.

A significant correlation between caries prevalence in preschool children and salivary proteins, including IgA, IgG immunoglobulins, PRP and histatin peptides, has been found. These saliva components may be used as biomarkers for ECC. To date, no clear association has been found between other salivary proteins and ECC risks, and the amount of total salivary proteins has not been proved to be useful in predicting caries risk.

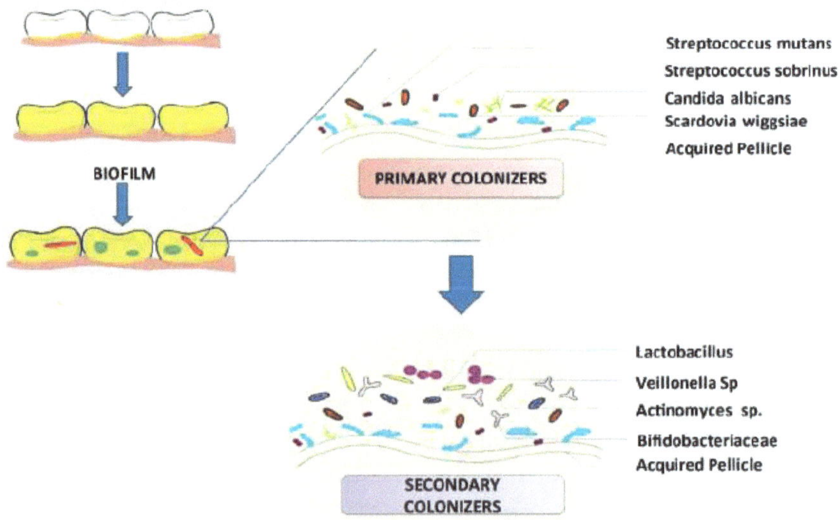

Fig (4). Predominant microorganisms in cariogenic biofilm in ECC.

Enamel Defects

In addition to saliva, the status of the 'host' can also be compromised if there is a disturbance in the development of the dental enamel. Such a disturbance can result in dental enamel that is low in mineral content (hypomineralization) or a decrease in thickness (hypoplasia). Enamel formation (amelogenesis) happens during the initial stages of growth and development from the second trimester of gestation until late childhood, and the process can be interrupted or compromised by febrile disease, medications, environmental pollutants, and malnutrition. In the situation that amelogenesis is compromised, leading to hypomineralized enamel, then the enamel may be more soluble in response to pH changes within the biofilm. If amelogenesis results in tooth morphology that is plaque retentive, such as in the case of deep pits and fissures, or in the presence of enamel hypoplasia, then the biofilm may have a physical niche and not be disturbed regularly by tooth-brushing, if a suitable substrate is present this can lead to caries development (Figs. **5** and **6**).

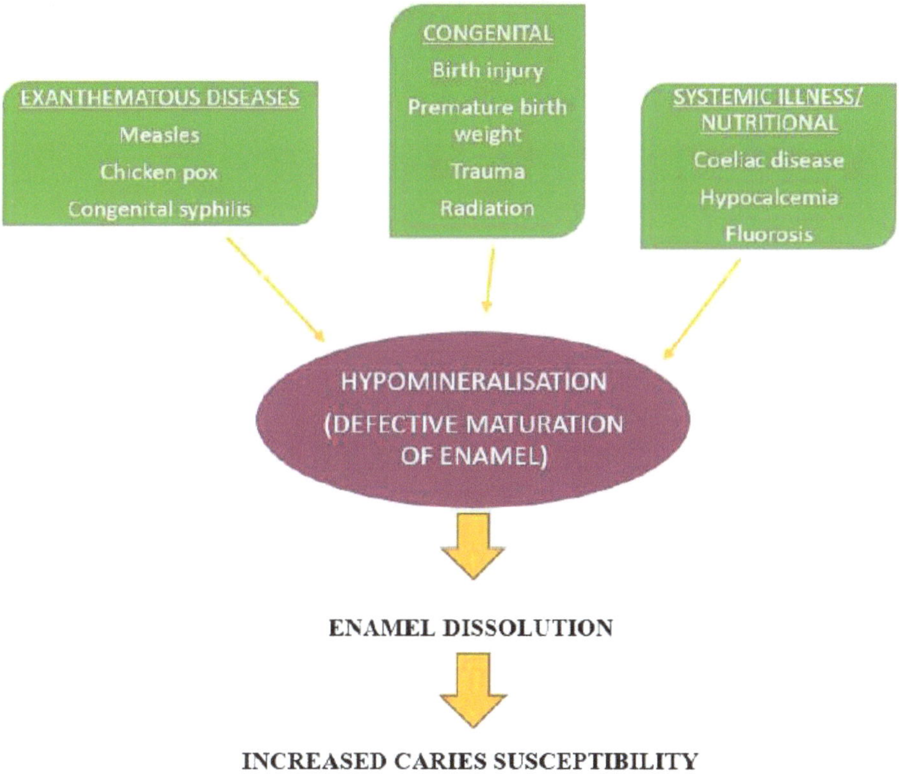

Fig (5). Hypomineralisation of enamel.

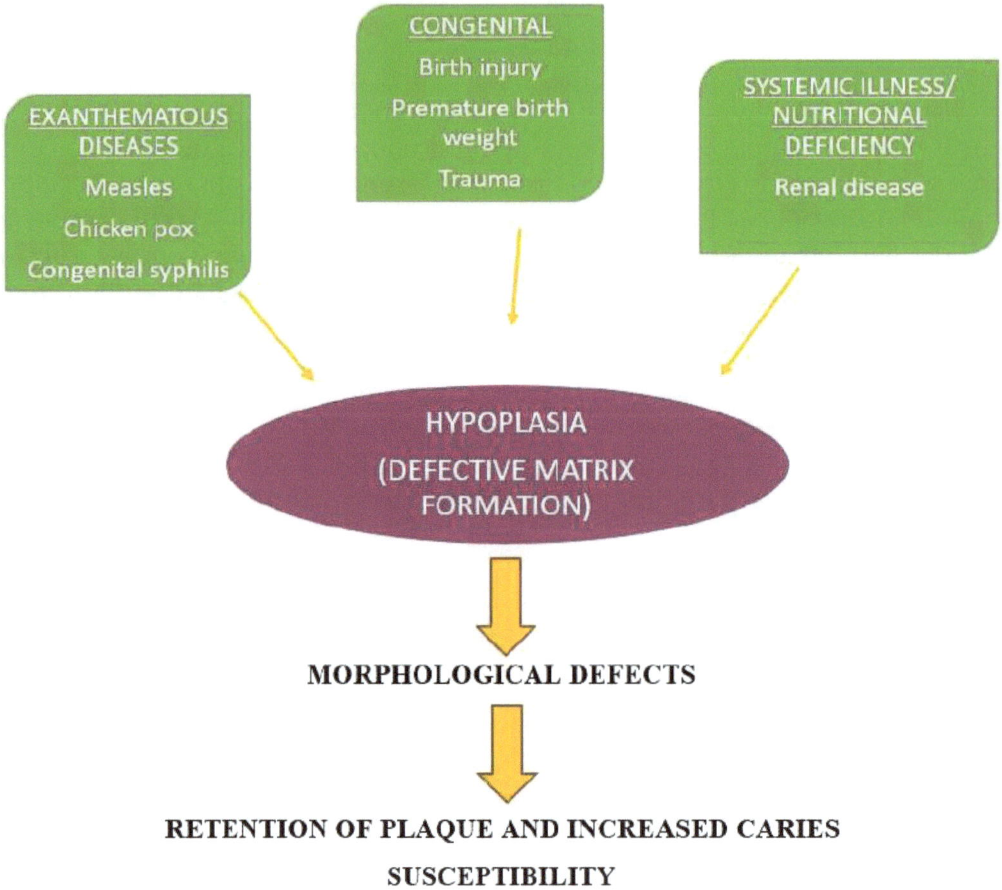

Fig (6). After effects of hypoplasia.

GENETIC FACTORS

Though a lot has been explored about etiology and progression of the disease of ECC, some grey areas are still there which keep the scientific community puzzled. It is not unusual to find children who are more susceptible while others are extremely resistant, regardless of the environmental risk factors to which they are exposed. It can be suggested that genetic variation in genes involved in enamel formation and genes involved in immune response may contribute to ECC, and that susceptibility is the result of gene-environment interactions [13].

Should the genotype play a significant role in moderating caries expression, then this could be an important target for therapeutic intervention at a molecular or genetic level in the future.

OTHER MODIFYING FACTORS

The Maternal-Child Link to ECC

Although there is a strong evidence-base for associations between maternal and child oral health, the causal relationship is less clear.

From a psycho-social point of view, the resistance of the host (child) to pathological factors is related to maternal nutritional status, psychological maternal stress, and maternal oral health literacy. Maternal caries experience is an independent risk factor for ECC in their children. However, good oral health practices rendered to the children by caregivers may reduce such risks. Mothers should be educated regarding the importance of good oral health behaviors and healthy eating habits for their children [14].

Both the mother and child are exposed to a majority of the same protective and pathological factors, and so the presentation of carious lesions will depend upon how the caries balance is managed in both individuals.

Socio Economic Status

Socioeconomic status may affect ECC in many ways. Low income can enhance the risk of caries due to poor awareness, compromised reach to dental care, oral hygiene neglect by parents and compromised overall health of children. All these factors can result in increased susceptibility to caries. However, on another side, it is not unusual to find out higher prevalence and dmft index in higher socioeconomic groups also. The reasons for that may be increased in-between meal snacking, more consumption of refined and processed food materials, frequent intake of sweetened beverages and sometimes dependence of the child on an untrained caregiver for all feeding and oral hygiene practices.

Parental Education and Awareness

Parental education level and dental awareness have a significant role in understanding the importance of primary dentition. Better awareness can encourage them to reach for prenatal counseling and effective infant oral health care. Unfortunately, a large population in our society tends to downplay the importance of primary teeth and thus resulting in higher caries prevalence in preschool children.

Oral Hygiene Practices

The oral hygiene practices in preschool children are usually not very satisfactory across various populations. While brushing twice a day is a highly effective means to reduce bacterial load, sometimes parents find it difficult to perform, especially in the evening or at night. Children usually are not very cooperative for oral hygiene practices around their sleep time which makes it challenging for the parents to thoroughly clean the oral cavity of their children after the last meal.

Additionally, children usually take milk just before their sleep time, which further complicates the matter and increases caries susceptibility drastically.

Low Birth Weight and Preterm Babies

Preterm and low birth weight babies are usually at more risk of defective enamel formation and higher levels of Streptococcus mutans. These make the infant more prone to ECC.

CLINICAL FEATURES

ECC is a specific form of primary tooth decay affecting the overall development of infants and toddlers. The development of ECC often follows a special pattern, usually affecting labial surfaces of maxillary incisors that are, otherwise, at lower risk for caries and lingual and buccal surfaces of maxillary and mandibular molars.

Initially, the lesions appear as a whitish area of decalcification along the gingival margin, which further becomes pigmented and spreads laterally and coronally.

Children in the early childhood age group have a special caries pattern which is different from older children. The teeth are affected according to their pattern of eruption. The teeth which have been present and exposed in the mouth for a longer time to the caries insult are affected more. The upper incisors are most vulnerable, while the mandibular incisors are protected by the tongue and by saliva from submandibular and sublingual glands. Caries on molars may start concurrently in the pit and fissure area and the gingival area of the buccal surface. This pattern of dental caries has been labeled variously as “bottle caries,” “nursing caries,” “baby bottle tooth decay,” or “night bottle mouth.” As per recent knowledge, improper nursing is not the only etiological factor. Therefore, the term “early childhood caries (ECC)” is used to describe any form of caries in infants and preschool children. The importance of preserving the integrity of the primary teeth can be realized from the fact that loss of these teeth can lead to space loss, masticatory deficiency, phonetic challenges, lack of pre-maxilla development and resulting malocclusion, development of para-functional habits and psychological problems that interfere with the personality and behavior of the child.

ECC begins as white-spot lesions in upper primary incisors along the gingival margin. If the disease is not intercepted, caries can progress and result in the complete destruction of the crown (Figs. **7a** - **7e**).

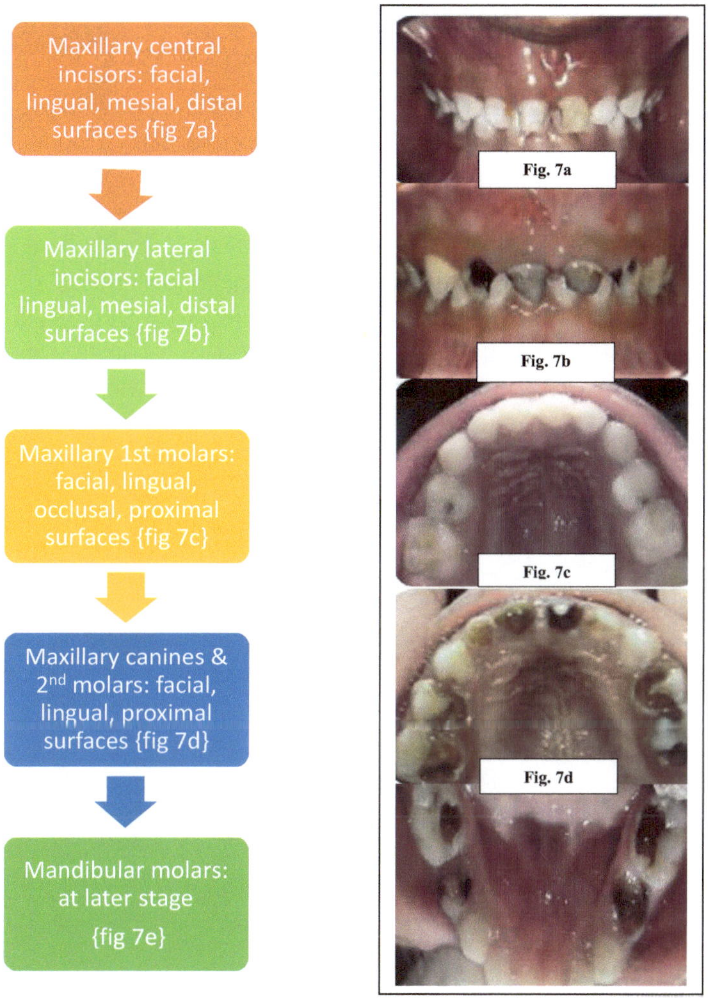

Fig. 7e

Fig. (7). Clinical features of ECC.

In the maxillary arch, the most highly involved decayed tooth is the central incisor, lateral incisor, first primary molar, second primary molar and followed by the canine. In the mandibular arch, the most highly involved tooth is the first primary molar, followed by the second primary molar, canine, central incisor, and lateral incisor. Regarding decayed surfaces (ds), the occlusal surface was most highly involved in the maxillary arch, followed by distal, mesial, buccal, lingual, labial, palatal, and incisal surfaces. In the mandibular arch, the occlusal surface was the most highly involved, followed by distal, buccal, lingual, and mesial surfaces. The pattern is the same as demonstrated by nursing caries [15].

CONSEQUENCES OF UNTREATED EARLY CHILDHOOD CARIES

ECC is recognized as a public health problem due to its high prevalence and the potential for negative health impacts if left untreated. For the past decades, diagnosis of caries has been made worldwide using the DMFT/dmft index. This traditional index provides details of caries and restorative and surgical treatment but fails to provide a clear picture of untreated dental caries, such as pulp involvement and dental abscess. The consequences of untreated carious lesions often lead to dental emergencies. It becomes essential to identify and use an index that measures and estimates the clinical consequences of untreated carious lesions among the population in epidemiological studies. A pufa/PUFA index has been developed to determine the severity of untreated carious lesions, and various stages of clinical findings of untreated carious lesions. It provides a better diagnosis of often missed untreated carious lesions. The index covers four different clinical stages of advanced caries providing a reality check on the often-unseen oral conditions. The pufa/PUFA score for the individual is counted cumulatively like the calculation of dmft/DMFT Score. Consequently, the score of pufa/PUFA can range from 0 to 20 for deciduous teeth and 0 to 32 for permanent teeth.

Code	Name	Description
P/p	Pulpal involvement	Recorded when the opening of the pulp chamber is visible or when the coronal tooth structures have been destroyed by the carious process and only roots or root fragments are left
U/u	Ulceration	Recorded when sharp edges of a tooth with pulpal involvement or root fragments have caused traumatic ulceration of the surrounding soft tissues, e.g., tongue or buccal mucosa
F/f	Fistula	Recorded when a pus releasing sinus tract related to a tooth with pulpal involvement is present
A/a	Abscess	Recorded when a pus containing swelling related to a tooth with pulpal involvement is present

EFFECTS OF UNTREATED CARIOUS LESIONS ON QUALITY OF LIFE OF THE CHILD

WHO has been recognized as an important sector of the Global Oral Health Program? Disease in the oral cavity during childhood can have a negative impact on the life of preschool children and their parents. Early childhood caries harms children's quality of life including pain in having hot and cold beverages, chewing and biting difficulties, reduced appetite, weight loss, sleeping difficulties, delayed growth, and development, change in behaviour like irritability and low self-esteem and decrease in school performance [16, 17].

EFFECTS OF UNTREATED CARIOUS LESIONS ON PARENTS' QUALITY OF LIFE

ECC can also affect them indirectly, for example, work-loss and monetary impact due to having to stay at home to take care of the child. These untreated carious lesions also cause an emotional and financial burden on parents as these lesions can lead to hospitalizations and emergency room visits, and high treatment costs.

EFFECTS OF UNTREATED CARIOUS LESIONS ON SUCCEDANEOUS TEETH

The consequences of ECC often include a higher risk of new carious lesions in both the primary and permanent dentitions, loss of school days, diminished ability to learn and diminished oral health-related quality of life.

Besides, it has been found that untreated carious lesions in primary teeth often lead to the developmental defects of their permanent successors. A primary tooth abscess may cause local sepsis around the developing permanent successor. Thus, interfering with normal development and resulting in enamel defects. Buccal surfaces of the incisors are more likely to be affected than the lingual due to the close approximation of the roots of the primary incisors to the former. If caries occurs in a primary tooth, the successor's tooth is more likely to have caries. Regardless of treatment, ECC is a risk factor for developing permanent first molar caries [18].

MANAGEMENT OF EARLY CHILDHOOD CARIES

Early Childhood Caries is a highly prevalent worldwide disease that has a high burden on society and has a major impact on parent's and children's quality of life. Caries is preventable, and the progression may be halted or slowed down by maintaining a balance between various behavioural and social factors like fluoride exposure, dietary habits, and oral hygiene practices. Now, it is well accepted that the management of caries needs a holistic approach rather than depending solely on surgical interventions. Different interventions are suggested for the management of ECC lesions, from active surveillance to extraction, depending on the disease process and the patient's risk of caries. Clinical decision-making for caries management should be based on the patient's risk levels, current oral health status, age, and the engagement of caregivers with preventive strategies.

PREVENTION

The prevention of ECC requires a multi-factorial approach due to its various etiological factors. The aims of prevention are targeted at

a. Early identification of patients who are at risk of ECC.
b. Preventing the progression of dental caries in children who are diagnosed with ECC.
c. Preventing the recurrence of dental caries in children who have been diagnosed with severe ECC.

SALIVA DIAGNOSTICS

Salivary samples can prove useful in providing information about etiological and predisposing factors:

- Host susceptibility: The rate of flow of saliva and its buffering capacity can indicate the potential for biologic repair.
- Bacterial challenge: Qualitative and quantitative assays of mutans streptococci can be indicators of a cariogenic environment [19].
- Diet: Levels of lactobacilli indicate sugar-induced biofilm stress.

Saliva malfunction has a key role in the caries balance, making it important to evaluate the normalcy or abnormality of secretion. The buffering capacity is also important for maintaining a neutral pH range in the oral biofilm. The chair-side buffer tests reflect the bicarbonate buffer system and identify saliva with normal (blue), intermediate (green) or poor (yellow) buffer capacity. Poor buffering may be associated with low saliva secretion and is considered an indicator of caries risk.

In addition to the diagnostic values of saliva tests, the outcome can be used as a patient-motivating tool [19].

CARIES RISK ASSESSMENT

Early identification of caries risk factors in children can reduce the lifetime burden of dental diseases. An assessment of caries risk during infancy periodically allows for early identification and understanding of a child's current and changing risk factors for ECC [20]. Based on the distribution of risk factors and protective factors, the health care provider can determine child's caries risk, explain the caries process and the causative factors to the parent, and develop in collaboration with the parent self-management goals to prevent or manage their child's caries risk [19] (Fig. **8**).

	High Risk	Moderate Risk	Protective
Risk (Biological) Factors			
Mother/primary caregiver has active cavities	Yes		
Parent/caregiver has low socioeconomic status	Yes		
Child has >3 between meal sugar-containing snacks or beverages per day	Yes		
Child is put to bed with bottle containing natural or added sugar	Yes		
Child has special health care needs		Yes	
Child is a recent immigrant		Yes	
Protective Factors			
Child receives optimally fluoridated drinking water or fluoride supplements			Yes
Child has teeth brushed daily with fluoridated toothpaste			Yes
Child receives topical fluoride from health professional			Yes
Child has dental home/regular dental care			Yes
Clinical Findings (Disease Indicators)			
Child has > 1 decayed/missing/filled surfaces	Yes		
Child has white spot lesions or enamel defects	Yes		
Child has elevated mutans streptococci levels	Yes		
Child has plaque on teeth		Yes	

Fig. (8). FCRA form for 0-5year old. (Adapted from American Academy of Pediatric Dentistry (AAPD). Guideline on caries-risk assessment and management for infants, children, and adolescents).

Management of the disease process should start in the first year of a child's life; and depending on the needs of the child includes primary, secondary, and tertiary prevention (Fig. **9**).

PRIMARY PREVENTION	SECONDARY PREVENTION	TERTIARY PREVENTION
• Prenatal oral health counseling • Infant oral health and concept of dental home • Diet and Nutrition Counseling • Oral Hygiene and use of fluoride • Non fluoride agents	•Fluorise varnish •Calcium-Based Strategies • Resin infiltration •Pit and Fissure sealant application	• Silver diamine fluoride • Conservative caries removal and restorative treatment. •Full coverage crowns

Fig. (9). Levels of Prevention.

PRIMARY PREVENTION

It includes:

1. Prenatal Oral Health Counseling- The goal of the prenatal counseling technique for early childhood caries prevention is to optimize parents'/caregivers' behaviour changes regarding the child's sugar consumption and oral hygiene. The use of motivational interviewing to improve health behaviours is based on the promise that an individual takes ownership and responsibility for his/her behaviour change.

2. Infant Oral Health and Dental Home- The bacteria often associated with early childhood caries are mutans streptococci, which metabolize sugars to produce acid that lowers the pH of oral plaque. Low pH for an extended period results in enamel demineralization, thus contributing to caries. Colonization often begins with a vertical transmission to a child from a primary caregiver/ mother. Prominent levels of mutans streptococci in a caregiver/mother and frequent snacking by the child increases the chance of mutans streptococci colonization and proliferation in children. The horizontal transmission also may occur during encounters with other family members or children in daycare centers or schools.

3. Dental Home - It is recommended that the first preventive dental visit and establishment of a dental home should be done not later than 12 months of age. A dental home is defined as an ongoing comprehensive relationship between the dentist and the patient/ parents. The four major components of a dental home are continuous access to care, quality oral health care, preventive care, and coordination of care with a timely referral when appropriate. Parents are advised to *"lift the lip"* once a month to look for early signs of decay on the surfaces of upper front teeth. Collaboration with parents and other health care providers to ensure all infants and toddlers have access to dental screening, counseling, and preventive procedures.

Early dental visits within 6 months of the eruption of the first tooth and no later than 12 months of age, to conduct a caries risk assessment which can potentially indicate those at risk even before the manifestation of caries lesions, should be encouraged (Fig.) [21].

4. Diet and Nutrition Counseling- Dietary counseling aims to help parents/caregivers improve their child's dietary behaviours to favor low- or non-cariogenic snacks, drink fluoridated water, and limit sugar-containing foods to mealtimes. Such dietary recommendations must be realistic and based upon the dietary norms of the family. The following factors are recommended to decrease caries risk in infants:

- The use of bottles and no-spill training cups should be discontinued by the age 12 months and open cups should be introduced.
- While breastfeeding is encouraged, it should not be done on-demand and at night during sleep, once babies are old enough to no longer need feeding every 3 hours to 4 hours.
- Avoid bedtime bottle or sippy cup with anything other than water.
- Limit sugary food, drinks, including fruit juices, to mealtimes.
- Encourage a balanced diet, healthy snacking, fruits, and vegetables.

5. Oral Hygiene and Use of Fluoride- The quality of tooth cleaning is important therefore, young children require assistance from an adult or caregiver. Gum pad cleaning should begin even before the first tooth erupts. The parents must clean the infant's gum pads with a damp cloth or gauze after every feed. After the first tooth erupts, the teeth should be brushed using a knee-to-knee position with two adults or by having an adult approach from behind the child's head, it should take no more than 1 minute to brush a young child's teeth.

Fluoride toothpaste containing at least 1000ppm is an effective, safe, and cost-effective prevention tool for children. The recommended fluoridated toothpaste for children younger than 2 years of age with medium and high caries risk is only a smear, while for children between 2-5 years of age a pea-sized amount of fluoride toothpaste is advised [22] (Fig **10**).

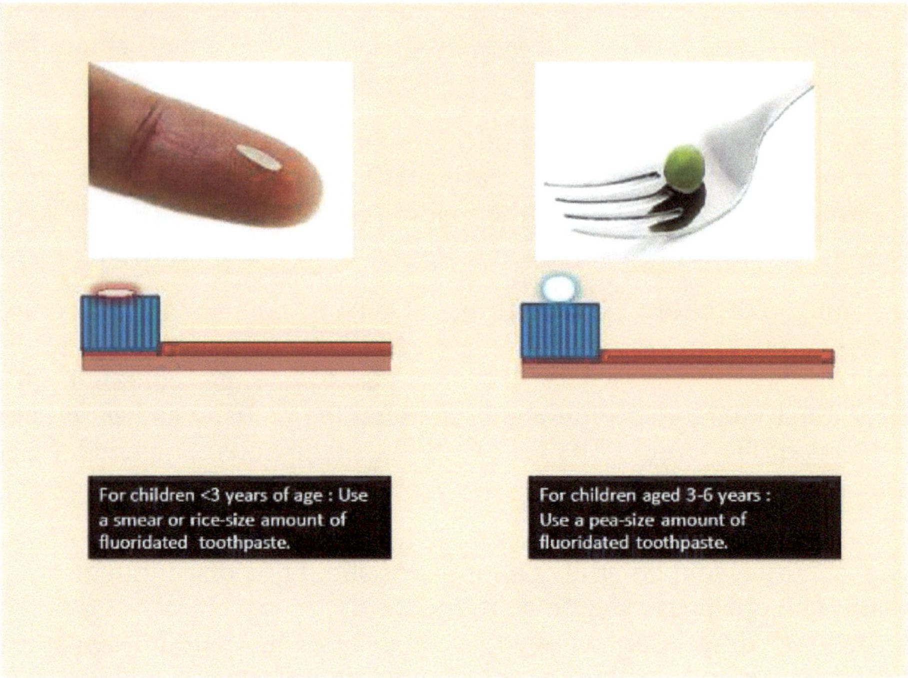

Fig. (10). Fluoride toothpaste recommendations for young children.

Water fluoridation is the most convenient and economical method for providing optimal fluoride benefits. The communities in areas with sub-optimal fluoride levels may require a fluoride supplement for high-risk groups.

NON-FLUORIDE AGENTS

Chlorhexidine- Chlorhexidine gluconate is effective against a wide variety of gram-negative and gram-positive organisms, aerobes, facultative anaerobes, and yeast. The drug has a strong affinity to oral structures. At lower concentrations, chlorhexidine interferes with cell wall transportation and metabolic pathways, whereas higher concentrations cause precipitation of the intracellular cytoplasm [19].

Povidone Iodine- It is a powerful germicidal agent effective against a wide range of bacteria, viruses, fungi, protozoa, and spores. It is evident that a 10% solution used causes moderate suppression of mutans streptococci in plaque and saliva.

Xylitol– It has a sweet taste and antimicrobial properties. Xylitol wipes can be used in infants to clean their teeth and gums.

REPLACEMENT THERAPY AND PROBIOTICS

Probiotics (derived from the Greek pro bios, for life) are defined by the World Health Organization as "live microorganisms which when administered in adequate amounts confer a health benefit on the host." Probiotics are present in the intestinal flora of healthy individuals and most of them belong to the lactobacilli and bifidobacterial groups

Three main routes of action by probiotics are:

1. Probiotic bacteria compete with other microorganisms for binding sites and nutrition in the biofilm.
2. Probiotic bacteria produce bacteriocins that inhibit the growth of various bacteria.
3. Probiotic bacteria stimulate the specific and nonspecific immune response by activation of T cells and through the production of cytokines that mediates the inflammatory process.

Probiotics influence the oral cavity and the caries balance locally and systemically [19]. Significant reduction of mutans streptococci can occur in saliva by regular consumption of probiotic tablets as an adjunct to daily use of fluoridated toothpaste in preschool children [23].

Secondary Prevention

Secondary prevention for ECC aims to arrest the progression of caries before the cavitation of lesions. In addition to primary prevention, secondary prevention includes more frequent fluoride varnish applications (duraphat, fluorprotector) and pit and fissure sealant application to occlusal surfaces of susceptible molars.

Pit and fissure sealants have been used for decades to prevent and control carious lesions on primary and permanent teeth. Teeth with anatomic grooves/ deep pits or fissures on occlusal surfaces trap food debris and promote bacterial biofilm, thus increasing the risk of developing carious lesions. Effectively penetrating and sealing these surfaces with sealants can inhibit the progression of non-cavitated carious lesions [22].

Calcium-Based Strategies - Remineralizing agents promote remineralization through an increase of bioavailable calcium and phosphate ions that become incorporated in tooth structure. Supplementing calcium and phosphates is likely to have a positive effect when effective fluoride levels are available at the same time [24].

Potential benefits have been shown for casein phosphopeptides, amorphous calcium phosphates, and other approaches. Inhibition of enamel and dentin demineralization, promotion of remineralization, and a slow-down of the caries process as well as regression of subsurface lesions have been reported for casein phosphopeptide–amorphous calcium phosphate (CCP-ACP) [24].

Other forms of calcium-based agents have also been tried and shown to have promising results. These include Tri-Calcium Phosphate, Calcium Silicophosphate, Calcium Sucrose Phosphate, Nano Hydroxyapatite, and Bioactive glass

Resin Infiltration— Resin infiltration of early lesions is a recent technique by which subsurface porosities in the lesion are filled with resin. It slows down or arrests the progression of white spot lesions, which makes it a promising agent for ECC management.

Tertiary Prevention

It can involve both non-invasive and invasive treatment protocols when there are cavitated lesions. Besides primary and secondary prevention approaches, silver diamine fluoride can be used to arrest cavitated lesions.

1. Silver Diamine Fluoride (SDF) arrests caries by the antibacterial effect of silver and remineralization of enamel and dentin. The black discoloration of teeth after application of SDF is the only reported side effect.

2. Conservative Caries Removal and Restorative Treatment-. It becomes necessary to prevent further tooth breakdown, pain and prevent unnecessary pulp exposures. Restorative treatment involves caries removal and considers various risk factors, protective factors as well as the age of the child. The choice of restorative material used is influenced by the site and extent of decay, a child's ability to cooperate caries risk status and the longevity of the restoration.

3. Conservative restorations are advised for children with lower caries risk, while high caries risk children require more aggressive treatment options.

In young children with an elevated risk of caries, there is good evidence that stainless steel crowns function better than multi-surface intraoral restorations. Preventive care based on caries risk is essential during follow-up visits.

4. Full Coverage Crowns: Full coverage crowns like zirconia and stainless-steel crowns may be necessary when restoring ECC in patients with high caries risk and extensive tooth structure loss (Fig. **11**).

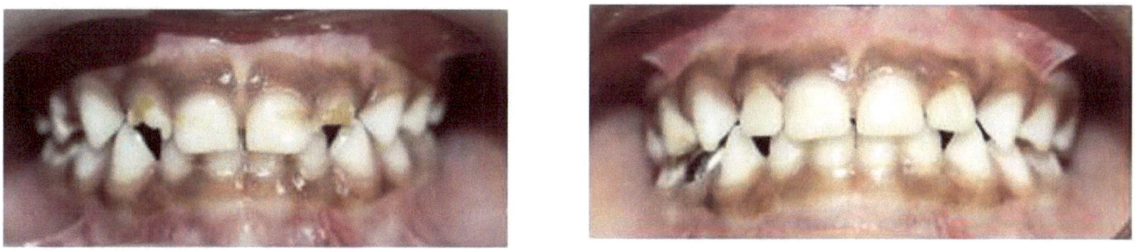

Fig. (11). Full coverage Zirconia crown on maxillary incisors.

Interprofessional Care assures that all infants and toddlers have access to oral health care. Children with their parents visit pediatricians, general physicians, and obstetricians much earlier than pediatric dental surgeons. A collaborative approach involving dental professionals with other health care providers can lead to more efficient prevention of ECC.

CONCLUSION

It can be concluded that ECC, as a highly prevalent childhood disease is a major burden for the health care system globally. Unfortunately, the prevalence of this disease is not showing a decline. The untreated carious lesions can lead to major consequences affecting the overall health and quality of life of children and their parents. The treatment of advanced lesions requires much energy, skill, and finances. On the other hand, timely and effective prevention approaches can reduce the burden significantly on the healthcare system.

CONSENT FOR PUBLICATION

Not applicable.

CONFLICT OF INTEREST

The author(s) declare no conflict of interest, financial or otherwise.

ACKNOWLEDGEMENT

Declared none.

REFERENCES

[1] Johnston T, Messer LB. Nursing caries: Literature review and report of a case managed under local anaesthesia. Aust Dent J 1994; 39(6): 373-81. [http://dx.doi.org/10.1111/j.1834-7819.1994.tb03110.x] [PMID: 7832687]

[2] Ismail AI, Sohn W. A systematic review of clinical diagnostic criteria of early childhood caries. J Public Health Dent 1999; 59(3): 171-91. [http://dx.doi.org/10.1111/j.1752-7325.1999.tb03267.x] [PMID: 10649590]

[3] Veerkamp JS, Weerheijm KL. Nursing-bottle caries: the importance of a development perspective. ASDC J Dent Child 1995; 62(6): 381-6.
[PMID: 8636472]

[4] National Oral Health Survey UK. 2013.

[5] Dülgergil ÇT, Dalli M, Hamidi MM, Çolak H. Early childhood caries update: A review of causes, diagnoses, and treatments. J Nat Sci Biol Med 2013; 4(1): 29-38.
[http://dx.doi.org/10.4103/0976-9668.107257] [PMID: 23633832]

[6] Nunes AMM, Alves CMC, Borba de Araújo F, *et al.* Association between prolonged breast-feeding and early childhood caries: a hierarchical approach. Community Dent Oral Epidemiol 2012; 40(6): 542-9.
[http://dx.doi.org/10.1111/j.1600-0528.2012.00703.x] [PMID: 22725605]

[7] Hu S, Sim YF, Toh JY, *et al.* Infant dietary patterns and early childhood caries in a multi-ethnic Asian cohort. Sci Rep 2019; 9(1): 852.
[http://dx.doi.org/10.1038/s41598-018-37183-5] [PMID: 30696871]

[8] Toh J, Yip G, Han W, *et al.* Infant Feeding Practices in a Multi-Ethnic Asian Cohort: The GUSTO Study. Nutrients 2016; 8(5): 293.
[http://dx.doi.org/10.3390/nu8050293] [PMID: 27187461]

[9] Loomba A, Damle SG, Dhindsa A, Loomba A, Beniwal V. Correlation between dental caries experience and mutans streptococci counts by microbial and molecular (polymerase chain reaction) assay using saliva as microbial risk indicator. Dent Res J (Isfahan) 2016; 13(6): 552-9.
[http://dx.doi.org/10.4103/1735-3327.197035] [PMID: 28182053]

[10] Damle SG, Yadav R, Garg S, *et al.* Transmission of mutans streptococci in mother-child pairs. Indian J Med Res 2016; 144(2): 264-70.
[http://dx.doi.org/10.4103/0971-5916.195042] [PMID: 27934807]

[11] Banas JA, Drake DR. Are the mutans streptococci still considered relevant to understanding the microbial etiology of dental caries? BMC Oral Health 2018; 18(1): 129.
[http://dx.doi.org/10.1186/s12903-018-0595-2] [PMID: 30064426]

[12] Chandna P, Srivastava N, Sharma A, Sharma V, Gupta N, Adlakha V. Isolation of *Scardovia wiggsiae* using real-time polymerase chain reaction from the saliva of children with early childhood caries. J Indian Soc Pedod Prev Dent 2018; 36(3): 290-5.
[http://dx.doi.org/10.4103/JISPPD.JISPPD_225_17] [PMID: 30246752]

[13] Abbasoğlu Z, Bussaneli D. G, Tanboğa İ, Henn I, W, Modesto A, Vieira A, R: Fine-Mapping of Xq25.1–27.2 Shows Association of Early Childhood Caries withGenetic Variants Depending on Dietary Habits, Protecting Children Who DrinkMilk before Going to Bed. Caries Res 2019; 53: 333-8.
[http://dx.doi.org/10.1159/000495975] [PMID: 30580329]

[14] Hariyani N, Do LG, Spencer AJ, Thomson WM, Scott JA, Ha DH. Maternal caries experience influences offspring's early childhood caries—a birth cohort study. Community Dent Oral Epidemiol 2020; 48(6): 561-9.
[http://dx.doi.org/10.1111/cdoe.12568] [PMID: 32776590]

[15] Kumar GR. Pattern and Severity of Early Childhood Caries among Preschool Children in Northern Region, Saudi Arabia: A Cross-Sectional Study. Pesqui Bras Odontopediatria Clin Integr 2019; 19e4622 [Internet].

[16] Policy on early childhood caries (ECC), classifications, consequences, and preventive strategies. Am Acad Pediatr Dentistr 2016; 39(6): 17-8.

[17] Singh N, Dubey N, Rathore M, Pandey P. Impact of early childhood caries on quality of life: Child and parent perspectives. J Oral Biol Craniofac Res 2020; 10(2): 83-6.
[http://dx.doi.org/10.1016/j.jobcr.2020.02.006] [PMID: 32181125]

[18] Songur F, Simsek Derelioglu S, Yilmaz S, Koşan Z. Assessing the Impact of Early Childhood Caries on the Development of First Permanent Molar Decays. Front Public Health 2019; 7: 186. [http://dx.doi.org/10.3389/fpubh.2019.00186] [PMID: 31338357]

[19] Svante Twetman" Treatment Protocols: Nonfluoride management of the caries disease process and available diagnostics. Dent Clin North Am 2010; 54(3): 527-40.

[20] American Academy of Pediatric Dentistry. Caries-risk assessment and management for infants, children, and adolescents. The Reference Manual of Pediatric Dentistry.Chicago, Ill.: American Academy of Pediatric Dentistry; 2020; pp. 243-7.

[21] Curto Manrique J, Malpartida-Carrillo V, Arriola-Guillén L. Efficacy of the lift-the-lip technique for dental plaque removal in preschool children. J Indian Soc Pedod Prev Dent 2019; 37: 162-6.

[22] Ng MW, Chase I. Early Childhood Caries: Risk-Based Disease Prevention and Management. Dent Clin North Am 2013; 57(1): 1-16. [http://dx.doi.org/10.1016/j.cden.2012.09.002]

[23] Hedayati-Hajikand T, Lundberg U, Eldh C, Twetman S. Effect of probiotic chewing tablets on early childhood caries – a randomized controlled trial. BMC Oral Health 2015; 15(1): 112. [http://dx.doi.org/10.1186/s12903-015-0096-5] [PMID: 26403472]

[24] Peters MC. Strategies for noninvasive demineralized tissue repair. Dent Clin North Am 2010; 54(3): 507-25.

CHAPTER 9

Craniofacial Growth and Development in Children

Arun M. Xavier[1,*], **H. Sharath Chandra**[2] and **M. Vijay**[3]

[1] *Department of Pediatric and Preventive Dentistry, Amrita School of Dentistry, Cochin, Kerala, India*

[2] *SJM Dental College and Hospital, Chitradurga, Karnataka, India*

[3] *Department of Orthodontics, CSI College of Dental Sciences and Research, Madurai, Tamil nadu, India*

Abstract: Human growth, development, and maturation are multifaceted processes that involve different aspects, including biological, physical, social, and intellectual aspects. Between conception and maturity, the size and complexity of the human body change dramatically. A multitude of changes in sensory, cognitive, and motor coordination are also associated with the development of an individual from infancy to adolescence and are related to brain growth and maturation. All the different facets of development are, however, interrelated. This chapter summarizes the various concepts, principles, theories, factors affecting growth and the parameters used to measure and assess maturity from time to time.

Keywords: Craniofacial Growth, Growth theories, Growth maturity, Growth assessment, Human Development.

INTRODUCTION

Growth involves an increase in size resulting from cell multiplication, expansion, and maturation of tissues. It implies development, from the time of birth to eventual senescence or death. It is an incredibly circuitous phenomenon, which involves large changes in body form, metabolism, and body processes, all occurring at different rates.

Complex mechanisms are involved in the regulation of craniofacial growth and development. The final morphology of the craniofacial bone is derived from the interactions between hormones, genes, nutrients, and environmental factors. These components grow and develop in a predictable, sequential, and orderly fashion throughout life, albeit with great variation in the amount and timing of

* **Corresponding author Arun M. Xavier:** Department of Pediatric and Preventive Dentistry, Amrita School of Dentistry, Cochin, Kerala, India; Tel: +919539084820; E-mail: arunmamachan@gmail.com

Satyawan Damle, Ritesh Kalaskar, Dhanashree Sakhare & Abdulkadeer Jetpurwala (Eds.)

growth (Nanda, 2000). However, any disturbances in this mechanism may result in a deviating growth pattern.

Understanding normal growth and its varying patterns from infancy to adolescence is essential to planning treatment involving dental and skeletal malocclusions as it may jeopardize post-treatment retention and stability.

Terminologies

Growth

- ***Todd*** (1931): An increase in size.
- ***Stewart*** (1982): Developmental increase in mass.
- ***Proffit*** (1986): Increase in size or number.
- ***Moyer*** (1988): Changes in the amount of living substance.
- ***Stedman*** (1990): Increase in the size of a living being or any of its parts, occurring in the process of development.
- ***Pinkham*** (1994): An increase, expansion, or extension of any given tissue.
- ***Moyer***: Quantitative aspect of biologic development per unit time.

Development

- ***Todd*** (1931): Increase in complexity; Progress toward maturity.
- ***Profit*** (1986): Development is in complexity.
- ***Moyers*** (1988): Naturally occurring unidirectional changes in the life of an individual from its existence as a single cell to its elaboration as a multifunctional unit terminating in death
- ***Stedman*** (1990): The act or process of the natural progression from a previous lower or embryonic stage to a later, more complex, or adult age.
- ***Pinkham*** (1994): Development addresses the progressive development of tissue.
- ***Enlow***: A maturational process involving progressive differentiation at the cellular and tissue levels

Factors Affecting Growth

The regulation of the rate, timing, form, and character of growth is orchestrated by the interactions between various genetic and environmental factors.

Enlow and Moyer classified factors into Natural or Disruptive. Goose and Appleton also listed certain factors affecting growth (Fig. **1**).

Genes and Heredity

The size of an organism, the rate and onset of growth and growth spurts are influenced by genes to a great extent. The genes within each cell are necessary to to produce an organism as a whole and to orchestrate the normal growth of the individual (Kohn, 1991).

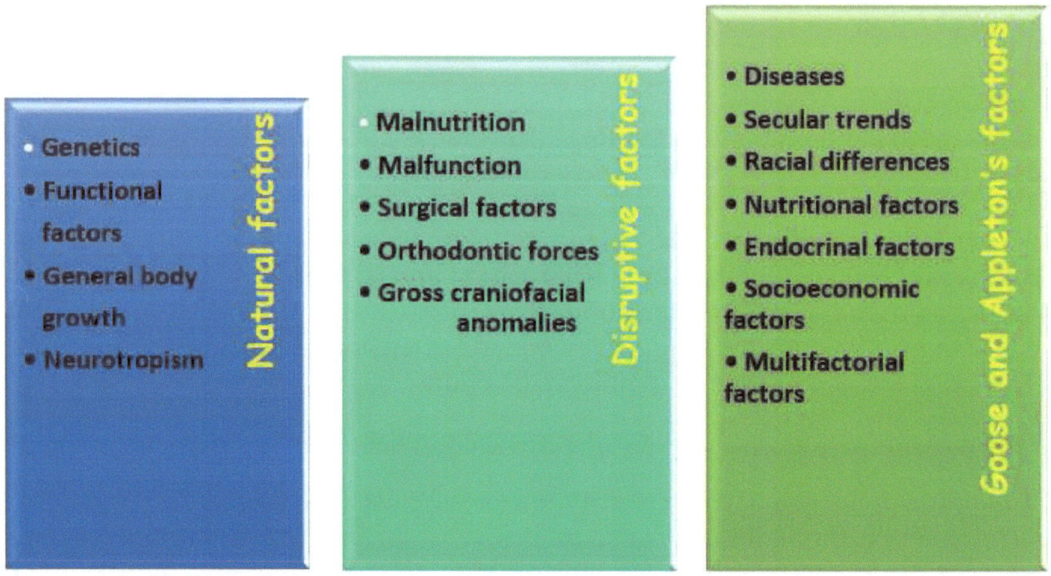

Fig. (1). Factors affecting the growth.

After birth, the infant's growth rate becomes independent of maternal factors and depends solely on his genetic makeup. A significant postnatal shift occurs after 1-2 years which is reflective of the mid-parental height of a child. During adolescence, the growth of a child correlates more with parental size. The size of parents should therefore be considered as the best marker for predicting the future size of a newborn baby.

Family Size and Birth Order

The family size may be correlated with the differences among different family members in size, maturation level, and intelligence. Studies have also concluded a first-born child usually weighs less at birth and has less stature but has a high IQ level (Belmont and Marolla, 1973).

Secular Trends

When race, socioeconomic status, nutrition, climate, and other differences lead to a change in growth, they are referred to as Secular trends (Hunter and Garn, 1969; Smith *et al*., 1986). Size and maturational changes in large populations have been shown to occur with time. *E.g.*, 15-year-old boys are 5 inches taller than 15-yea--olds of 50 years back.

Socioeconomic Factors

The socioeconomic status of the family is related to the growth potential. Children living in favourable socioeconomic conditions tend to be larger, display different types of growth (height, weight ratio) and show a variation in the timing of growth (Bardley and Corwyn, 2002).

Climate and Seasonal Variations

Growth also varies according to seasons and is faster in springs and summers as compared to winters (Woitge *et al*., 1998). Similarly, growth in terms of height is faster during the spring, while an increase in weight occurs faster during autumn.

Nutrition

Malnutrition during childhood causes a delay in overall growth and growth spurts [1]. It may affect all aspects of growth, including size, body proportions, and the onset of growth events. During short periods of malnutrition, growth waits for good nutrition to return to a faster pace until the genetically determined curve is approached again (Dressino, 1997). Catch-up growth appears when a favourable nutritional regimen is supplied early enough. This is seen in both sexes; females are better buffered against the effects of malnutrition (de Fonseca, 2017).

Hormones

Thyroid hormone affects the intramembranous and endochondral ossification in the skull. A deficiency may manifest as patent or persistent fontanelles, patent sutures, delayed dentition, Wormian bones and deafness, while an excess results in premature fusion of the calvarial sutures and cranial base synchondroses. This indicates that thyroid hormones have a pivotal role in the growth and development of the craniofacial skeleton, and the skull is exquisitely sensitive to changes in available T3 (Leitch *et al*., 2020) [2].

Sex hormone levels can affect both craniofacial growth and bone metabolism. Omori *et al*., (2019) stated that both increased and decreased levels of estrogen influence the maxilla and mandible dimensions. Table **1** summarizes the hormones responsible for growth [3].

Table 1. Hormones related to growth.

Groups	Hormones
Group 1: Affect skeletal growth	• Growth Hormone (anterior pituitary) • Insulin (β cells of Langerhans) • Thyrotropic hormone
Group 2: Cause long bone ossification	• Parathormone
Group 3: Cause pubertal growth spurt	• Androgens • Progesterone and estrogen
Group 4: Miscellaneous	• Prolactin hormone (anterior pituitary)

Growth Factors

Growth factors or growth stimulants are peptides responsible for transmitting signals that regulate cell activity *via* several mechanisms such as mitogenic, migration, differentiation, and gene regulation, occurring simultaneously in different tissues, thus promoting growth and development. They also promote the regeneration of supporting tissues and increase osseous tissue formation (Spears and Kathy, 2005) [4].

Muscular Functions

Muscle tissues affect the vascular supply as a force element to the bone, which in turn is responsible for proper bone growth. Masticatory muscle hyperfunction results in increased transverse growth of the maxilla, anterior growth rotation pattern of the mandible, well-developed angular, coronoid, and condylar process and a broader base of the dental arches owing to increased sutural growth and bone apposition (Daly, 2004). Most patients with myotonic dystrophy have deteriorated craniofacial morphology with vertical growth pattern, high incidence of distal occlusion, anterior open bite, lateral crossbite and crowding (Killaridis, 1995).

Exercise and Adult Physique

Exercise may be useful for the development of motor skills, an increase in muscle mass, general well-being, and fitness, but has no favourable effect on linear growth (Torun and Viteri, 1994).

Illness

Serious prolonged debilitating illnesses have a marked effect on the growth process of a child, while minor illnesses do not (Sinnema, 1983). However, after the period of illness, "catch-up growth" brings back the child to the predetermined growth curve.

Psychological Disturbances

Children experiencing stress display inhibition of growth hormone secretion and thereby inhibition of growth, the severity of which depends on the severity of the psychological disturbances (Aguia, 1991).

GENERAL PRINCIPLES OF GROWTH AND DEVELOPMENT

Continuity

As a child develops, the already acquired skills and the new skills become the basis for further achievement. Most children follow a similar, continuous process from conception to death which not only involves maturity in body size and functioning but also behaviour. Development depends on the growth and maturity of individuals who interact with the environment. As in maturation, for a child to write/draw, he must develop the manual (hand) control to hold a pencil.

Sequentiality

Development in the prenatal period follows a genetic sequence, appearing at fixed intervals with pertinent characteristics. At both prenatal and postnatal stages, the path of development follows a proximodistal direction, wherein the spinal cord grows first, followed by the rest of the body.

- Arms development precedes the development of hands
- Hands and feet develop before the development of fingers and toes.

Cephalocaudal development occurs from head to feet.

- **Fetal period (2nd month IU):** During this stage head measures about 50% of the total body length; the cranium is larger than the face while the limbs and trunk remain underdeveloped.

- **At birth:** Proportion changes due to faster growth rate of limbs and trunk, which results in decreased head proportion to 25-30% of the entire body, and legs represent approximately one-third of the total body length.
- **In adulthood**: There is a progressive reduction of the relative size of the head to about 12% and legs represent half the total body length (Fig. **2**).

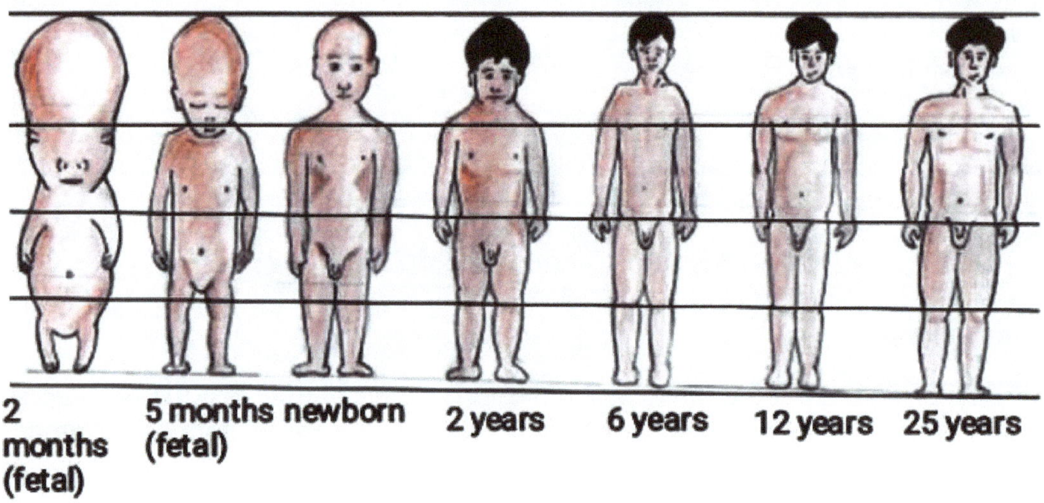

Fig. (2). Cephalocaudal gradient of growth.

The brain and associated tissues mature faster than the face and grow rapidly after birth. Nearly one-half of the postnatal growth of the brain occurs in the first year and nearly three fourth by 3 years. An infant's skull compared to that of an adult show that the infant has a relatively larger cranium and a smaller face. The mandible being away from the brain tends to grow later than the maxilla.

Generality to Specificity

In all areas of development, general activity always precedes specific actions and occurs from large muscle movements to fine (smaller muscle) movements. The infant's first motor movements are generalized, unidirectional and reflexive, like waving arms or kicking before being able to reach out and pick up objects easily without much effort.

Differentiality

Not all tissue systems of the body grow at the same rate as described in Scammon's growth curve explained later in this chapter. Mental abilities like verbal, numerical, spatial, *etc*., develop at different ages. Creative imagination develops rapidly and reaches its peak in early adolescence.

Variability

Variability is merely the extreme of normal variation and should not be categorized as normal and abnormal but should be defined in terms of deviation from the usual pattern. It is expressed in quantitative terms.

No two individuals are ever exactly alike (except monozygotic twins). A wide range of differences can be found in the population of similar age, sex, race, and socioeconomic background.

The overall principles of bone growth summarize the nature of growth patterns and variability in an individual (Fig. **3**).

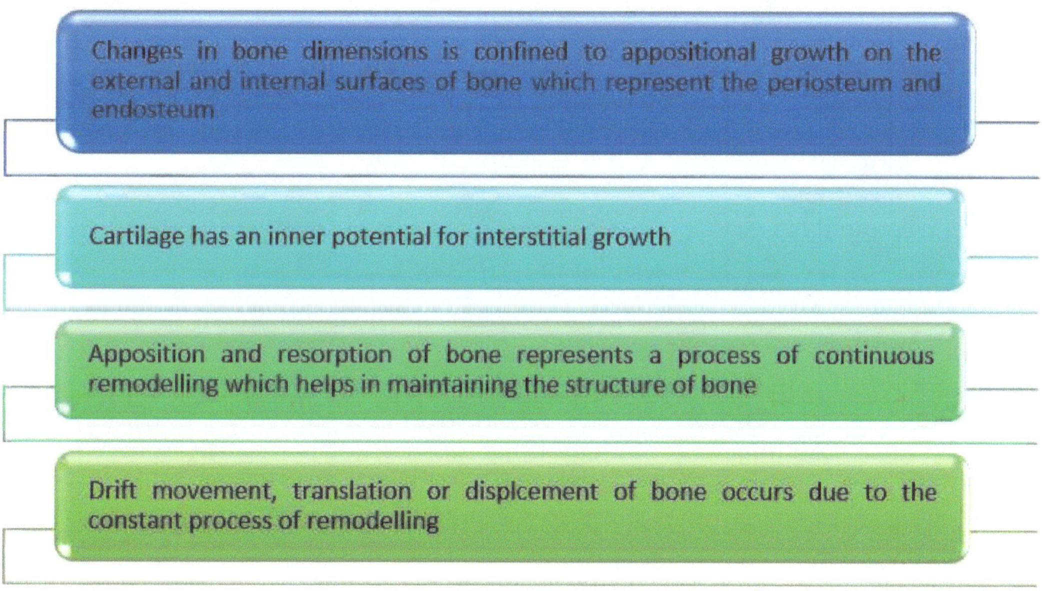

Fig. (3). Principles of bone growth.

Growth Spurts

Growth does not occur uniformly at all ages. The greater increment of growth is contributed by growth sites located in certain regions of the body. These growth sites may be active at one period causing a sudden acceleration of growth, termed a Growth Spurt [5].

Periods of growth spurts: It occurs at four stages (Fig. **4**).

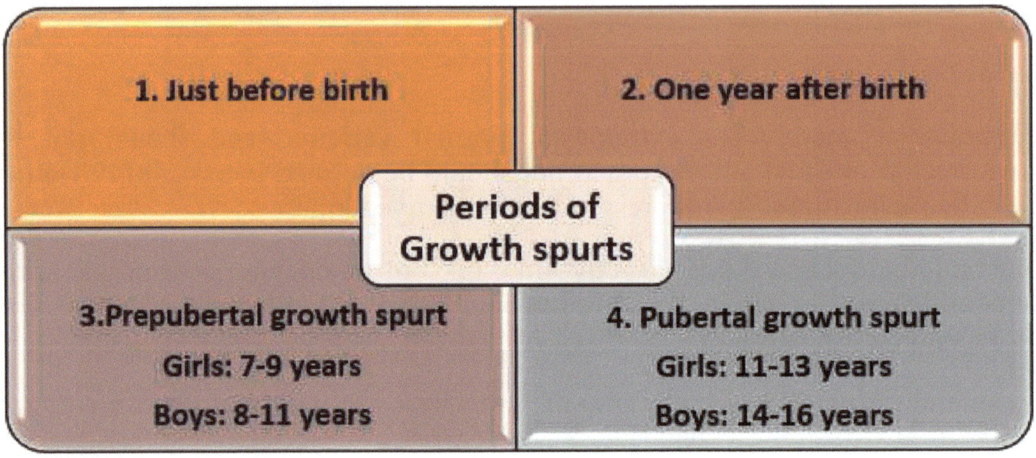

Fig. (4). Different periods of Growth Spurts.

Importance of Growth Spurts:

- Determine the predictability and direction of growth,
- Excellent indicator for timing of orthodontic treatment
- Patient management
- Overall treatment time.

Orthodontic Correction Considerations

- Orthodontic treatment may be considered earlier in girls as their growth spurt occurs earlier than in boys.
- Interceptive orthodontic procedures can be best considered during prepubertal growth spurts as there is a change in growth direction from vertical to horizontal.
- Arch expansion and rapid skeletal expansion can be planned during periods of maximum growth.
- Class III tendency with mandibular prognathism should be treated before a prepubertal growth spurt.
- Malocclusion requiring orthognathic correction should only be undertaken after the growth spurt is completed [6].

Differential Growth

Body proportions change considerably from the newborn to the grown-up adult at various proportions from time to time. They proceed at different speeds reflecting the changing morphology and individuality of the child as they grow older (Marshall 1977). This pattern of growth is referred to as differential growth.

Scammon's curves were named after Richard Everingham Scammon (1883-1952). Scammon used tissue and organ weights at each age to characterize the growth of the body into four basic curves that included the general (physical dimension), neural, genital, and lymphoid curve (Fig. 5) [7].

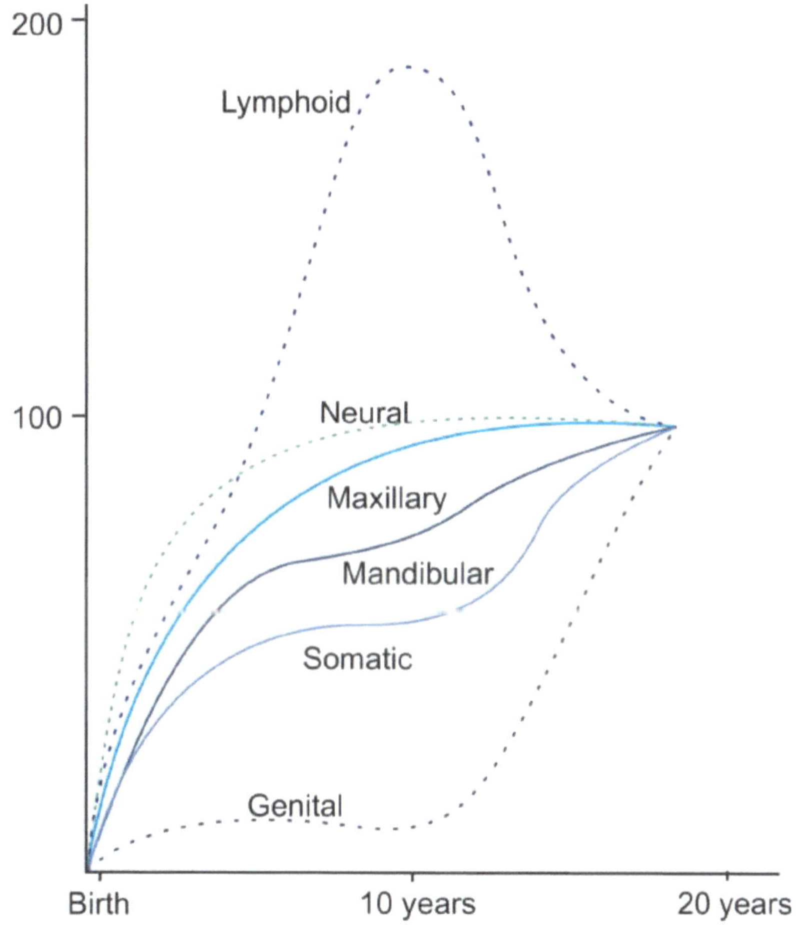

Fig. (5). Scammon's growth curve.

Lymphoid Curve: Represents lymphoid tissues that grow rapidly to reach 200% of the adult size between 10-13 years of age. This is an adaptive mechanism that protects children from infections. Later its size matures to 100% in early adulthood. The growth of the thymus, adenoids (pharyngeal and tonsillar), lymph nodes, and intestinal lymphatic masses are included in this curve.

Neural Curve: It rises during early childhood as the neural tissues grow rapidly. It includes the brain, spinal cord, optic apparatus, upper face, and vertebral column. The size of the cranium depends on brain growth and attains its approximate adult size (90%) by 8 years of age. This growth is accompanied by other internal structures thus enabling the 8-year-old child to perform mental processes at the pace of an adult. The maxilla also follows a similar growth pattern, with growth potential ceasing earlier. Hence skeletal problems involving maxillary deficiency may be treated at an early age.

The General Curve: Represents general/somatic tissues typically show an S-shaped growth curve. The curve steadily rises from birth to five years, followed by a plateau between 5-10 years and later accelerates during puberty before slowing down in adulthood. It includes a bony skeleton, musculature, respiratory organs, digestive organs, kidneys, and blood volume. The mandible follows a somatic growth pattern, with growth potential extending up to early adulthood.

Genital Curve: It includes the primary sex apparatus (ovary and testis) and all secondary sex characters/traits. The genital curve has a small rise in the first year of life and is then quiescent up to around 10 years of age. However, it shows rapid acceleration during puberty.

Cranial Base Synchondroses

The development of a union between two bones by the formation of either hyaline cartilage or fibrocartilage is referred to as Synchondrosis. Cranial base synchondroses are regarded as important growth centers of the craniofacial skeleton (Fig. **6**). A growth site differs from a growth center (Table **2**). Any factor that adversely affects these centers has a bearing on the growth pattern of the individual.

It is usually transient till the intervening cartilage becomes progressively thinner and ultimately becomes obliterated and converted into bone before adult life.

A growth site differs from a growth center (Table **2**). Cranial base synchondroses are regarded as important growth centers of the craniofacial skeleton. The different types include intersphenoidal, intraoccipital, spheno-occipital and sphenoethmoidal synchondroses (Fig. **6**). Due to the late ossification at around 20 years of age, the spheno-occipital synchondrosis plays an important role in the post-natal cranial base growth. Lengthening of the cranial base between the foramen magnum and Sella turcica is the contributory effect of the drift and remodeling happening in this synchondrosis.

The spheno-ethmoidal synchondrosis is known to fuse at 6 years, the intraoccipital synchondrosis at 3-5 years of age and the intersphenoid synchondrosis ossifies immediately before birth.

Table 2. Growth Site *versus* Growth Center.

Growth Site	Growth Centre
• Located where growth takes place • Transplanted growth sites do not continue to grow • Marked response to external influences • Does not control the overall growth of bone; however, are responsible for exaggerated growth • All growth sites are not growth centres • Theories of growth are not based on growth sites	• Located where genetic control of growth takes place • Transplanted growth centres continue to grow • Lesser response to external influence and increased response to functional needs • Cause growth of major part of the bone • All growth centres are growth sites • Certain theories of growth are based on the expression of growth centres

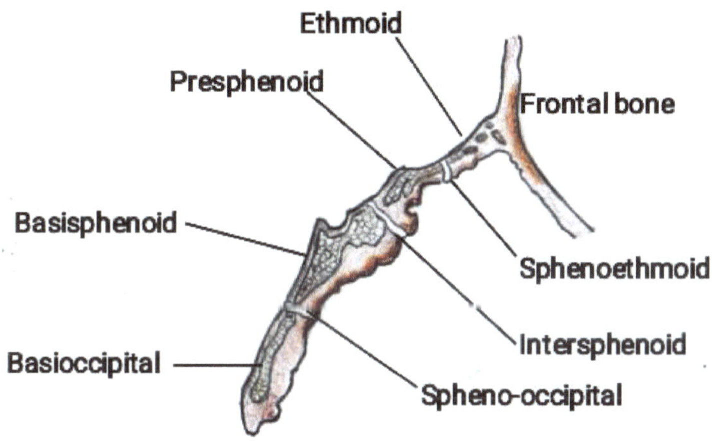

Fig. (6). Synchondroses of the cranial base depicting the growth sites.

Fontanelles

The space between the bones of an infant's skull where the sutures intersect is covered by tough membranes that protect the underlying soft tissues and brain. These are referred to as "soft spots". Six fontanelles are present during infancy, the most notable being the anterior and posterior fontanelles (Fig. 7). The others include the paired mastoid and sphenoid fontanelles.

The anterior fontanelle is the junction between the two frontal and parietal bones. It is the largest fontanelle and remains soft until about 18-24 months of age.

The posterior fontanelle forms the junction of the two parietal bones and the occipital bone. It usually closes first, before the anterior fontanelle.

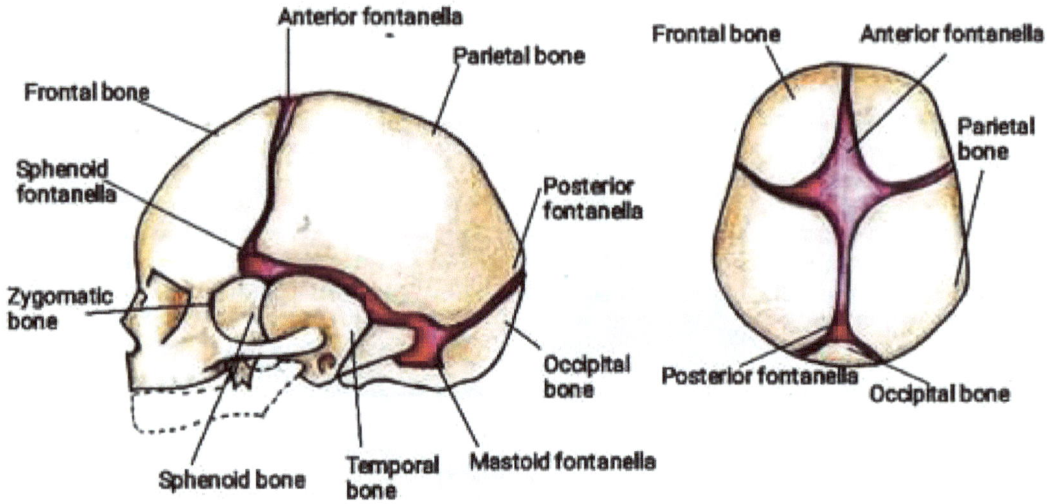

Fig. (7). Fontanelles in the skull of a newborn.

Theories of Craniofacial Growth

Several theories have evolved over the years to understand the complex nature of craniofacial development. None of these theories have, however been able to explain growth completely, and hence current understanding of growth is explained by a combination of different growth theories and concepts.

The major theories/concept that have been postulated over the years are:

1. Bone Remodeling theory – Brash,1930
2. Genetic theory – Brodie, 1940
3. Sutural dominance theory – Siecher and Weinmann,1941
4. Cartilaginous theory – James Scott, 1950
5. Functional Matrix theory – Moss,1962
6. Van Limborgh Multifactorial Hypothesis, 1970s
7. Cybernetics – Petrovic, Stutzman, 1974
8. Synthetic Hypothesis, 1988
9. Functional Matrix Hypothesis Revisited, 1997
10. Growth Relativity Hypothesis, 2000

Other Theories Related to Craniofacial Growth are:

1. Enlow's Expanding V principle
2. Enlow's counterpart principle
3. Neutrophic process in orofacial growth

Bone Remodelling Theory

It was proposed by Brash. According to him, all craniofacial skeletal growth occurs exclusively by the process of remodeling – selective addition and resorption of bone at surfaces [8]. This theory failed to explain the role of other structures such as sutures, synchondroses, and the mandibular condylar cartilage in the growth of the craniofacial skeleton.

Genetic Theory / Genetic Blueprint

Was proposed by Allan G. Brodie in 1941. According to Brodie, the recurring pattern of facial configuration is genetically determined. However, the primary genetic regulation decides only a few characteristics and does not affect development [8].

Cartilaginous Theory / Scott's Hypothesis, Nasal Septum Theory, Nasocapsular Theory

Cartilaginous theory was put forward by James Scott, in 1956. There is intrinsic growth potential in the cartilage and periosteum, acting as growth centers. The cartilage is a pressure-adapted tissue, and the growth of nasal septum cartilage provides the forces that displace the maxilla downward and forward.

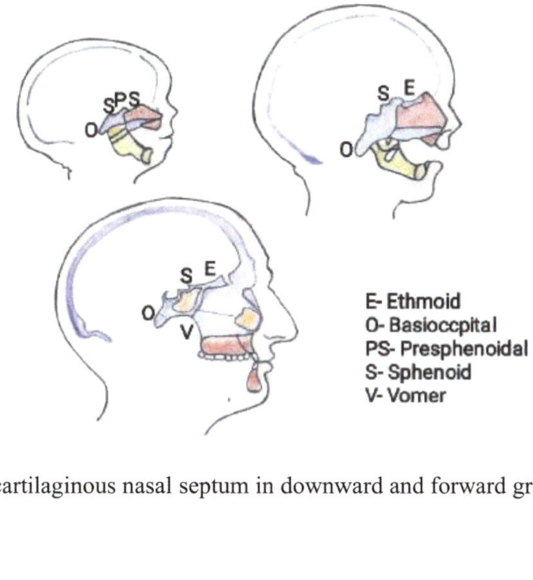

Fig. (8). Possible role of cartilaginous nasal septum in downward and forward growth of maxillary complex.

The hyaline cartilage has certain properties that allow it to determine growth in the cranial base and the nasal areas. This establishes a template for the face to be formed intramembranously around the cartilage (Figs. **8** & **9**). Disturbances in the nasal septum led to midfacial deformities. Condylar cartilage of the mandible is the pacemaker for the growth of the mandible, and the remodeling of the ramus and other surface changes are secondary to the primary cartilage [8].

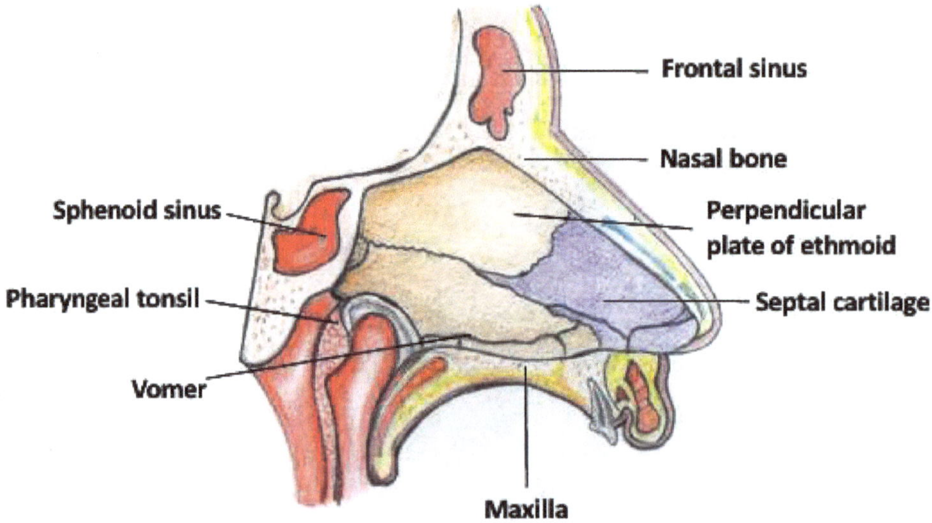

Fig. (9). Nasal septum cartilage and related structures.

The sutural growth is passive and secondary to cartilaginous growth.

Nasal septum is the major contributor to maxillary growth and the nasoseptal cartilage is attributed to be responsible for the growth of the whole nasomaxillary complex (Fig. **9**). Disturbances in the nasal septum led to midfacial deformities. Condylar cartilage of the mandible is the pacemaker for growth of the mandible and the remodeling of the ramus and other surface changes are secondary to the primary cartilage [8].

Limitations

Condylar cartilage does not have intrinsic growth potential and it gets affected by external stimuli like functional appliances. In case of injury, mandibular condyle resorbs. Neither transplantation experiments nor removal of condyle could support that the cartilage of the mandibular condyle is an important center. The role of environmental factors and muscle forces was neglected.

Sutural Growth Theory / Sicher's Hypothesis, Sicher's Sutural Dominance Theory

Sutural growth theory was put forward by Sicher and Weinmann in 1941. This theory is also called dominance theory because the proliferation of connective tissue and the replacement by bone in the sutures was considered as the primary factor in bone growth (Fig. **10**).

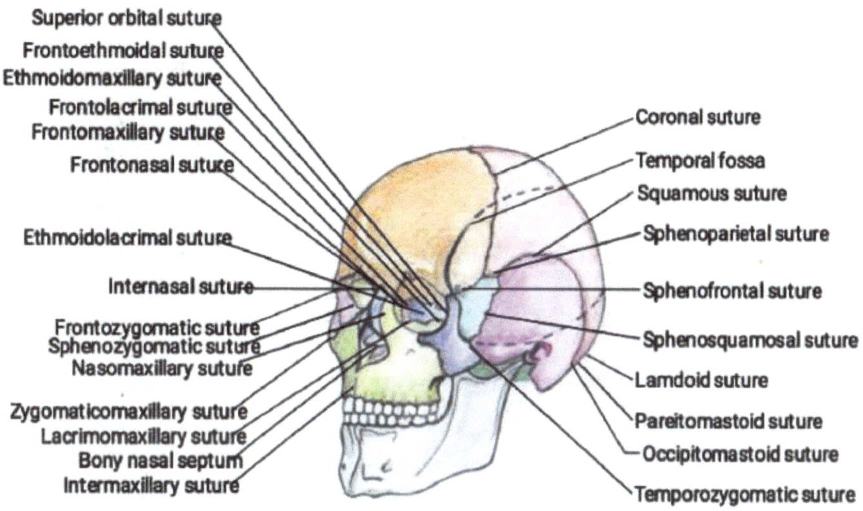

Fig. (10). Sutures and corresponding bones of craniofacial region.

Principle: Sutures were responsible for the majority of the craniofacial growth, predicted by studies conducted using vital dyes. Sutures were the primary growth centers. It was seen that when sutures are pulled apart, bone fills in, and if sutures are compressed, there is impeded growth [9].

1. All the bone-forming elements like cartilage, sutures, and periosteum act as growth centers.
2. All paired parallel sutures that attach nasomaxillary complex to the cranial vault and base of the cranium are responsible for the growth of the whole nasomaxillary complex.

Limitations

1. Removal of facial sutures had no effect on the growth of the skeleton.
2. Suture is a tension-adapted area, and any unusual pressure on the suture-initiated bone resorption, but not a bone deposition.

3. The differences in the development of the skull in microcephaly and hydrocephaly could not be correlated with the size of sutures.
4. The shape of sutures is dependent on external stimuli (*e.g.*, palatal expansion).
5. Growth takes place even in cases of the untreated cleft palate where there is an absence of suture.

Sutures do not act as primary growth centers and are just growth sites. The sutural growth is secondary in response to functional needs, according to which the shape of the sutures varies.

Functional Matrix Hypothesis (FMH)

Melvin Moss proposed functional matrix theory in 1969, based on the work of Van der Klaaus. He proposed that the development of the face is a result of functional needs and is mediated by soft tissues embedded in the jaws, *i.e.*, the regulation for growth is in the adjacent soft tissues rather than the cartilage or bone. This is the most strongly accepted theory, which proclaims the soft tissue's superiority over skeletal development [9].

According to this theory, all skeletal tissues and organs' origin, development, shape, location, and maintenance are often secondary, compensatory, and mandatory responses to temporally and operationally prior events occurring in related non-skeletal tissues, organs, or functioning spaces (functional matrices).

The "functional cranial part" refers to the tissues and spaces that work together to perform a single operation. It is divided into two components, the functional matrix, and the skeletal unit. The interactions between the functional matrix and skeletal units result in the growth and development of the craniofacial unit (Fig. **11**).

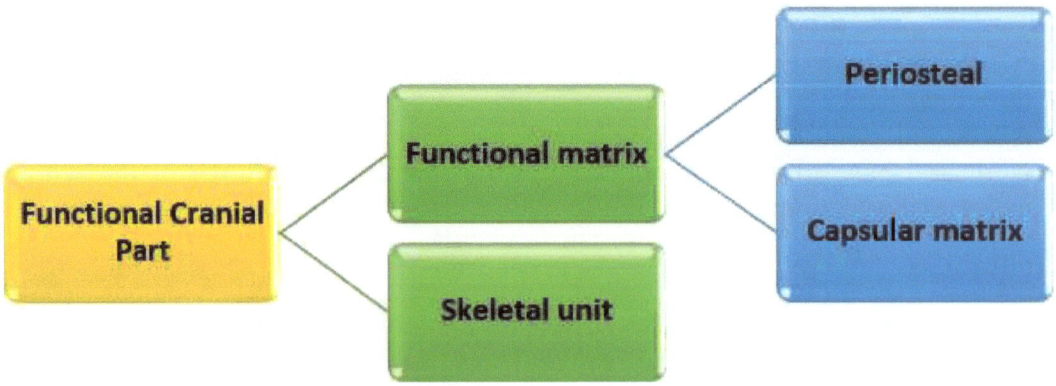

Fig. (11). Components of Functional Cranial Part.

Functional Matrix: It is a complete mass of soft tissues associated with a single function consisting of muscles, glands, nerves, vessels, fat, teeth, and the functioning spaces.

a) Periosteal Matrix: It is made up of all non-skeletal units and has a direct effect on the bone *via* the periosteum, which is limited to a small part of the bone, known as the "Microskeletl a micro skeletal unit."

E.g., Teeth, muscles, blood vessels, nerves, and glands.

All the periosteal matrices act by the process of bone deposition and resorption. This matrix alters both the size and shape of the bone and produces a secondary compensatory transformation.

b) Capsular Matrix: It includes the capsule that surrounds the soft tissues, organs, and spaces.

E.g., Capsule of the scalp (surrounds the neural mass), the orofacial capsule (surrounds the nasopharyngeal spaces), and capsule of supporting tissues of the eye (surrounds the orbital mass).

They function on their associated skeletal units indirectly and passively, causing a secondary compensatory translation in space. When their enveloping capsule moves in space, the facial skeletal units move passively and secondarily.

Skeletal Unit: It is the sum of all the skeletal tissues associated with a single function that provides protection and support to the functional matrix. It comprises of bone, cartilage, and tendinous tissue.

There are two types of skeletal units, micro skeletal unit and macroskeletal. (Fig. **12**)

a. Micro Skeletal Unit: It is comprised of several contiguous skeletal units. The maxilla and mandible are comprised of several such micro skeletal units, including the condylar process, coronoid process, alveolar process, and angle of the mandible.

b. Macro Skeletal Unit: When adjoining portions of several neighboring bones are united to function as a single cranial component, it is called a macro skeletal unit. The entire endocranial surface of the calvarium, orbit, core of the maxilla and mandible are examples of macro skeletal units. The capsular expansion causes the macro skeletal unit to passively change its position, leading to bone translation.

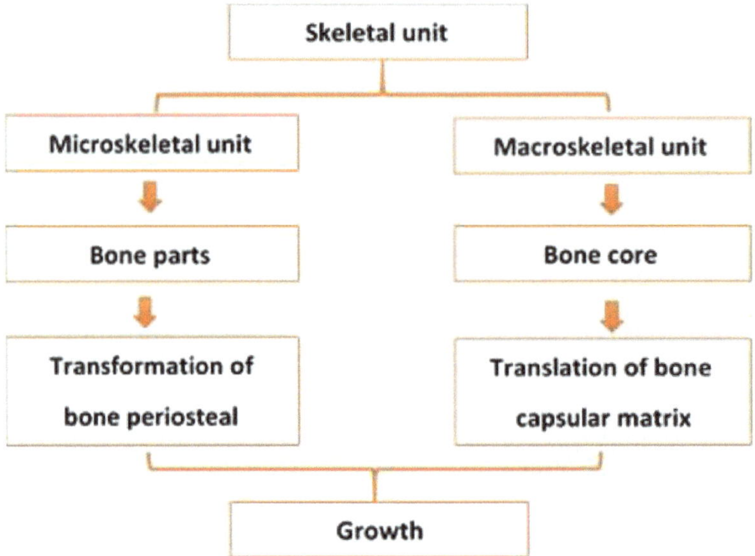

Fig. (12). Skeletal components in Functional Cranial Part.

Intraoral and/or extraoral appliances may be used to fix malocclusions in orthodontics that appear to change the functional matrix. Changes in the micro skeletal unit are caused by changes in the periosteal matrix, whereas changes in the macro skeletal unit are caused by changes in the capsular matrix.

***Limitations*:** In patients with hydrocephaly, the cranial vault is bigger while the brain size is smaller.

Neurotropism

Behrent and Moss proposed this theory in 1976. Soft tissues influence skeletal growth by functional stimuli, according to the functional matrix theory. The neurotropism mechanism is involved in the transmission of the functional stimuli to the skeletal unit interface physiology of neurotropism because the nervous system, apart from conducting efferent and afferents, is also concerned with the integrity of body structures. It is non-impulsive, involving axoplasmic transport providing long-term interactions between neurons and innervated tissues, which homeostatically regulate the morphological, compositional, and functional integrity of those tissues.

Neurotropism is of Three Types

According to functional matrix theory, the nerve influences cell gene expression. *Via* neuromuscular trophism, the periosteal matrices control the size and shape of the microskeletal units. Similar factors are most likely present in the capsular matrix, which governs the location of the macroskeletal unit passively (Fig. **13**).

Van Limborgh Multifactorial Hypothesis / Van Limborgh's Composite Hypothesis

Van Limborgh, in the 1970s, put forward a multifactorial theory which is a combination of three theories: functional matrix theory, sutural theory, and the genetic theory.

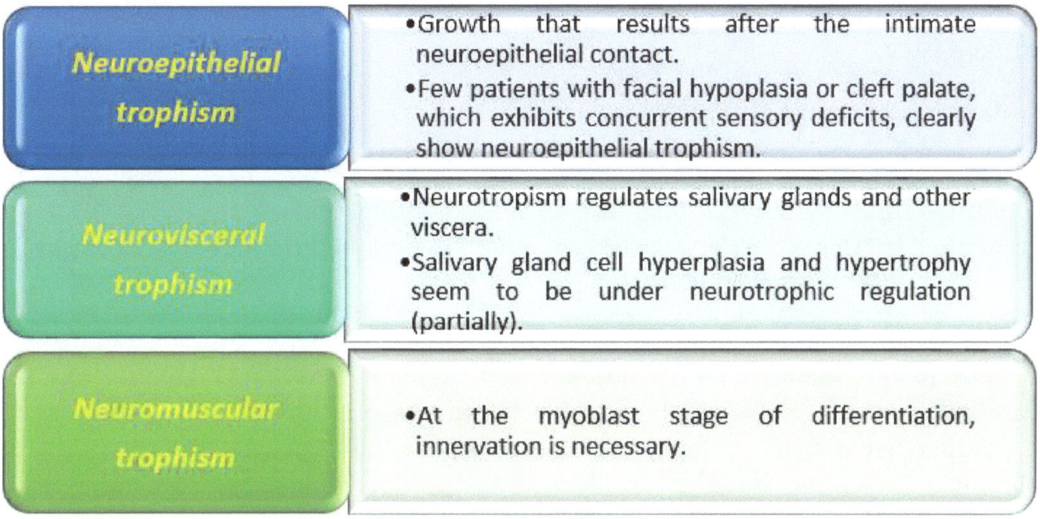

Fig. (13). Types of Neurotropism.

According to this theory, primary intrinsic stimulation of growth is present in cartilage and periosteum, while the secondary factors are the local feedback and inner communication mechanisms between the cells and the tissues.

It indicates that intrinsic genetic factors are a major concern, with modeling, resorptive and depository alterations, changes under the influence of muscles and other environmental factors. He proposed five controlling factors of growth that includes local genetic, local, and general epigenetic, local, and general environmental factors.

The chondrocranial growth (cranial base) is mainly controlled by intrinsic genetic factors. Desmocranial growth (cranial vault) is mainly affected by local epigenetic and environmental factors, with some intrinsic genetic factors. Cartilaginous part of the skull is the growth center. Skull cartilages influence the growth of the Sutures. The growth of adjacent structures influences the growth of the periosteum. Non-genetic environmental factors govern the growth of the sutures and periosteum.

Servo System Theory / Cybernetics Theory

Based on the cybernetic principles, the servo system theory was put forward by Alexander Petrovic in 1974. According to this theory, craniofacial growth is controlled by a series of changes occurring in the craniofacial skeleton and dentition, which, in turn, starts a feedback mechanism, to stimulate further growth changes. The cybernetics form of command controls the primary cartilage, while the direct and indirect effects of the cell's multiplication influence the secondary cartilage [9].

Application of Servo System

The effect of somatotrophic hormone on the cartilage growth of the nasal septum, spheno-occipital synchondrosis, and other synchondroses, follows a cybernetic command pattern. Secondary cartilages, such as the condyle, develop in response to local and environmental factors.

The constant reference input is the maxillary dental arch, and the controlled variable is the mandibular dental arch. It sends retro discal signals *via* the stimulation of the retrodiscal pad and lateral pterygoid muscles if there is a disturbance between the respective positions of the maxillary and mandibular arch and affects the output signal (final sagittal position of the maxillary arch).

Limitations: It is more useful as a research tool and is difficult to explain the growth of most of the parts of the body with servo system theory.

Enlow's Expanding 'V' Principle

The concept of expanding "V" principle was put forward by Enlow. Many facial and cranial bones have V-shaped regions/configurations (Fig. **14**). The growth occurs toward the wider end of V with selective deposition along the inner and wide ends of V and resorption on the outer aspect. Thus, as the remodeling continues, there is an increase in size and simultaneous movement of the bone in the shape of expanding V.

This mechanism is seen at the end of long bones, maxilla, zygomatic bone, coronoid region, angle and body of the mandible, and palate. Growth of the palate is one of the best examples of expanding 'V' principle. Deposition occurs on the palatal periosteal surface, and resorption occurs on the side of the nasal floor. In this way, the palate expands in the lateral direction and moves downward.

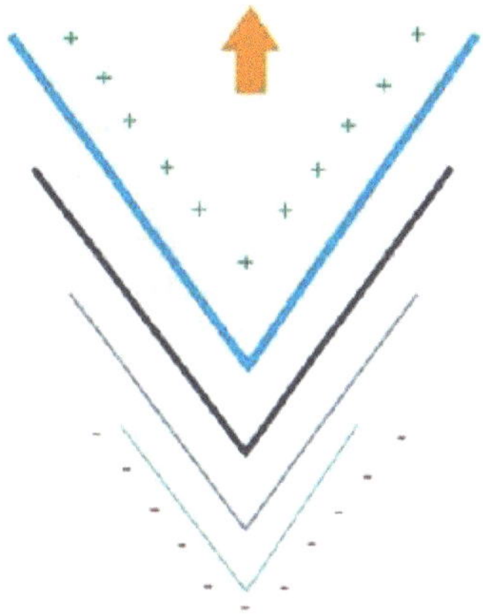

Fig. (14). Schematic representation of Enlow's V principle.

Enlow's Counterpart Principle / Growth Equivalents Concepts

The growth of any craniofacial structure is related and can be compared with certain other specific structural and geometric counterparts (growth equivalent) in the craniofacial complex. A dimensionally balanced growth occurs when each regional part and its counterpart enlarge to the same extent. Imbalance can be produced by the difference in the amount of growth, direction of growth, and the time of growth between the counterparts and can result in either protrusion or intrusion of the part of the face (Fig. **15**).

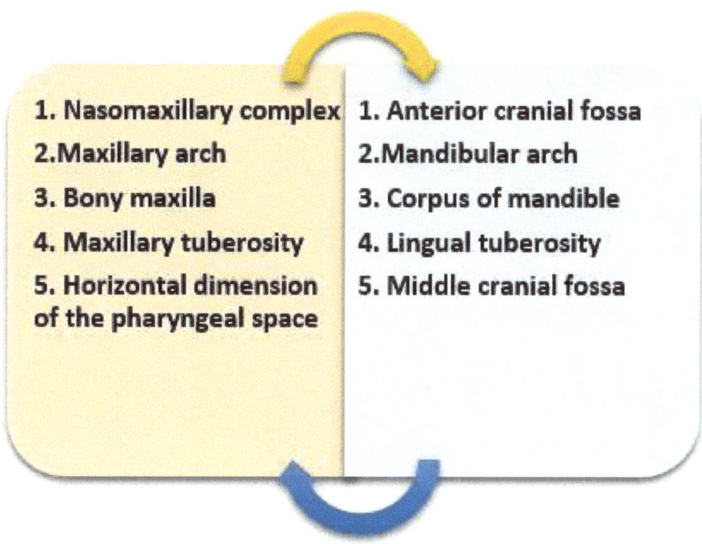

Fig. (15). Regional Counterparts in growth by Enlow.

Functional Matrix Hypothesis Revisited (1997)

FMH was first put forth by Melvin Moss based on his study on the regulatory roles of intrinsic (genomic) and extrinsic (epigenetic) factors in cephalic growth. The initial version stressed upon epigenetic primary and became peer accepted. With advances in the biomedical, bioengineering and computer sciences, more comprehensive explanatory versions of FMH were proposed. Thus, functional matrix theory was revisited and based on:

- *The role of mechano-transduction*
- *The role of osseous connected cellular network*
- *The genomic thesis*
- *The epigenetic antithesis and the resolving synthesis*

According to this concept, the mechanical stimulus is pursued by the specialized cells by a process called mechanoperception. These signals are then transmitted through the tissues by way of mechanoconduction or mechanotransmission. Finally, these signals are transmitted to the genome of the bone, where protein synthesis takes place. These signals alter the protein metabolism depending upon the severity and longevity of the mechanical stimulus. Thus, Moss FMH revisited theory states that the ultimate growth controlling factor of the craniofacial skeleton depends on two factors: genetic factors and environmental factors.

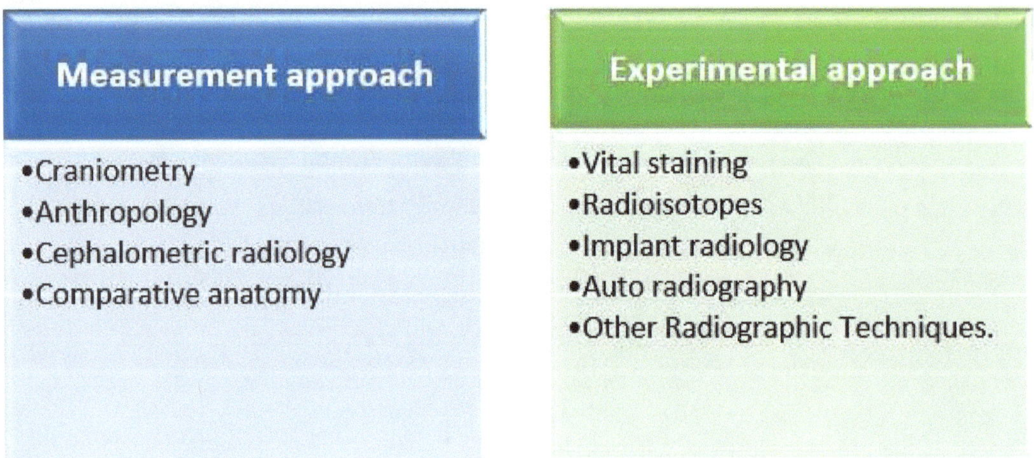

Fig. (16). Approaches to study growth.

Methods of Studying Physical Growth

Growth can be studied by two approaches: the measurement approach and the experimental approach (Fig. **16**).

Growth Assessment Parameters

The different types of ages explained by Krogman (1960) give an overview of the overall development of a child Fig. **17**).

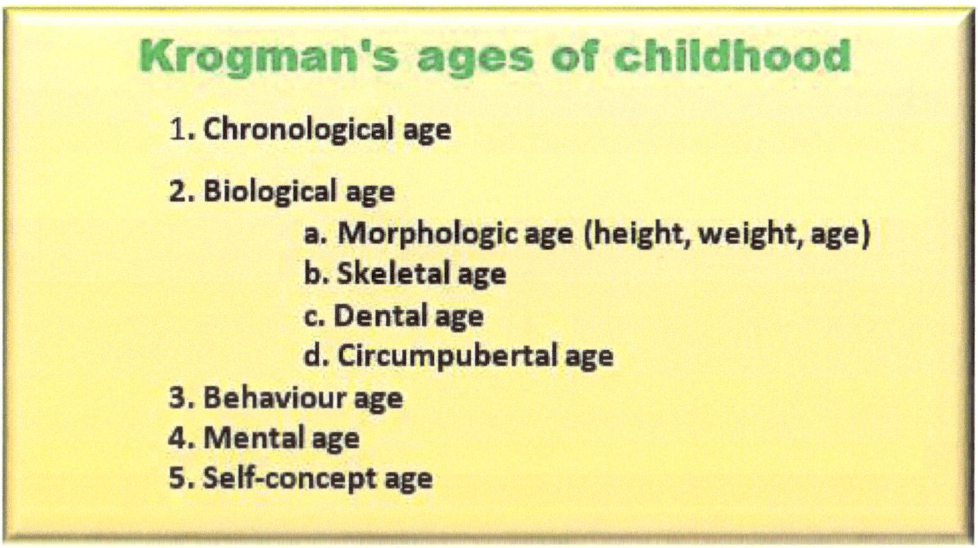

Fig. (17). Childhood ages by Krogman.

Chronological Age

- It is the most commonly and easily determined developmental age parameter, determined from the child's date of birth.
- Each child with the same chronological age has his/her characteristic growth pattern and time clock, which is affected by disease and various environmental factors.
- Chronological age, however, is neither an accurate indicator of development nor a good predictor of growth potential [7].

Somatotypic Age

- It gives an overview of the developmental pattern of a is not an accurate scale to predict age or growth.
- Sheldon (1954) classified individuals based on somatotype into three categories: Endomorph, Ectomorph, and Mesomorph (Figs. **18** & **19**).

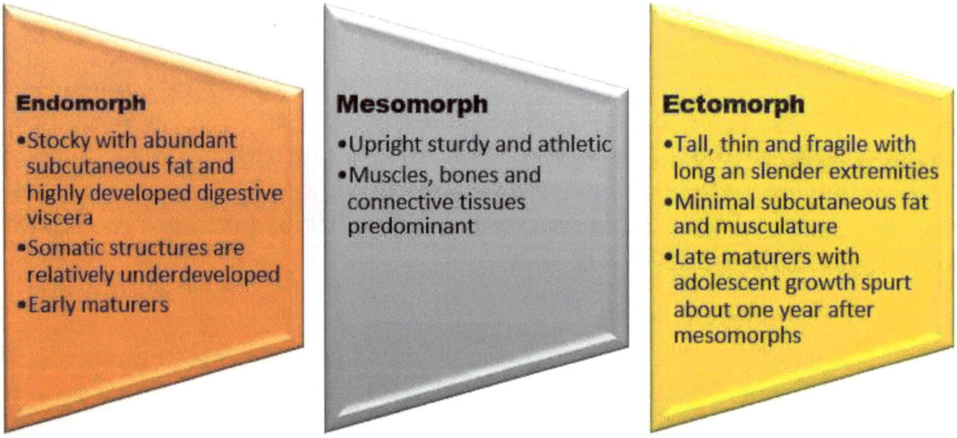

Fig. (18). Somatotype differences.

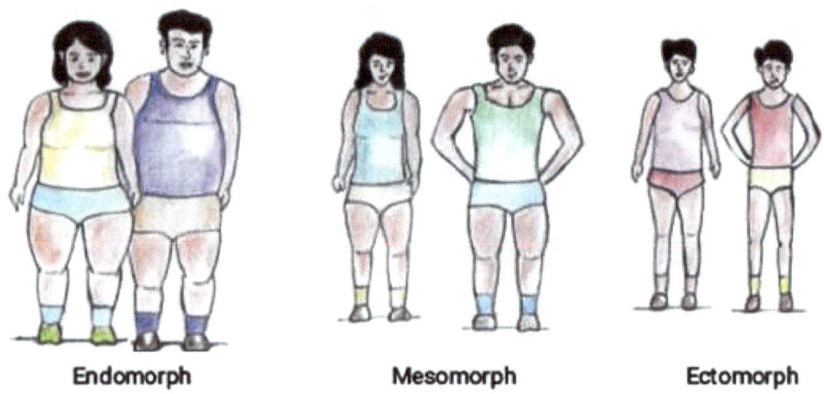

Fig. (19). Three categories of somatotypes.

Sexual Age

With the onset of puberty, different hormonal changes yield characteristic body changes. Secondary sexual features include pubic hair growth, genital organ growth acceleration, the appearance of breast buds, and distribution of body fat occurs [10].

Facial Age

It is an important parameter and a predictor of future growth. Measurement of facial age can be done using anthropometric measurements, facial growth velocity curve, and cephalometric radiographs.

Skeletal Age

The assessment of skeletal maturation can be used as an indicator of developmental age, as skeletal age was found to highly correlate with developmental age (Staneseu 1977). Skeletal age is mostly based on the ossification of endochondral bone [10].

Hand and Wrist Radiographs

The numerous small bones in hand–wrist region follow a pattern in ossification and union of the epiphysis with diaphysis. The bones are assessed in the order of Distal radius, ulna, carpals, and metacarpals – proximal, middle, and distal phalanges (Fig. **20**) [7].

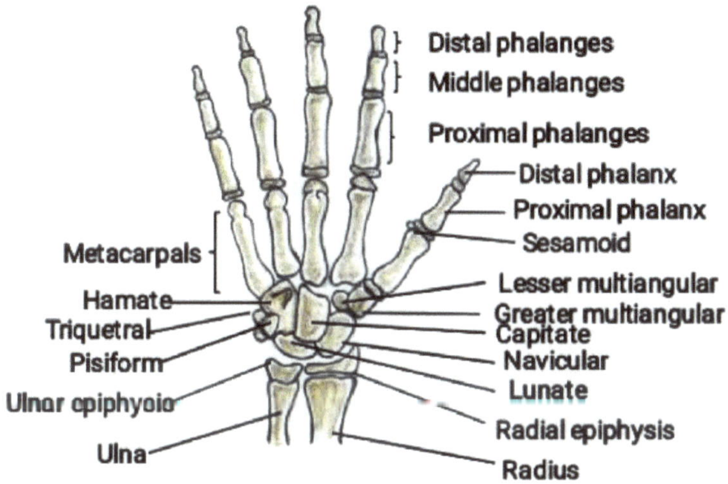

Fig. (20). Hand-wrist radiograph.

Determination of Skeletal Age

Greulich and Pyle (1959) published an atlas of standard hand and wrist films at various stages for males and females. The hand and wrist radiograph of the child can be compared with the atlas standards of nearest age and sex to determine the skeletal maturity of that individual [11]. Tanner and Whitehouse *et al.,* (1975) suggested the RUS (radius, ulna, short bones) score rates, the carpel bone method, and The Tanner and Whitehouse (TW2) method, to determine the skeletal age. Taranger *et al.,* (1976), Bjork, Helm *et al.,* (1967), and Björk, Grave and Brown Method (1976) devised other methods to determine skeletal age.

Indications of Hand and Wrist Radiographs

1. Patients who exhibit severe discrepancy between dental and chronological age
2. Predict future skeletal maturation rate and status
3. Predict pubertal growth spurt
4. Predict the skeletal age of patients whose growth is affected by infection, trauma *etc.*
5. Assess growth status and skeletal maturity in patients with skeletal malocclusion, necessitating orthognathic surgery.

Dental Age

In addition to bone age, dental age is also often used to determine somatic maturity. Dental age is determined by various methods (Fig. **21**).

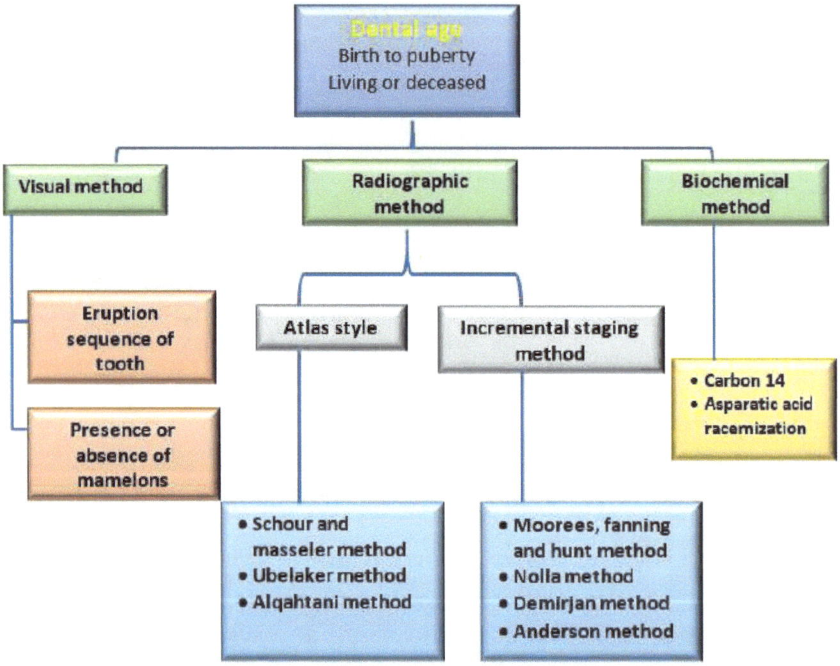

Fig 21. Different methods of determination of dental age.

The simplest and least accurate dental age indicator involves recognizing the teeth clinically present in the oral cavity in comparison to dental eruption charts. The sequence and timing of eruption are genetically determined. Teeth eruption is usually faster in girls than in boys. Mandibular canine calcification coincides with puberty [10].

Computerized Growth Forecasting

Schuhof and Bagha (1975) utilized the science of biomathematics to the concept of growth of the craniofacial complex. This is called computerized growth forecasting. Ricketts (1950) put forth the clinical usefulness and applicability of growth prediction [12].

Cranial base prediction in a normal child – 2mm/year, expressed by 1mm forward growth of nasion and 1mm backward growth of basion (Bjork 1955) (Fig. **22a**). Growth prediction in the mandible can be predicted with the help of two axis: Condylar axis and Corpus axis (Fig. **22b**). In Maxillary growth prediction, N-A angle remains the same, and the Skeletal convexity can be determined by the relationship of point A with the facial plane (Fig. **22c**).

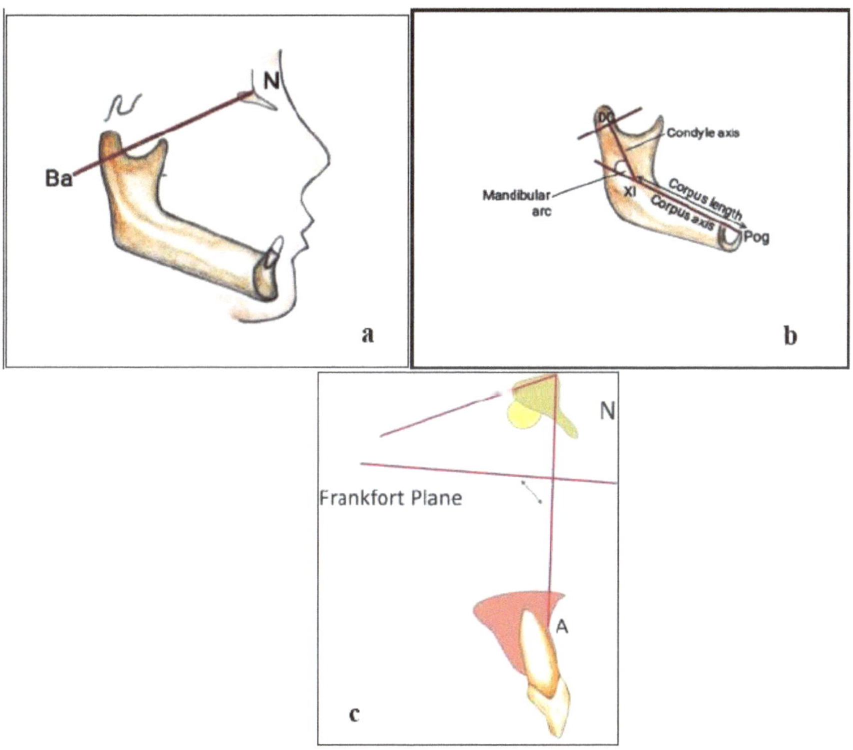

Fig. (22). a. Prediction of cranial-base, b. Prediction of Mandibular growth, c: Prediction of Maxillary growth.

CONCLUSION

The amount of relative growth in the facial skeleton from early childhood to adolescence significantly varies. Thus, sound knowledge of these growth-related changes is necessary for planning dentofacial treatment. Every individual should be considered independent for these growth considerations, and hence group norms to determine the range of deviation must be treated cautiously to address individual needs. Considering the periods of catch-up growth, orthodontic treatment outcomes may require long-term retention and stability to prevent future growth alterations, if any.

CONSENT FOR PUBLICATION

Not applicable.

CONFLICT OF INTEREST

The author(s) declare no conflict of interest, financial or otherwise.

ACKNOWLEDGEMENT

Declared none.

REFERENCES

[1] da Fonseca MA. Malnutrition and oral health in children. Curr Oral Health Rep 2017; 4(2): 92-6. [http://dx.doi.org/10.1007/s40496-017-0130-6]

[2] Leitch VD, Bassett JHD, Williams GR. Role of thyroid hormones in craniofacial development. Nat Rev Endocrinol 2020; 16(3): 147-64. [http://dx.doi.org/10.1038/s41574-019-0304-5] [PMID: 31974498]

[3] Omori MA, Matsumoto MAN, Bezerra Segato RA, Bezerra da Silva LA, Filho PN, Kuchler EC. The effect of estrogen on craniofacial dimensions: A systematic review. Dentistry 3000 2019; 7(1): 21-6. [http://dx.doi.org/10.5195/d3000.2019.84]

[4] Spears R, Svoboda KKH. Growth factors and signaling proteins in craniofacial development. Semin Orthod 2005; 11(4): 184-98. [http://dx.doi.org/10.1053/j.sodo.2005.07.003]

[5] Sanders JO, Qiu X, Lu X, *et al.* The Uniform Pattern of Growth and Skeletal Maturation during the Human Adolescent Growth Spurt. Sci Rep 2017; 7(1): 16705. [http://dx.doi.org/10.1038/s41598-017-16996-w] [PMID: 29196711]

[6] Leigh SR. Evolution of human growth spurts. Am J Phys Anthropol 1996; 101(4): 455-74. [http://dx.doi.org/10.1002/(SICI)1096-8644(199612)101:4<455::AID-AJPA2>3.0.CO;2-V] [PMID: 9016361]

[7] Songra G, Mittal TK, Williams JC, Puryer J, Sandy JR, Ireland AJ. Assessment of growth in orthodontics. Orthodontic Update 2017; 10(1): 16-23. [http://dx.doi.org/10.12968/ortu.2017.10.1.16]

[8] Manlove AE, Romeo G, Venugopalan SR. Craniofacial Growth: Current Theories and Influence on Management. Oral Maxillofac Surg Clin North Am 2020; 32(2): 167-75. [http://dx.doi.org/10.1016/j.coms.2020.01.007] [PMID: 32151371]

[9] Castaldo G, Cerritelli F. Craniofacial growth: evolving paradigms. Cranio 2015; 33(1): 23-31. [http://dx.doi.org/10.1179/0886963414Z.00000000042] [PMID: 25547141]

[10] Patel K. Age assessment methods: A review. Int J Prev Clin Dent Res 2018; 5(2): 77-83.

[11] Greulich WW, Pyle SI. Radiographic atlas of skeletal development of the hand and wrist. 2nd ed., Stanford: Stanford University Press 1959.
[http://dx.doi.org/10.1097/00000441-195909000-00030]

[12] Kasinathan G, Kommi PB, Kumar SM, Yashwant A, Arani N, Sabapathy S. Evaluation of Soft Tissue Landmark Reliability between Manual and Computerized Plotting Methods. J Contemp Dent Pract 2017; 18(4): 317-21.
[http://dx.doi.org/10.5005/jp-journals-10024-2038] [PMID: 28349911]

CHAPTER 10

Growth and Development of Maxilla and Mandible

Bhavna Gupta Saraf[1,*], **Dhanashree Sakhare**[2] and **Parag Kasar**[3]

[1] *Department of Pedodontics and Preventive Dentistry, Sudha Rustagi College of Dental Sciences and Research, Faridabad, Haryana, India*

[2] *Lavanika Dental Academy, Melbourne, Australia*

[3] *Chief Pediatric Dentist at Deep Dental Clinic, Nerul, Navi Mumbai, India*

Abstract: Growth is defined as the normal changes in the amount of living substance. Development refers to all the naturally occurring unidirectional changes in an individual's life, from its existence as a single cell to its elaboration as a multifunctional unit terminating in death. It encompasses the normal sequential events between fertilization and death. Note that development to the biologist refers to the individual in contradistinction to species. The life of the individual does not start as a gamete or zygote, but as primordial germ cells that give rise to gametes. In some invertebrates and plants, life starts from almost any cell which is properly stimulated and maintained. The term multifunctional unit emphasizes the elaboration of multiple functions rather than multiple cellularities. Unidirectional changes continue until death. Therefore, development is a result of a combination of growth, differentiation, and translocation: These terms are not synonymous.

Keywords: Postnatal, Prenatal, Development, Growth, Mandible, Maxilla.

INTRODUCTION

Every dentist especially Pediatric Dentists needs a thorough knowledge of craniofacial growth and development. Even for those who have worked with children, it is difficult to comprehend conditions observed in adults without understanding the process that produced these problems.

Scope

- Differentiate whether growth changes are normal or pathological.
- Follow the child's growth over a period using growth charts.

* **Corresponding author Bhavna Gupta Saraf:** Department of Pedodontics and Preventive Dentistry, Sudha Rustagi College of Dental Sciences and Research, Faridabad, Haryana, India; Tel: +91 9899124779; E-mail: guptabhavna2000@yahoo.com

Satyawan Damle, Ritesh Kalaskar, Dhanashree Sakhare & Abdulkadeer Jetpurwala (Eds.)

- Since we deal with not only the development of dentition but the entire dentofacial complex, we should be able to manipulate facial growth for patient benefit.
- Orthodontic treatment continued growing children, during the growth period. Growth does not always take place uniformly. There seem to be periods when a sudden acceleration of growth occurs, this sudden increase in growth is termed growth spurts.

Prenatal Growth and Development of Maxilla and Mandible-Maxilla

Development of the maxilla includes the development of:

1. Maxilla proper

2. Premaxilla

3. Accessory cartilages.

1. Maxilla Proper

It develops in the mesenchyme of the maxillary process of the mandibular arch as intramembranous ossification. it has a centre of ossification, which appears in a band of fibro cellular tissue immediately lateral to and slightly below the infraorbital, giving off its anterior superior dental branch. The ossification center lies above that part of the dental lamina from which develops the enamel organ of the canine [1].

The Ossified Tissue Appears as a Thin Strip of Bone. It Spreads in Different Directions as:

- Backward: Below the orbit toward the developing zygomatic bone.
- Forward: Toward the future incisor region.
- Upward: To form the frontal process of the maxilla.

As a result of this pattern of bone deposition, a bony trough formed (infraorbital groove) where the infraorbital nerves lie. The inner and outer edges of this groove grow up, meet, and fuse forming a canal that encloses the nerve & opens anteriorly at the infraorbital foramen [2].

- **Downward:** To form the outer alveolar plate for the maxillary tooth germs [2].
- **Toward the midline**: Ossification spreads with the development of the palatal process in the substance of the united palatal folds to form the hard palate. At the union between the palatal process and the main part of the developing

maxilla, a large mass of bone is produced. From this region & on the inner side of the dental lamina & tooth germs, the inner alveolar plate of deciduous canines and molars develops.

Development of the maxillary sinus: At 4 MIU a small depression of the mucosa of the lateral wall of the nasal cavity. In its gradual extension, the sinus comes into relation with the maxilla above the level of the palatal process & hollow out the interior of the bone, separating its upper orbital surface from its lower or dental region.

2. Premaxilla

Two Centres of Ossification for the Premaxilla:

A. **The palate-facial centre:** Appear at the end of 6 WIU. It starts close to the external surface of the nasal capsule, in front of the anterior superior dental nerve and above the germ of the lateral deciduous incisor. From this center bone formation spreads:

1. Above the teeth germ of the incisors.

2. Then downward behind them- To form the inner wall of their alveoli & palatal part of the premaxilla.

B. **The prevomerine center (paraseptal centre):** It begins at about 8-9 WIU along the outer alveolar wall. It is situated beneath the anterior part of the vomer bone, and it forms that part of the bone that lies mesial to the nasal paraseptal cartilage. At 8 WIU union occurs between the maxilla and premaxilla [3].

3. ACCESSORY CARTILAGES

Unlike the mandible, the development and growth are little affected by the appearance of secondary cartilages:

- The accessory cartilaginous center appears in the region of the future zygomatic or molar process, and this undergoes rapid ossification & adds considerable thickness to the bulk of this part.
- Also, small areas of the secondary cartilaginous center appear along the growing margin of the alveolar plate.
- In the middle line of the developing hard palate between the two palatine

processes.

The developing brain and pericardium are the main elements on the ventral side of the embryo around the fourth week of the IUF.

STOMATODEUM divides these bulges (future mouth). The Buccopharyngeal membrane forms the stomodeum floor (Fig. **1**).

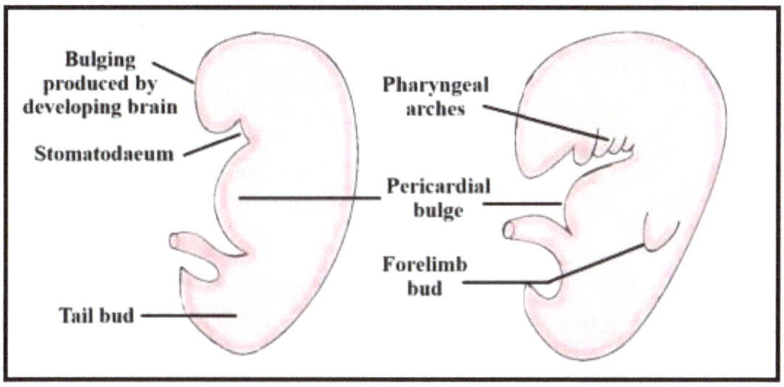

Fig. (1). Formation of Stomodeum.

Soon, the mesoderm that covers the developed forebrain spreads and forms a downward projection that overlaps the top of the stomodeum.

The FRONTONASAL PROCESS is the downward projection. The lateral wall of the stomodeum forms the mandibular arch. At the dorsal end, the arch gives a bud. The maxillary process is called that bud. The maxillary process grows in the central part of the jawbone arch (mandibular process). The frontonasal process overlaps the stomodeum from above, the mandibular process from below, and the maxillary process from either side. The ectoderm that overlays the frontonasal process shows bilateral localized thickenings over the stomatodeum. This is known as NASAL PLACODES. The placodes quickly sink into a nasal pit. (Fig. **2**) [4].

6 branchial arches are formed in the region of the head and neck (Fig. **3**) .5th arch disappears soon. Each arch gives rise to-

- Muscles
- Connective tissue
- Vasculature
- Skeletal and neural components

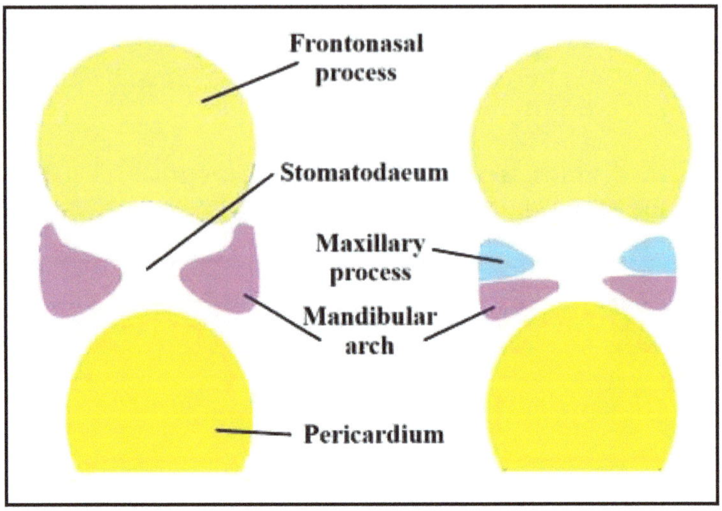

Fig. (2). Formation of Maxillary and Mandibular Process.

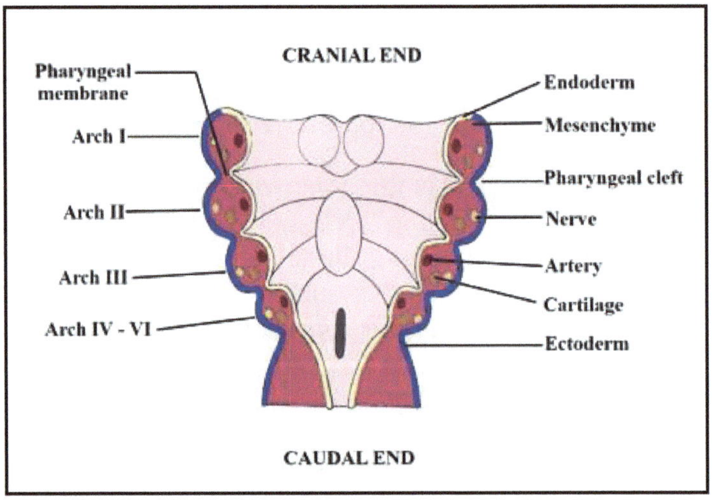

Fig. (3). Development of Pharyngeal Arch.

The Frontonasal Process (Fig. **4**) is divided into two parts by the development of nasal pits:

1. Median Nasal Process

2. Lateral Nasal Process

The maxillary process grows medially and joins the lateral nasal process first, then the medial nasal process.

The nasal pits get closer together as the frontonasal process narrows from side to side.

The maxillary process fusion line and median nasal process give rise to naso-lacrimal duct.

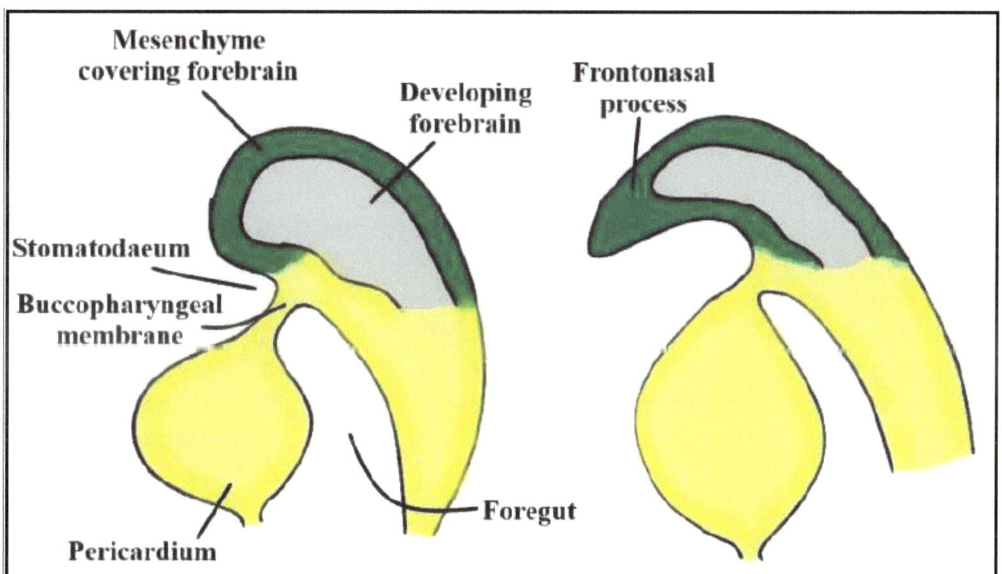

Fig. (4). Formation of Frontonasal Process.

The maxillary prominence enlarges and promotes the medial nasal prominence towards each other. At the fusion line, the nasolacrimal groove develops. The medial nasal prominence moves in the middle fuses with each other and forms the intermaxillary segment, which forms the origin of the upper lip, philtrum, maxillary incisors, and the primary palate. Sagittal maxillary and mandible growth rates are presented in this philosophy as a function of STH - somatomedin and testosterone levels. In each LPM activity level, the slope of a straight line for condylar cartilage growth and mandible lengthening is greater than that required for maxillary growth (except after resection of lateral pterygoid).

For the normal level of STH-somatomedin and the normal contractile activity of LPM, the maxillary and condylar cartilage lines grow straight on an M [5].

Since the level of testosterone varies between T2 and T3, the growth rate of the condylar cartilage varies from C2-C3, in part because of the servo system's regulation.

DIVISIONS OF DEVELOPMENTAL SCIENCE

Growth and developmental studies do not exist apart from other biologic disciplines or their techniques. Studies of developmental events require the knowledge and methods of gross and microscopic anatomy, psychology, physiology, genetics, anthropology, and other disciplines.

Molecular Biology

During the 1920s and 1930s, physical scientists developed a fantastic array of examples, including the electron microscope. During the same time, in the field of biochemistry, important advances were being made in concepts and the precision of methods. When it became possible to elucidate the detailed roles or specific molecules in living systems through these new tools of biochemistry and biophysics (the tidy of physical phenomena in living processes), an exciting new era in biology began. We are amid a biological revolution that is as important for man as the atomic revolution. The discovery of RNA and DNA and deciphering the genetic code are among the most exciting events in the history of science. Molecular biology includes such fast-developing new disciplines of molecular genetics, biophysics, and genetic engineering [6].

Developmental Biology

Because a fertilized egg starts with a single microscopic cell and eventually, by development, becomes an adult comprising millions of cells, the biologists who study this fascinating series of events represent several areas of speciality. The field of developmental biology includes workers from cellular biology, embryology, teratology, reproductive biology, perinatal biology, and other disciplines. Developmental oral biology is the area of research and teaching concerned with craniofacial growth and development.

PRINCIPLES AND THEMES OF DEVELOPMENT

Principles

No principles or mechanisms of development are unique to embryos, the face, man, or even mammals. For this reason, principles and mechanisms of development are best understood through principles, and mechanisms of development are best understood using a generalized model system. As a model of himself, man can be used only descriptively, not experimentally. Much that we have learned about human development has been learned by the formulation of such general models during studies of species other than a man.

SHIFTS FROM COMPETENT TO FIXATION

Undifferentiated cells can become any of various cell types through development, but after they become fixed and cannot ordinarily become another type. This is like the student entering the university who still has the chance to be a physician, engineer, philosopher, or dentist. However, advanced standing usually "fixes" one's career, and it is more difficult to change.

SHIFTS FROM DEPENDENT TO INDEPENDENT

The development brings greater independence to most levels of the organization. The dependent foetus becomes a less dependent child who finally develops into an independent adult.

The Ubiquity of Genetic Control Modulates by Environment

At all levels, the genetic control of development is constantly being modified by environmental interactions which persist through life.

Control of maxillary growth-STH-somatomedin, testosterone, and oestrogen play primary roles in the extrinsic control of the upper jaw. There are direct effects on the growth of spheno-occipital synchondrosis and nasal septal cartilage, the lateral masses of the ethmoid bone, and between body and greater wings of sphenoid by stimulating skeletal cell multiplication rate.

MANDIBLE

Meckel's Cartilage

The cartilage of 1st arch is called Meckel's cartilage (Fig. 5). It provides a template for guiding the growth of the mandible. It develops on the 41st- 45th day of I.U.L. It extends from the otic capsule to Midline or Symphysis. The mandibular branch of the trigeminal nerve appears 1st at about 2/3rd length of Meckel's cartilage level. This nerve bifurcates into the medially lingual nerve and laterally inferior alveolar branches. It then further bifurcates into incisive and mental branches more anteriorly.

In the 6th week of IU's life, in the bifurcation area of the inferior alveolar nerve, each half of the mandible forms an ossification centre. Osteogenesis is then induced at the ossification centre by neurotrophic factors caused by the nerve.

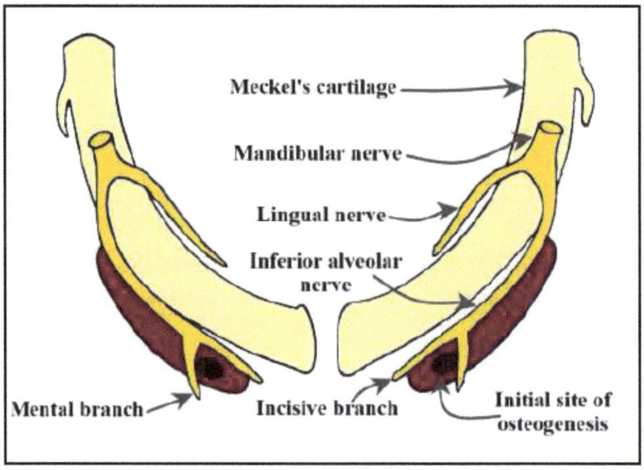

Fig. (5). Development of Mandible from Meckel's Cartilage.

Meckel's Cartilage Ossification (Fig. 6)

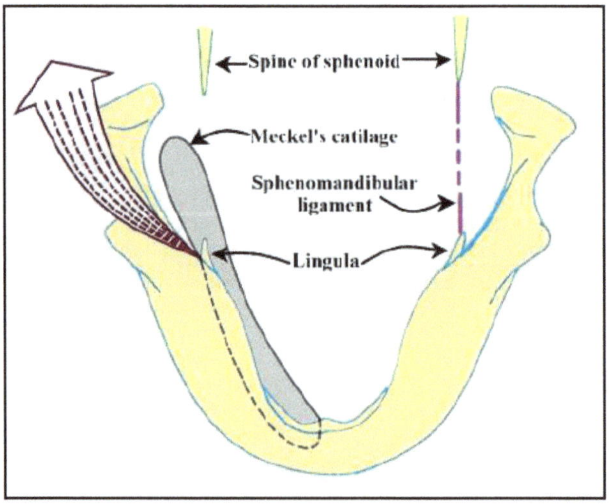

Fig. (6). Ossification of Meckel's Cartilage.

From the center of ossification, bone formation spreads

- Anteriorly - towards the midline
- Posteriorly – till the place where the mandibular nerve divides into the lingual and inferior alveolar branch and forms the body of the mandible.

Bone formation posterior to this division forms the ramus of the mandible. Ossification spread later into the ramus of the jaw, turning away from the Meckel's cartilage. The lingula in the adult mandible marks this point of divergence. A large part of the Meckel's cartilage is disappeared, and the remaining part develops into:

1. Incus & Malleus.

2. Spine of the sphenoid bone.

3. Anterior ligament of malleus.

4. Spheno – mandibular ligament.

OSSIFICATION OF THE MANDIBLE (TABLE 1).

Table 1. Ossification of the mandible.

ENDOCHONDRAL	INTRAMEMBRANOUS
• Cartilage template is replaced by endochondral bone • Indirect bone growth • Slow expansion	• Direct deposition of osseous tissue in periosteal membrane • Direct bone growth • Rapid expansion

ENDOCHONDRAL BONE FORMATION

The appearance of three secondary cartilages strongly affects further growth of the mandible until birth, namely:

A. Condylar cartilage

B. Coronoid cartilage

C. Symphyseal cartilage

A. Condylar Cartilage

In the fifth week of intrauterine life, a mesenchymal condensation area is seen above the central part of the mandible that develops (Fig. 7).

It develops in cone-formed cartilage at about ten weeks.

At about 4 months it migrates downwards and fuses with mandibular ramus and persists until the second decade ends [7].

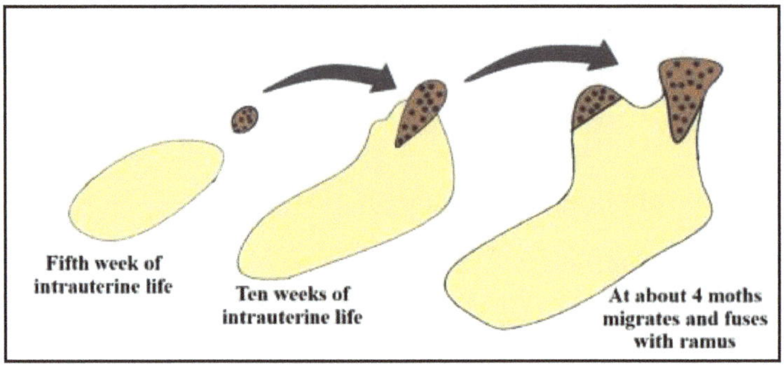

Fig. (7). Endochondral Bone Formation (Condylar Cartilage).

B. Coronoid Cartilage

Secondary accessory cartilage appears in the region of the coronoid process at about 10- 14 weeks of intrauterine life (Fig. **8**). Cartilage growth is believed to grow as a response to developing temporalis muscle. This cartilage becomes incorporated into expanding intramembranous bone of the ramus & disappears by birth.

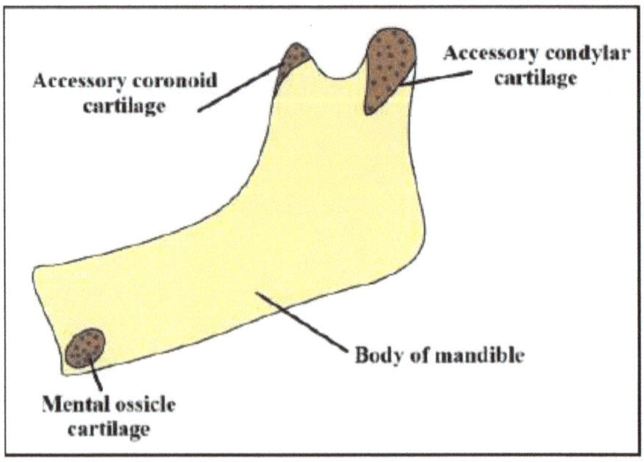

Fig. (8). Endochondral Bone Formation (Coronoid Cartilage).

C. Symphyseal Cartilage

These are two in number. Generally, appear in between the two ends of Meckel's cartilage. At about the 7th month of IUL, these undergo ossification and form mental ossicles. Later, these ossicles merge with the symphysis region. Ossification of symphysis will be completed by the end of 1 yr. after birth.

Postnatal Growth of Maxilla and Mandible Maxilla

Functions of Maxilla-

A. Significant role in chewing
B. A Substantial part of the airway.
C. Fill the voices with resonance
D. Speech and expression of the face.

Growth of The Maxilla

1. Sutural growth

2. Alveolar process development

3. Subperiosteal bone formation

4. Enlargement of the maxillary sinus

5. Bone resorption and bone deposition

1. ***Sutural Growth*** –It continues till 10 years of age and then becomes less significant. The maxilla articulates with the other bones of the skull by 4 main sutures: a) Fronto maxillary suture. b) Zygomaticomaxillary suture. c) Zygomaticotemporal suture. d) Pterygopalatine suture. All these sutures are parallel to each other and directed from upward anteriorly to downward posteriorly. So, growth at these sutures will shift the maxilla forward and downward.

2. ***Alveolar process development***- It will add to the height of the maxilla. Eruption of teeth, especially the permanent set, serves much in this direction, while the eruption of the upper permanent molars adds to the length of the arch.

3. ***Subperiosteal bone formation***- Occurs throughout life and serves as the main factor for the growth of the maxilla.

4. ***Enlargement of the maxillary sinus***- It plays a key role in the growth of the body of the maxilla. The sinus, which occupies the body of the maxilla, expands by bone resorption on the sinus side and bone deposition on the facial surface of the maxillary process. A process is known as pneumatization [8].

5. ***Bone resorption & bone deposition***- Occurs also in other sites than the sinus. Bone resorption at the floor of the nasal cavity compensated by bone deposition on the oral surface of the palate will aid in the enlargement of the nasal cavity and consequently increase the height of the maxilla, which also occurs in other sites than the sinus. Bone resorption at the floor of the nasal cavity compensated by bone deposition on the oral surface of the palate will aid in the enlargement of the nasal cavity and consequently increase the height of the maxilla [4].

Growth Centers

1 – Maxilla Proper Above canine fossa (6th week)

2 – Premaxilla (incisive)

- Above incisive fossa (7th week)
- Ventral margin of the nasal septum (10th week)

Growth Sites

- Sutures
- Maxillary Tuberosity
- Alveolar process
- Nasal septum
- Lateral wall – surface apposition

Mechanisms

- Displacement
- Growth at sutures
- Surface remodelling

Bone remodelling: Process of Bone Deposition and Resorption

Cortical drift: Combination of bone deposition and resorption resulting in growth movement towards deposition surface

Displacement: Movement of whole bone as a unit

I. Primary displacement
II. Secondary displacement

Displacement - Maxilla is attached to the cranial base by several sutures. Thus, the growth of the cranial base has a direct bearing on the nasomaxillary growth.

Primary displacement – Forward direction (Fig. **9**) Growth of maxillary tuberosity in a posterior direction. The Maxilla is carried anteriorly. The amount of forwarding displacement equals the amount of posterior lengthening. Structures of the nasomaxillary complex are displaced forward as the cranial base lengthens and the anterior lobe of the brain grows. Then the Middle cranial fossa grows.

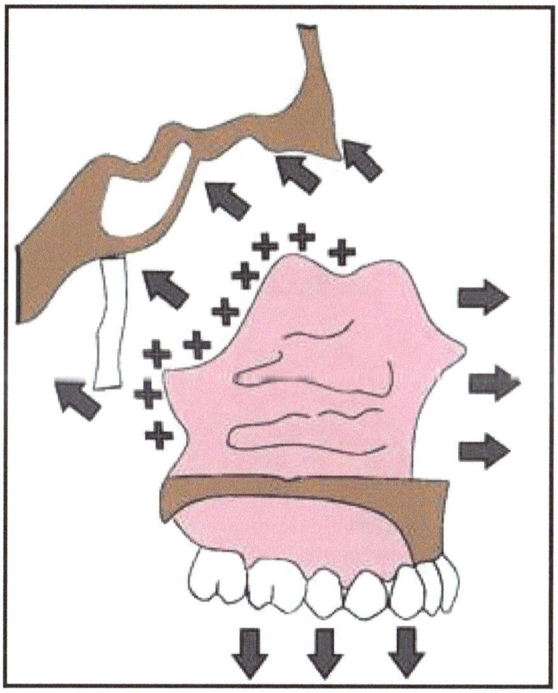

Fig. (9). Primary Displacement.

Secondary displacement of Naso-maxillary complex: downward and forward direction (Fig. **10**) as the nasomaxillary complex attach to the cranial base by mean of no. of sutures, and these sutures are oblique and parallel to each other [13]. The maxilla is repositioned downward and forward as growth occurs at these sutures. Then space opens at suture attachment, new bone is then formed on either side of the suture. The overall size of the bones on either side increases, hence tension-related bone formation occurs at the sutures. Growth of surrounding soft tissue transform the maxilla downward and forward, opening space at its superior and posterior suture attachments, and new bone is added on both sides of the sutures [9].

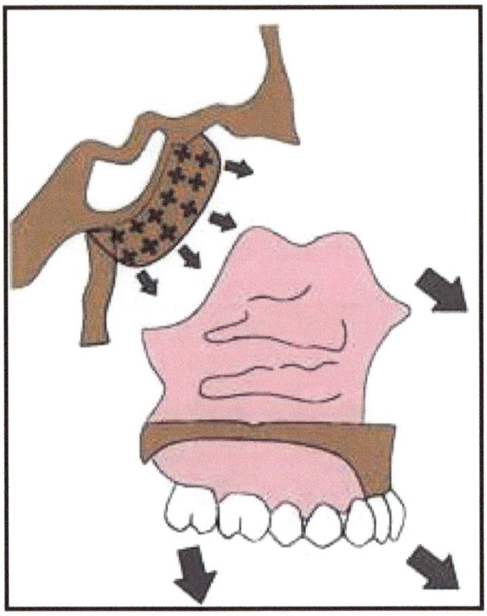

Fig. (10). Secondary Displacement.

Surface Remodeling

Surface remodelling by bone deposition and resorption occurs to bring about:

a. Increase in size
b. Change in shape of the bone
c. Change in the functional relationship [10]
   - **resorption**– lateral surface of the orbital rim
   - **Deposition** – medial rim of orbit and on the external surface of the lateral rim
   - the floor of orbit (growth in superior, lateral, anterior direction)
   - **Deposition** – posterior margin of maxillary tuberosity.
   - Hence lengthening of dental arch and enlargement of the anteroposterior dimension of the entire maxillary body
   - **Resorption** – lateral wall of the nose (increase in the size of nasal cavity), the floor of the nasal cavity.
   - **Deposition**– on the palatal side. (Hence increase in maxillary height)

- **Resorption** – anterior surface, medial surface of the zygomatic bone
- **Deposition**– posterior surface, lateral surface of zygomatic bone (hence zygomatic bone moves in the posterior direction, face enlarges in width)
- **Deposition**– anterior nasal spine prominence
- Endosteal surface of the labial cortex
- Periosteal surface of the lingual cortex
- **Resorption** – periosteal surface of the labial cortex.
- As teeth start erupting, bone **deposition** occurs at alveolar margins. (Increases maxillary height and depth of palate)
- Entire wall of the maxillary sinus except the mesial wall undergoes **resorption**. (Increases size of the maxillary sinus)

Mandible

Mandibular Growth after 1st Year of Life

The growth is more selective and has a definitive sequence –

Growth in width is completed first

Then, growth in length and

Finally, growth in height is completed.

Mandibular Remodeling

Remodelling in various anatomical units (Fig. **11**).

- Ramus
- Lingual Tuberosity
- Body of the mandible
- Condylar process
- Condylar neck
- Coronoid process
- Angular process
- Mandibular foramen
- Alveolar process
- Mental foramen
- Chin

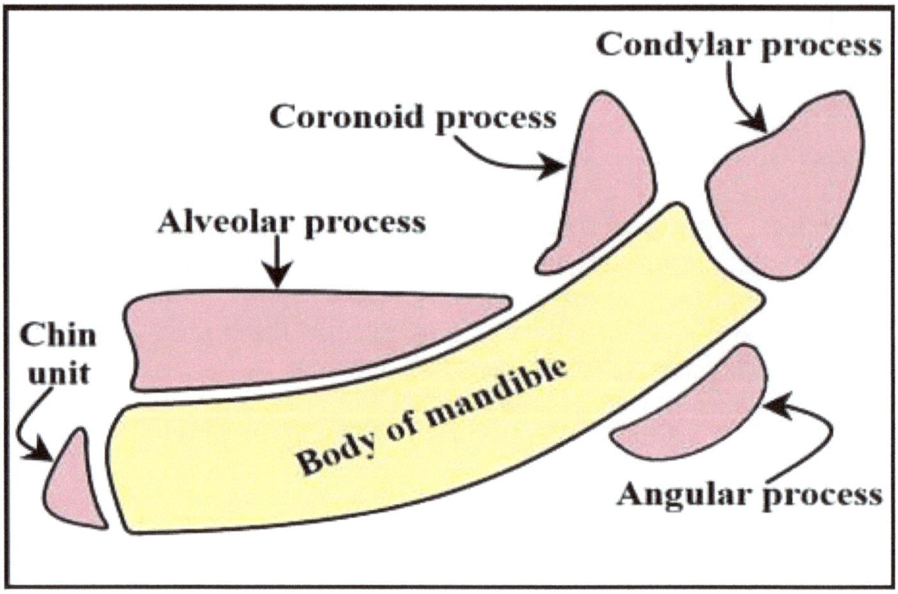

Fig. (11). Mandibular Remodeling.

Growth At Ramus

- Resorption in the anterior part of the ramus.
- Deposition in posterior region.

Results in

The drift of the ramus in a posterior direction.

This resorptive nature is usually described as "making room for the last molars."

- Superior part of ramus below sigmoid notch-lingual-deposition, Buccal-resorption
- Lower part of the ramus below the Coronoid Process-Buccal-deposition, Lingual-resorption
- This leads to the growth of ramus in posterior, superior and lateral positions.

Just as maxillary tuberosity in the maxilla, lingual tuberosity in the mandible is the growth site.

Lingual Tuberosity

Just as maxillary tuberosity in the maxilla, lingual tuberosity in the mandible is the growth site. It grows posterior and medial by bone deposition. The resorptive field below tuberosity makes it more prominent. This resorptive field below termed as Lingual fossa

Body of the Mandible

The increase in width of the mandible occurs primarily due to resorption on the inside and deposition on the outside (Fig. **12**). It increases in length occurs due to drift of the ramus posteriorly and an increase in height occurs due to eruption of the teeth [10].

The Mandibular Condyle

It is a major site of growth. Endochondral growth occurs at the condyle because of condylar cartilage. Condyle grows upwards & backwards, resulting in downward and forward growth of the mandible. Selective remodelling of condyle follows Enlow 'V' principle. Condylar growth reaches a peak at pubertal growth spurt (12-15 yrs).

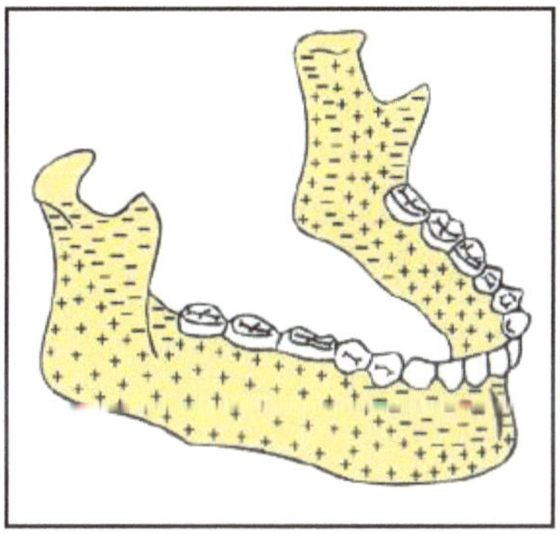

Fig. (12). Body of Mandible.

Condylar Neck

Since the circumference of the condyle is greater than the circumference of the neck, the lingual and buccal sides of the neck have resorptive surfaces. In the mandible of an adult, both the outer and inner surfaces of the cortices of the condylar neck are composed of endosteal bone. This is another example of the ***V principle*** [11].

Coronoid Process

The deposition is present on the lingual side and resorption on the buccal surface. It follows V Principle.

Antegonial Notch

A single field of surface resorption is present on the inferior edge of the mandible at the ramus corpus junction. This forms the Ante gonial notch (Fig. **13**). In Vertical growth, it is deep and in horizontal growth is shallow [12].

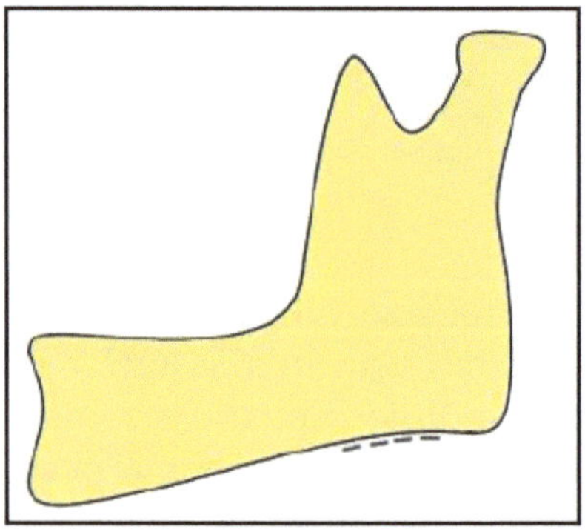

Fig. (13). Antegonial Notch.

The Mandibular Foramen

With the remodelling of the ramus posteriorly, the mandibular foramen maintains its position by deposition in the anterior rim and resorption in the posterior rim (Fig. **14**). It also shifts posteriorly and maintains its central position on the medial surface of the ramus.

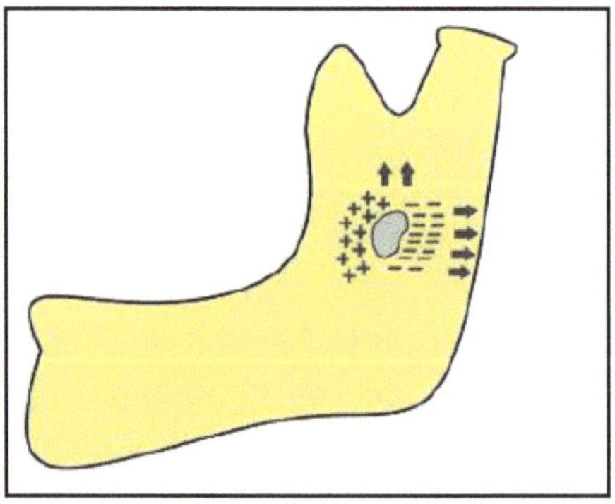

Fig. (14). Bone Remodeling at Mandibular Foramen.

The Alveolar Process

As teeth erupt, the alveolar process develops and increases in height by bone deposition at the margins. If teeth are absent, the alveolar process fails to develop. If teeth are extracted, the alveolar process resorbs [13].

Mental Foramen

In new-born, mental foramen points forward. At 5 years of age, mental foramen points upwards. In adults, mental foramen points backward. This is because of the difference in the growth rate of the buccal and lingual periosteum of the body of the mandible.

The Chin

In infancy, the chin is usually underdeveloped. As age advances the growth of the chin becomes significant. Mental protuberance is formed by bone deposition during childhood. Its prominence is accentuated by resorption in the alveolar region above it.

Recent Advances to Study the Growth and Development of Mandible

- Genex 3D camera
- 3D digital photogrammetric images
- 3D digitizer screening
- Aid with metallic implants
- 3D facial imaging system [14]

Age Changes in Maxilla and Mandible in mandible (Table 2)

Table 2. Age Changes in Maxilla and Mandible in Mandible.

-	AT BIRTH	ADULT	OLD AGE
MENTAL FORAMEN	Near the lower border	Midway between upper and lower borders	Upper border
ANGLE OF MANDIBLE	Obtuse (nearer 180°)	Right angle	-
CORONOID AND CONDYLAR PROCESSES	Coronoid Process is larger and above the level of the Condyloid Process.	The condyloid process is above the level of the coronoid process	The condyloid process is above the level of the coronoid process but in extreme old age and bent backward.
MANDIBULAR CANAL	Lies a little above the mylohyoid line	Runs parallel with the mylohyoid line	Runs close to upper or alveolar border
SYMPHYSIS MENTI	Present: the bone remains in two halves united by fibrous tissue	Represented by a faint ridge only in the upper part	Absent

In Maxilla

At Birth

- Transverse and anteroposterior diameter>vertical diameter
- Well-marked frontal process
- Body consists of little more than alveolar process tooth sockets –close to the orbit
- Maxillary sinus is a mere furrow on the lateral wall of the nose

In Adults

- Vertical diameter is more due to –

Developed alveolar process

Increased size of the maxillary sinus

In Old

- Infantile condition
- Resorption of alveolar bone

Applied Aspects of Development of Maxilla and Mandible (Table 3)

Table 3. Anomalies associated with Maxilla and Mandible.

Congenital Anomalies	Developmental Anomalies
Agnathia	Infantile Cortical Hyperostosis
Micrognathia	Achondroplasia
Facial Hemihypertrophy	Torus mandibular
Facial Hemiatropy	Stafnes Cyst
-	Odontogenic Cyst
-	Odontogenic Tumour

A cleft palate occurs if the palatal shelves fail to fuse or may happen if the tongue fails to descent due to under-development of the mandible

4th ----8th week of IUL ------ cleft in the primary palate

8th ----12th week of IUL ------- cleft between the hard and soft palate

Reasons

- Defective growth of palatine shelves
- Failure of elevation of shelves
- Failure of fusion of shelves
- Post fusion rupture of shelves
- Micrognathia as in robin complex
- Microstomia
- Macrostomia
- Binders Syndrome
- Orofacial Digital Syndrome
- Treacher Collins Syndrome and Robin Sequence
- Achondroplasia
- Downs Syndrome
- Marfans Syndrome
- Turners Syndrome
- Kleinfelters Syndrome
- Pierre-Robin Syndrome

Recent Updates on Growth and Development

Even though development alteration is significant from the start of orthodontics, the perspectives on its clinical value have differed enormously after a certain time. To orthodontists in the late nineteenth, development adjustment was simple since it was expected that development was constrained by natural factors and was judged as effective because the dental impediment improved. By mid-century, cephalometrics had shown that the progressions delivered by the treatment techniques of that time were tooth development, not changed development.

The components that direct post-natal development of the craniofacial intricate and eventually decide the size and state of our countenances are not surely known. Hippo flagging is an overall instrument to control tissue development and organ size, and even though realized that Hippo flagging capacities in neural peak particular and designing during embryogenesis and before birth, its job in postnatal craniofacial development stays tricky. *In vitro* and *in vivo* studies exhibited that FoxO6 initiates Lats1 expression, expanding Yap phosphorylation and enacting Hippo flagging. Craniofacial explicit articulation of FoxO6 postnatally controls Hippo flagging and cell multiplication. Together, these outcomes distinguish a FoxO6-Hippo administrative pathway that controls skull development, odontogenesis, and face morphology [2, 3].

The morphological development pattern of the maxilla and mandible in infants can be assessed quantitatively utilizing 3D investigation. Information about the growth of kids and their orofacial development designs during the predental period can be applied as a record for symptomatic standards [15-17].

CONCLUSION

Hence, craniofacial skeleton growth influences the occlusal relations, jaw, and orofacial functions. Cartilage tissues, including those of spheno-occipital synchondrosis, play a significant role as important growth sites for the respective anatomical components that are the craniofacial skeleton, and nasal septal cartilage in the nasomaxillary complex and condylar cartilage in the mandible. The maxilla and mandible form the lower part of the facial skeleton, which serves vital functions in our daily lives. Jawbones function as anchors for teeth, which are necessary for mastication and speech. Jaw and tooth development are linked not only by their common origins in cranial neural crest cells but also by the regulatory mechanisms and factors that they share. Therefore, it is necessary to study the growth and development and its molecular regulation to better understand a defect and further facilitate its treatment.

CONSENT FOR PUBLICATION

Not applicable.

CONFLICT OF INTEREST

The author(s) declare no conflict of interest, financial or otherwise.

ACKNOWLEDGEMENT

Declared none.

REFERENCES

[1] Suda N. Growth of maxillo-facial region and related anomalies. Clin Calcium 2017; 27(10): 1357-62. [PMID: 28947685]

[2] Sun Z, da Fontoura CSG, Moreno M, *et al.* FoxO6 regulates Hippo signaling and growth of the craniofacial complex. PLoS Genet 2018; 14(10): e1007675. [http://dx.doi.org/10.1371/journal.pgen.1007675] [PMID: 30286078]

[3] Wang J, Martin JF. Hippo pathway: an emerging regulator of craniofacial and dental development. J Dent Res 2017; 96(11): 1229-37. [http://dx.doi.org/10.1177/0022034517719886] [PMID: 28700256]

[4] Premkumar S. Textbook of orthodontics-e-book. Elsevier Health Sciences 2015.

[5] Kihara T, Kaihara Y, Iwamae S, *et al.* Three-dimensional longitudinal changes of maxilla and mandible morphology during the predental period. Eur J Paediatr Dent 2017; 18(2): 139-44. [PMID: 28598185]

[6] Mizoguchi I, Toriya N, Nakao Y. Growth of the mandible and biological characteristics of the mandibular condylar cartilage. Jpn Dent Sci Rev 2013; 49(4): 139-50.

[http://dx.doi.org/10.1016/j.jdsr.2013.07.004]

[7] Yuan Y, Chai Y. Regulatory mechanisms of jaw bone and tooth development. Curr Top Dev Biol 2019; 133: 91-118. [http://dx.doi.org/10.1016/bs.ctdb.2018.12.013] [PMID: 30902260]

[8] Kotagal S, Bicknese AR, Eswara M, *et al.* Developmental Disorders. Atlas of Clinical Neurology. Cham: Springer 2019; pp. 1-52.

[9] Davidovitch M, Eleftheriadi I, Kostaki A, Shpack N. The use of Bjork's indications of growth for evaluation of extremes of skeletal morphology. Eur J Orthod 2016; 38(6): 555-62. [http://dx.doi.org/10.1093/ejo/cjv084] [PMID: 26609074]

[10] Martinez-Maza C, Rosas A, Nieto-Díaz M. Postnatal changes in the growth dynamics of the human face revealed from bone modelling patterns. J Anat 2013; 223(3): 228-41. [http://dx.doi.org/10.1111/joa.12075] [PMID: 23819603]

[11] Allouch GM. Applied anatomy on the maxilla and mandibular regions of the bovine with special reference to its important in regional anesthesia. Int. J. Food, Agricult. Veter. Sci 2014; 4: pp. (3)58-64.

[12] Proffit WR, Fields HW, Larson B, Sarver DM. Contemporary orthodontics-e-book. Elsevier Health Sciences 2018.

[13] Singh SP, Verma S. Orthodontics: current principles and techniques. 2017.

[14] Cobourne MT, DiBiase AT. Handbook of Orthodontics E-Book. Elsevier Health Sciences 2015.

[15] Singh G, Ed. Textbook of orthodontics. JP Medical Ltd 2015.

[16] Tak HJ, Park TJ, Piao Z, Lee SH. Separate development of the maxilla and mandible is controlled by regional signaling of the maxillomandibular junction during avian development. Dev Dyn 2017; 246(1): 28-40. [http://dx.doi.org/10.1002/dvdy.24465] [PMID: 27756109]

[17] Baais A, Mushtaq M. Postnatal growth of maxilla and mandible. AkiNik Publications 2018.

CHAPTER 11

Development of Dentition and Occlusion in Children

Pratik Kariya[1,*] and **Bhavna Dave**[1]

[1] *Department of Pediatric and Preventive Dentistry, K. M. Shah Dental College, and Hospital, Sumandeep Vidyapeeth Deemed to be University, Vadodara, Gujarat, India*

Abstract: The development of dentition and occlusion is an integral part of craniofacial growth as the formation, eruption, exfoliation, and exchange of teeth occur during this period. It is an assimilation of facts, predictions, and studies in static and dynamic situations, the factors influencing them, and their clinical implications. The development of dentition and occlusion is a dynamic concept. The first sign of tooth development appears late in the third week of intrauterine life. An ideal occlusion is the perfect interdigitation of the upper and lower teeth, which results from a developmental process consisting of three main events, jaw growth, tooth formation, and eruption. Development of occlusion starts before the eruption of first teeth in the oral cavity and lasts lifelong thereafter.

Keywords: Anomalies, Dentition, Development, Growth, Occlusion, Terminal planes.

INTRODUCTION

The development of dentition and occlusion is a dynamic concept. The formation of teeth, dentition development, and craniofacial growth are closely related to prenatal and postnatal development periods. The development, emergence, resorption, and shedding of deciduous teeth and the development and emergence of permanent teeth constitute a continuous series of maturational events from before birth to adulthood available for assessment of dental maturation and even for prediction of growth in individuals.

Evolution of Dentition

During evolution, the jaws and teeth display several significant changes (Fig. **1**). The literature revealed that when the reptilian evolved into mammalians, the

* **Corresponding author Pratik Kariya:** Department of Pediatric and Preventive Dentistry, K M Shah Dental College, and Hospital, Sumandeep Vidyapeeth Deemed to be University, Vadodara, Gujarat, India;
E-mail: prateek.kariya@gmail.com

dentition moved from Polyphydont (having many successive sets of teeth, as fishes and other lower vertebrates compared diphyodont)to Heterodont. (having teeth of different types *e.g* in mammals).

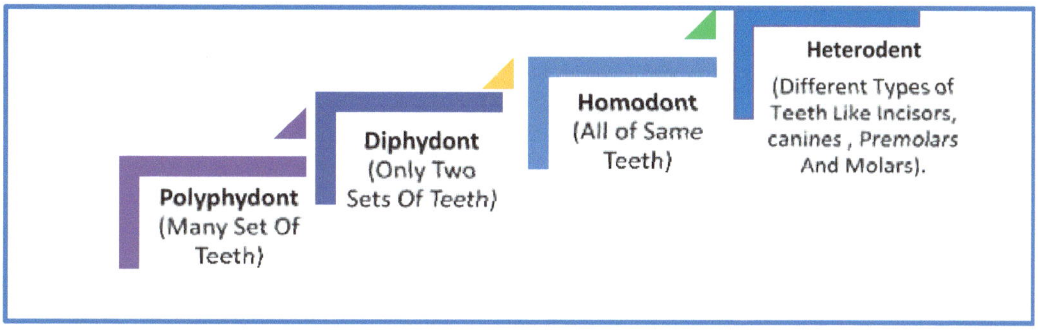

Fig. (1). Evolution of dentition.

There are four stages of Tooth Evolution:

1. The reptilian stage (Haplodont)
2. Early mammalian stage (Triconodont)
3. Triangular stage (Tritubercular Molars)
4. Quadritubercular molars.

1) The reptilian stage (Haplodont) is represented by the simplest tooth form-single cone type confined to single hinge movement of the jaw

2) Early mammalian stage (Triconodont) exhibits three cusps in the line of development of posterior teeth. One larger original cusp is located between a smaller cusp anteriorly and another posteriorly.

3) Triangular stage (Tritubercular Molars)- According to the study of evolutionary tooth development, three triconodont lines evolved to three cones shaped with teeth still by-passing each other more or less when the jaw is opened or closed. Dogs and other carnivorous (predatory) animals have the tritubercular molar type of dentition.

4) Quadritubercular stage shows projection on the triangular form that finally occludes with the antagonist of the opposing jaw. The articulation of the jaws changed accordingly as an accommodation to the changes in the tooth form and anatomy.

Characteristics of Human Dentition

The teeth of vertebrates characterize depending upon the following:

1. Mode of attachment
2. Number of successive sets
3. Type or Shape of teeth.

- **Based on the Mode of Attachment to Jaw:**

Acrodont-- Teeth are attached to the jaw (without socket) by connective tissue.

Pleurodont-- Teeth are directly embedded (fused) inside the jaw.

Thecodont-- Teeth bases enclose into a bony socket.

- **Based on the Number of Successional Teeth sets:**

Polyphyodont-- Teeth replaces throughout life. *E.g.*, shark (Unlimited set of successional teeth sets)

Diphyodont-- Two sets of teeth, *e.g.*, human beings (One set of Successional teeth set)

Monophyodont-- One set of teeth, *e.g.*, sheep, goat. (No Successional set of dentitions)

- **Based on the Type or Shape of Teeth**

Homodont– Dentition consists of similar types of teeth.

Heterodont– Dentition consists of different kinds of teeth, *e.g.*, Incisor, Canine, Premolar, Molar

Thus, Human Dentition characterizes Acrodont, Diphyodont, and Heterodont.

Development of Dentition-

Dentition refers to the natural teeth in the jawbones. It is defined as the type, number, and arrangement of teeth, or it relates to all the upper and the lower teeth collectively. Humans exhibit two sets of dentitions during their lifetime, Deciduous and Permanent (Diphyodont). Teeth development usually begins in the 5th to 6th week of IU life. Deciduous teeth generally develop between 6-30 months after birth, depending on the type of tooth. Crown completion and mineralization are completed before the eruption, while root formation continues for 18 months.

Ameloblast that forms the enamel is lost on eruption, so no further enamel remodeling is possible. It is a permanent record of environmental and genetic factors during its development. With age, the enamel undergoes physiological wear and some pathological destruction.

A). Development during Prenatal Period

Tooth development, (odontogenesis) appears in many stages, for both dentitions. Odontogenesis is a continuous process and has no limitation, *i.e* beginning or end.

Beginning of primary dentition development:

During the 3rd week of IUL, teeth development initiates to form odontogenic epithelium, which proliferates in the 5th week to create the dental lamina. This invagination will develop into tooth buds.

During the 5th week of IUL

The inferno-lateral border of the maxillary arch & the superolateral border of the mandibular arch show Localized Proliferation.

Oral ectoderm

↓

Resulting in the Horseshoe shaped formation of a band of tissue

Dental lamina

↓

Tooth bud

It has three main overlapping phases listed below:

1) Beginning of the Primary Dentition Development

The development of teeth begins in the third week of intrauterine life from odontogenic epithelium. In the fifth week, it proliferates to form the dental lamina. The dental lamina forms invaginations that develop into tooth buds.

2) The Formation of the Successional Lamina

Dental lamina plays a vital role in developing dentition. The deciduous teeth develop from the dental lamina's direct proliferation, while the permanent molars develop from distal proliferation.

All other permanent teeth develop from the lingual extension of the dental lamina, termed the successional lamina. The dental lamina's lingual extension, also called the successional lamina, develops from the fifth month in utero (permanent central incisor) to the tenth month after birth (2nd premolar).

Permanent molars develop from the proliferation of distal extension of the dental lamina. They are known as accessional teeth.

3) Initiation of the Permanent Dentition

Behind the second primary molars, the distal proliferation of the dental lamina forms the tooth germs of the permanent molars. Development of the first permanent molars initiates in the fourth month in utero.

Morphological Changes in the Dental Lamina Occur in the Following Phases (Table 1):

- Initiation of the entire deciduous dentition starts during the second month in utero
- Initiation of the 1st permanent molar takes place around the fourth month in utero.
- The entire permanent dentition initiation starts during the fifth month in utero and lasts till 4-5 yrs. after birth.
- Initiation of the 2nd permanent molar occurs around the first year after birth.
- Initiation of the 3rd permanent molar occurs between four to five years after birth.

Table 1. List of some important polymers and their roles.

Age	Tooth Bud formation
8-10 weeks (IUL)	All the deciduous teeth
4th month (IUL)	Permanent first molar
5th month (IUL)	Permanent central incisor to first premolar
10th month	Permanent second premolar
1 year	Permanent second molar

- There are mainly four morphogenic stages of tooth development which includes:
  - Bud stage
  - Cap stage
  - Bell stage
  - Hertwig's epithelial root sheath and root formation
  - Formation of enamel and dentin matrix

Bud stage-

▪ This stage is the initial stage of tooth formation, where the enamel organ resembles a tiny bud.

▪ The enamel organ consists of peripherally located low columnar cells and centrally located polygonal cells.

▪ The area of condensation immediately below the enamel organ is the dental papilla. The dental papilla and the dental sac are not well defined during the bud stage.

▪ The dental papilla cells form the dentin and the pulp, while the dental sac cells form the cementum and periodontal ligament (Fig. **2a**).

▪ The cap stage characterizes shallow invagination on the undersurface of the bud.

▪ The outer cells of the cap covering the convexity are cuboidal and are called the outer enamel epithelium.

▪ The cells lining the concavity of the cap become tall columnar and are known as the inner enamel epithelium.

▪ The central area of the enamel organ between the outer and inner enamel epithelium, which initially consisted of polygonal cells, acquires more inter-cellular fluid, and forms a cellular network called the stellate reticulum.

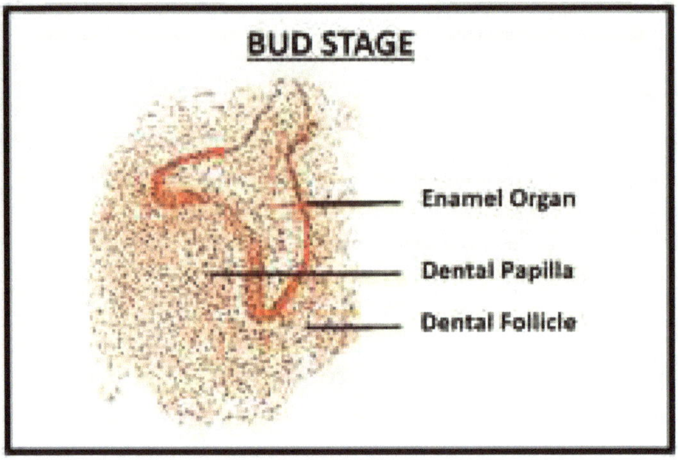

Fig. (2a). Bud stage.

▪ The stellate reticulum reveals a branched network of cells (Fig. **2b**).

Bell stage-

This stage is further divided into:

• Early Bell Stage

• Advanced Bell stage

Early bell stage-

Continued uneven growth - bell shape.

Layers:

• Inner Enamel epithelium

• Stratum Intermedium

• Stellate Reticulum

• Outer Enamel Epithelium

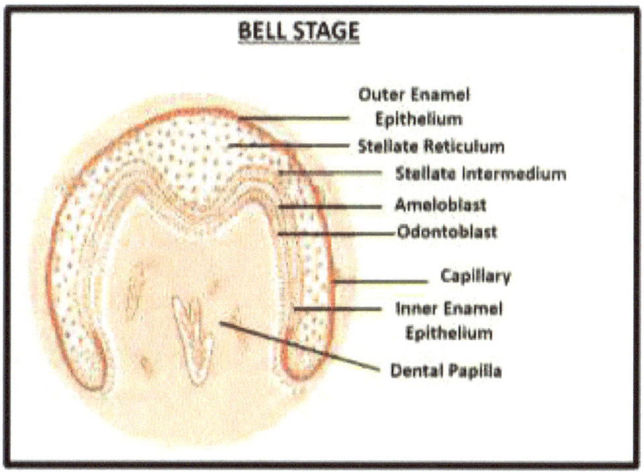

Fig. (2b). Cap stage.

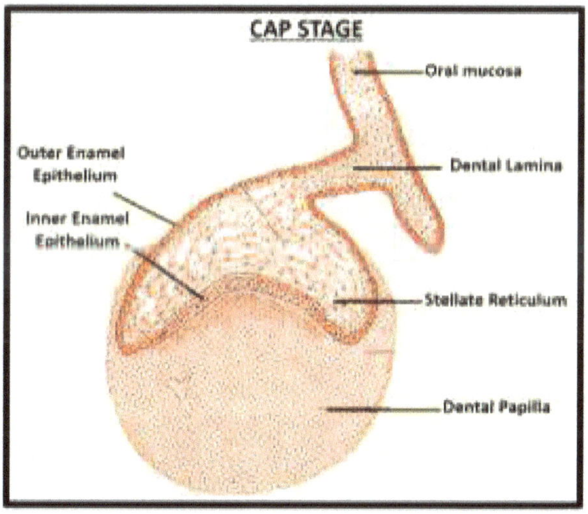

Fig. (2c). Bell stage.

Researchers believed that the shape of the crown is due to pressure exerted by the growing dental papilla cells on the inner enamel epithelium. However, this pressure is opposed equally to the pressure exerted by fluid present in the stellate reticulum. The folding of enamel organs in different crown shapes is due to varying rates of mitosis & difference in cell differentiation time.

Inner Enamel Epithelium: Single layer of cells - tall columnar cells - Ameloblasts

Stratum Intermedium: A few layers of squamous cells between the IEE & Stellate Reticulum are essential for enamel formation.

Stellate Reticulum: Expands further - continued accumulation of intracellular fluid.

Advanced Bell Stage-

Characterized: commencement of Mineralization & Root Formation

Formation of dentin:

- Layer along future DEJ - future cusps proceeds pulpally & apically
- Enamel over the dentin in the future incisal & cuspal areas
- The cervical portion of the enamel organ –
- Hertwig's Epithelial Root Sheath (HERS) outlines the future root (size, shape, length & number of roots) (Fig. **2c**).

B). Status of Development at Birth

The teeth are in different stages of development at birth. In the primary dentition, the incisors exhibit almost complete crown development, and the canines and primary molars exhibit lesser growth. Only the First permanent molar Mineralization is evident at birth.

C). Development of Postnatal Period

It involves completion of the crown and initiation of root formation in primary teeth. At the end of the first year, crown formation of all primary teeth is completed and associated with the emergence of teeth in the oral cavity.

A number of changes take place in the development of teeth-

a. **Initiation-** The 1st sign of tooth formation is the development of the dental lamina from the oral epithelium. Development of bud stage enamel organ appears during initiation. These cells form a sheet of epithelial cells that pushes into the underlying mesenchyme around the perimeter of both the maxillary and mandibular jaws. Due to this, twenty areas of enlargement will appear that form tooth buds for the twenty primary teeth.

b. **Proliferation-** There will be an increase in the size and shape of developing tooth germs and cells that can differentiate into various structures based on stimulation that helps form teeth. In this stage, the first sign of cellular arrangement will initiate. The mesenchymal tissue will form an enamel organ, dental papilla that will differentiate into dentin and pulp, and the dental sac that will differentiate and give rise to cementum and PDL.
c. **Histodifferentiation-** In this stage, formative cells of tooth germ undergo many morphologic and functional changes and give the potential to multiply the cells. The peripheral cells of the dental papilla will differentiate into odontoblast, which will form dentin. It also contains four different types of cells present in the enamel organs.
d. **Morpho-differentiation-** A complete morphological formation of a tooth takes place in this phase. Dentinoenamel junction and Cementoenamel junction develop by continuous enamel, dentin, and cementum deposition by ameloblast, odontoblast, and cementoblast.
e. **Apposition** – The deposition of a matrix of dental hard tissue is called apposition. It characterizes regular and rhythmic deposition of the extracellular matrix, which itself is incapable of further growth. The period of activity and rest alternate at definite intervals during tooth formation. It signifies fulfillment of the plans outlined at the stages of histodifferentiation and morpho-differentiation, so this stage has an additive effect. After the crown attains its final shape in the early bell stage, the inner enamel epithelium will stop proliferating except for the cells at the cervical loop. The first layer of dentin is deposited at the cusp tips, which progresses cervically by reversal of polarity. The columnar cells of the inner enamel epithelium will elongate, and the nucleus moves adjacent to Stratum intermedium. The boundary between the odontoblast and inner dental epithelium defines the future DEJ [1].

It is crucial for every dentist treating children to understand the growth and development of dentition properly. Nolla CM in 1952 gave a meaningful concept of normality, involving an individual's growing child, which aids the dentist to assess and track the development of a children's dentition (Table **2**) [2].

Table 2. Nolla's Stages of tooth Development.

Nolla's Stages of tooth Development		
Stage 00	**Absence of crypt**	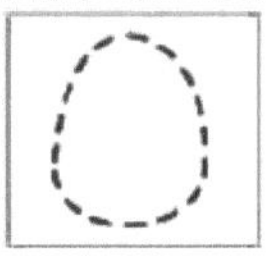

(Table 2) cont.....

Nolla's Stages of tooth Development		
Stage 01	**Presence of crypt**	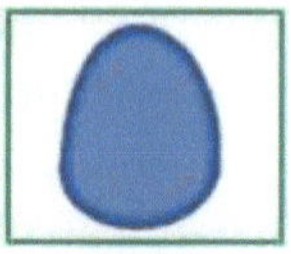
Stage 02	**Initial calcification**	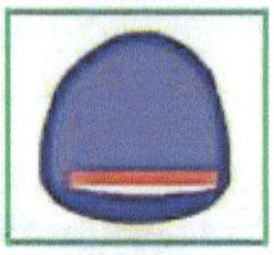
Stage 03	**1/3 of the crown completed**	
Stage 04	**2/3 of the crown completed**	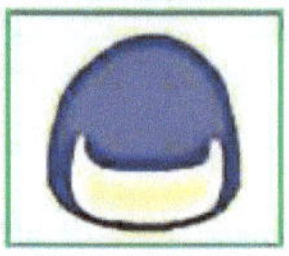
Stage 05	**Crown almost completed**	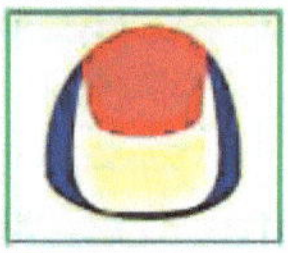
Stage 06	**Crown completed**	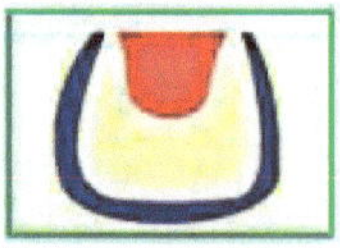
Stage 07	**1/3rd root completed**	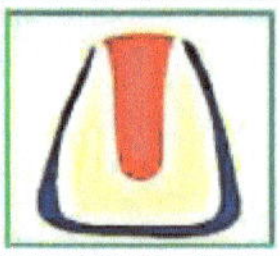
Stage 08	**2/3rd root completed**	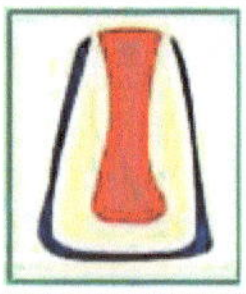
Stage 09	**Root almost completed, open apex**	
Stage 10	**The apical end of root completed apical foramen closed**	

Hertwig's Epithelial Root Sheath and Root Formation

- Root development begins after the dentin and enamel formation reaches the future cementoenamel junction.
- The outer and inner enamel epithelium join and form a sheath that helps mold the shape of the root.
- This sheath is called the "Hertwig's Epithelial Root Sheath and will help form radicular dentin.
- As the first layer of dentin is formed, the epithelial layer loses its structural continuity, and the persisting remnants are called the cell rest of Malassez.
- The roots are not completely formed at the time of the eruption. It continues to form for a few months to several years after the tooth erupts in the oral cavity. Its formation will differ for single and multi-rooted teeth (Fig. **3**).

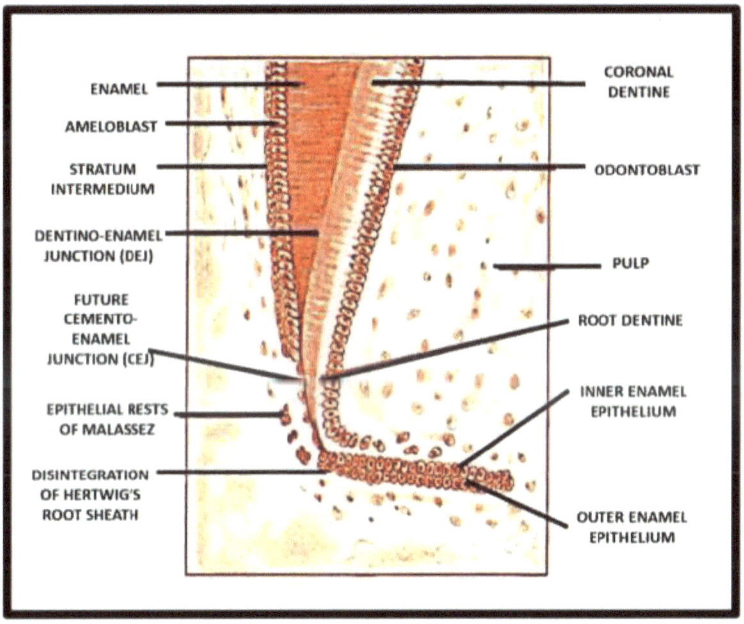

Fig. (3). Root formation (multi-rooted tooth).

NOLLA in 1952, described the various stages of tooth development as follows:

Eruption of Teeth

Tooth eruption is when developing teeth emerge through the soft tissues of the jaws and the overlying mucosa to enter the oral cavity, contact the teeth of the opposing arch, and function in mastication.

The term “eruption” is derived from the Latin word “erupptione” which means output with momentum, and the Greek word “Erumpere”, which means to break out. The eruption is a dynamic and continuously ongoing process that ends with losing teeth from the oral cavity. The eruption sequence can be explained as the Eruption of deciduous teeth, their exfoliation followed by eruption of permanent dentition, and lastly, loss of teeth from the oral cavity. It is an orderly, sequential, and age-specific event and is considered an important milestone during a child's development. Tooth eruption is a process in tooth development in which the teeth enter the mouth and become visible. A tooth moves from its developmental position within the jaws to emerge in the oral cavity. The primary teeth begin erupting into the oral cavity from 6 months of age and continue until two and half years. The first tooth may erupt as late as 13 months, and the last primary tooth may erupt as late as around three years. These are considered normal variations. If the teeth fail to erupt even beyond this age, it is necessary to check the presence or absence of teeth with the help of radiographs. Another possible reason could be an extremely thick fibrous gum pad that does not facilitate the tooth's eruption. In this case, surgical intervention may be required.

Two types of Eruption

***Active Eruption*:** Active eruption is the eruption of teeth into the oral cavity from its developmental position towards the occlusal plane. It is a natural path of eruption of all the teeth as they emerge from the gingiva and continue erupting until they contact the opposing tooth.

***Passive Eruption*:** After the active eruption of teeth is completed, Passive eruption starts. It is the movement of the gingiva apically or away from the crown of the tooth to the level of Cementoenamel junction (CEJ) after the tooth has entirely erupted into the occlusal plane to expose the entire clinical crown.

Patterns of Eruptive Tooth Movements

1) ***Pre-Eruptive Tooth Movement-*** Primary teeth have space between them mesiodistally and labiolingually, and the developing permanent teeth utilize this space. If there is no spacing between them, the successor teeth become crowded. There will be a labial and cortical drift of tooth follicles within the bone. The crowding is relieved by the growth of the infant's jaw by an increase in the height and width of the jaws. The growth for the mandible will be in an outward and upward direction while downward in the maxilla. Permanent teeth undergo complex tooth movement. Permanent teeth develop lingually to the primary teeth germ, and as the primary teeth develop, they move to the apical position.

2) ***Eruptive Tooth Movement-*** Eruptive movements begin soon after root begins to form. Eruption starts in the "pre-emergent spurt phase." Two processes are necessary:

a. There must be resorption of bone and primary tooth roots overlying the crown of the erupting tooth.
b. Then, the eruption mechanism must move the tooth in the direction where the path has been cleared.

3) ***Post-Eruptive Tooth Movement-*** It occurs primarily to maintain the position of erupted teeth. Teeth emerge into the oral cavity when 2/3rd of its root development is complete. Then, it emerges and erupts rapidly to approach the occlusal level, where it is subjected to masticatory forces.

The stage of a relatively rapid eruption from the time a tooth first penetrates the gingiva until it reaches the occlusal level is called the post-emergent spurt. The oral cavity of a neonate includes gum pads, neonatal jaw relationship, and dentition status.

Theories of Tooth Eruption-

There are various theories for the eruption of teeth as the teeth start erupting in the oral cavity when the crown is completely developed, and root formation is taking place.

1. Growth Displacement Theory

According to this theory, roots are growing in the apical direction while the tooth erupts in the opposite direction, *i.e.*, the root impinges on a fixed structure, creating an apically directed force translated into the eruptive movement of the tooth.

2. Tissue Fluid Theory

According to this theory, a local increase in tissue fluid pressure in the periapical region leads to tooth eruption.

3. Contraction Bone Formation

According to this theory, the selective resorption and deposition of bone bring about tooth eruption.

4. Contraction of a periodontal ligament

Formation and renewal of PDL can be a factor in tooth eruption because of the traction power of the fibroblast. Contraction of fibroblast situated near the PDL create pressure that favors tooth eruption.

5. Myofibroblast Contraction

The myofibroblast contraction theory proposes that the fibroblasts possess contractile filaments which are in contact with one another to permit the summation of contractile forces. They exhibit fibro nexus by which the forces are transmitted to the collagen fiber bundles of PDL, bringing the tooth movement.

Histology of Tooth Movement

Histologically, in the pre-eruptive tooth movement, the walls of the bony crypt undergo remodeling, and there is eccentric growth of the tooth germ. A few significant changes are seen in the periodontal ligament during the eruptive phase. There exists a close relationship between fibroblast cell components, fibronectin, a sticky glycoprotein, and collagen fibers surrounding the tooth. A constant change in the relation of these components contributes to the eruptive force. The eruption of successional teeth has an additional aspect to it. As the primary teeth erupt, they remain connected to the secondary tooth germ by the gubernacular canal, containing the gubernacular cord filled with remnants of the dental lamina. This is said to act as a guide for the erupting permanent tooth. The development of human dentition is shown in Figs. (**4** and **5**).

Resorption of alveolar bones by osteoclasts is essential for tooth eruption. ClC-7 is highly expressed in the ruffled membrane of osteoclasts and is responsible for acidifying resorption lacuna. ClC-7 may affect tooth development by directly targeting tooth cells and regulating tooth eruption through DFC mediated osteoclast pathway (Figs. **4** and **5**), (Table **3**), [3, 4].

Table 3. The process of Tooth Development.

Dental Lamina	Bud Stage	Cap Stage	Bell Stage	Advanced Bell Stage	Eruption
→	→		→		→
Initiation	Morphogenesis		Cell Differentiation		Matrix Secretion

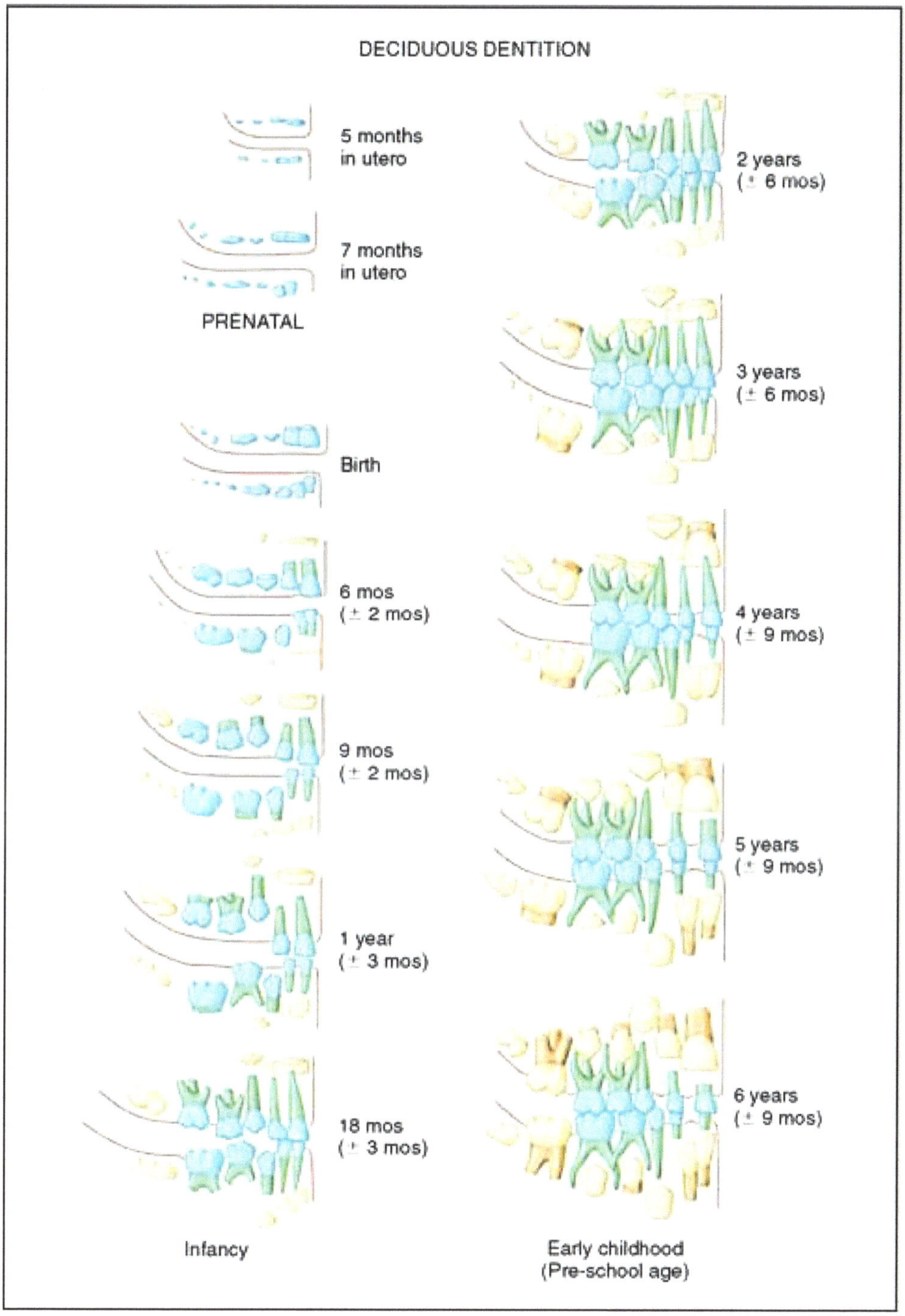

Fig. (4). Stages of tooth development in primary dentition.

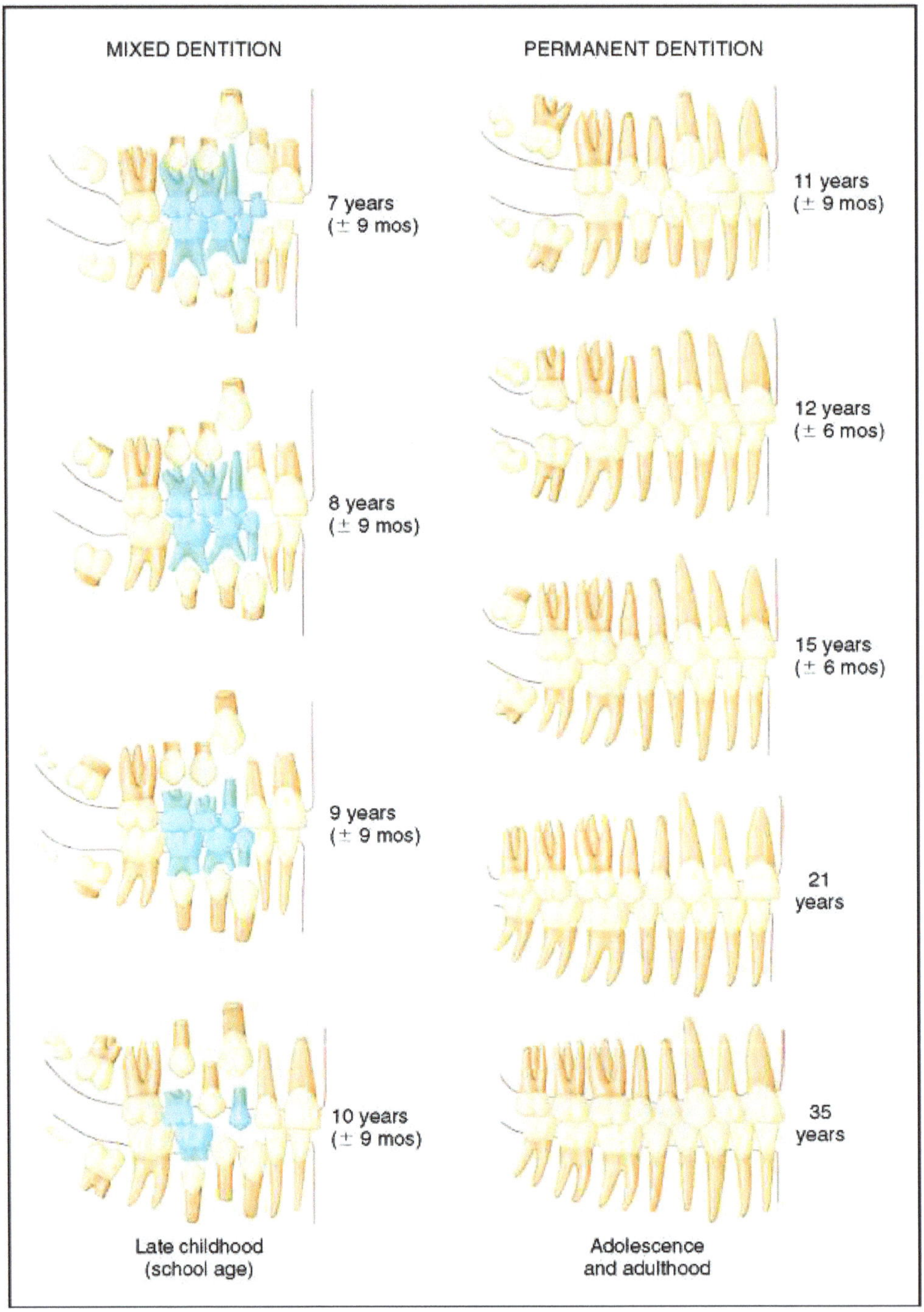

Fig. (5). Stages of mixed and permanent dentition.

Factors Affecting Eruption

1. Genetic Factors

Various processes can occur during foetal development that can result in lifelong effects on health. For example, variation in the age of emergence of the primary dentition is influenced by preconception factors that act on the foetus and affect it throughout pregnancy and infancy.

2. Environment Factors

- Maternal smoking
- Ethnic age group
- Malnutrition
- Ethnic age group
- Weight and height at the time of birth and early foetal life
- Metabolism and nutrition
- Maternal breastfeeding

A polymorphism in the timing of the first primary tooth eruption has been seen in this modern era. Changes in lifestyle in various modes like frequencies of breastfeeding, mode of breastfeeding, dietary habits, hormonal changes, and timing of initiation of soft food, bottle feeding has a significant impact on the timing and pattern of the eruption of first primary teeth [5].

Chronology of Primary and Permanent Dentition

Chronology is a list of events in the order in which they happened. Chronos means time, and logos means to study. It is defined as the study that deals with the timings of various stages of tooth development, starting with the initiation of the first dental tissue laid down to the emergence of teeth in the oral cavity and its completion of calcification [5 - 7] (Tables **4** & **5**).

Table 4. Chronology of primary dentition.

Primary Teeth	Calcification begins at	Formation completes (Months)	Eruption Maxillary (Months)	Eruption Mandibular (Months)	Exfoliation Maxillary (Years)	Exfoliation Mandibular (Years)
Central incisor	4th foetal month	18-24	6-10	5-8	7-8	6-7
Lateral incisor	4th foetal month	18-24	8-12	7-10	8-9	7-8
Canine	4th foetal month	30-39	16-20	16-20	11-12	9-11

(Table 4) cont.....

Primary Teeth	Calcification begins at	Formation completes (Months)	Eruption Maxillary (Months)	Eruption Mandibular (Months)	Exfoliation Maxillary (Years)	Exfoliation Mandibular (Years)
1st molar	4th foetal month	24-30	11-18	11-18	9-11	10-12
2nd molar	4th foetal month	36	20-30	20-30	9-12	11-13

Table 5. Chronology of permanent dentition.

Permanent Teeth	Calcification begins at	Crown (enamel) complete at (Years)	Root completion (Years)	Eruption Maxillary (Years)	Eruption Mandibular (Years)
Central incisor	3-4 month	4-5	9-10	7-8	6-7
Lateral incisor	Maxilla- 10-12 month Mandible- 3-4 month	4-5 4-5	11 10	8-9	7-8
Canine	4-5	6-7	12-15	11-12	9-11
1st premolar	18-24	5-6	12-13	10-11	10-12
2nd premolar	24-30	6-7	12-14	10-12	11-13
1st molar	At Birth	3-3.5	9-10	5.5-7	5.5-7
2nd molar	30-36 months	7-8	14-16	12-14	12-14
3rd molar	Maxilla-7-9 yr. Mandible-8-10 yr.	-	-	17-30	17-30

Developmental Anomalies of Teeth

Developmental disturbances mean an abnormality where the pathology starts in the embryonic stage of human life before the formation of dentition. The development of a tooth is a complex process wherein there is a series of interactions between the ectoderm and ectomesenchyme. Disturbance of the epithelium and mesenchymal interactions can markedly alter the normal odontogenesis leading to the developmental anomaly of teeth. Depending on the developmental stage in which the alteration has occurred, different abnormalities could happen, *e.g.*, number, structure, size, or shape. Developmental dental anomalies are marked deviations from the usual colour, contour, size, number, and degree of development of teeth (Table **6**).

Table 6. Self-correcting anomalies in pre-dentate period.

S. No	Self-Correcting Anomaly	Correction
1	Anterior Open bite	Eruption of Primary incisors
2	Retrognathic Mandible	Differential growth of mandible during the first year of life
3	Infantile Swallow	Introduction of food (Weaning) Eruption of Primary Incisors

Development of Occlusion

- The development of occlusion is a genetically and environmentally conditioned process that shows plenty of individual variations to develop an acceptable occlusion.
- Guidance of eruption and development of the primary, mixed and permanent dentitions is an integral component of comprehensive oral healthcare for all pediatric dental patients.

Definition

Occlusion is defined as the way the teeth meet when the lower jaw (mandible) and upper jaw (maxilla) come together.

An ideal occlusion is the perfect interdigitation of the upper and lower teeth, which results from a developmental process consisting of three main events, jaw growth, tooth formation, and eruption.

Normal occlusion is desirable as it allows oral functions to operate correctly, provides the best aesthetics, and is helpful in the prevention of disease. Deviation from normal occlusion is termed malocclusion. Malocclusion may result in functional and parafunctional imbalance leading to dental disorders, chewing, speech, and aesthetics (especially facial profile) problems.

Centric Occlusion (CO) can be described as the occlusion the patient makes when they fit their teeth together in maximum intercuspation.

Periods of Developing Occlusion

The development of Occlusion can be divided into the following periods:

1. Pre dentate period
2. Deciduous dentition period
3. Mixed dentition period
4. Permanent dentition period.

1. *Pre-Dentate Period*

The pre-dentate period refers to a period just after birth till the first teeth erupt in the oral cavity. This is the period when the neonate does not have any teeth. The alveolar arches at the time of delivery are called gum pads. It usually lasts for six months after birth and may continue until 13 months in delayed eruption cases.

The pre-dentate period of occlusal development can be explained under the following heading:

a). *Gum Pads*

At the time of birth, the alveolar processes are known as gum pads, which are pink, firm & are covered by a dense layer of fibrous periosteum. They are horseshoe-shaped and develop into two parts- the labiobuccal portion and lingual portion and are separated from each other by a groove called a **dental groove.**

The gum pads are divided into ten segments by **transverse grooves**. Each of these consists of one developing deciduous tooth sac, and the gingival groove separates the gum pads from the palate and the floor of the mouth. Lastly, the transverse groove between the canine & 1st deciduous molar segment is called the **lateral sulcus**.

- The maxillary arch is horseshoe shape, while the mandibular arch is U-shaped.
- The maxillary arch is extended buccally, labially, and posterior to the mandibular arch.
- Gum pads are pink, firm, and covered by a layer of dense periosteum.
- Dental groove-the gum pads are divided into labial and lingual by a groove called a dental groove.
- The labial portion develops first, followed by the lingual part.
- Transverse Groove- The Gum Pads are divided into ten segments by transverse grooves. Each Segment has one developing primary tooth sac.
- The lateral sulcus is a transverse groove between the canine and 1st molar extending to the buccal side of the gum pad. It helps predict inter arch relation.
- Gingival Groove separates the maxillary gum pad from the palate and defines the limit of the palate both anteriorly and laterally by three straight boarders.
- At the rest position, there is an open bite in the anterior region of gum pads covered with the tongue. There is contact only in the molar region, and space is in the anterior region. This is called infantile open bite, which helps in sucking and is considered normal.

• The mandibular jaw is positioned distally and is referred to as mandibular retrognathism. Further, during the first year, the mandibular arch growth catches with the development of the maxillary arch based on a different growth pattern (Fig. **6**).

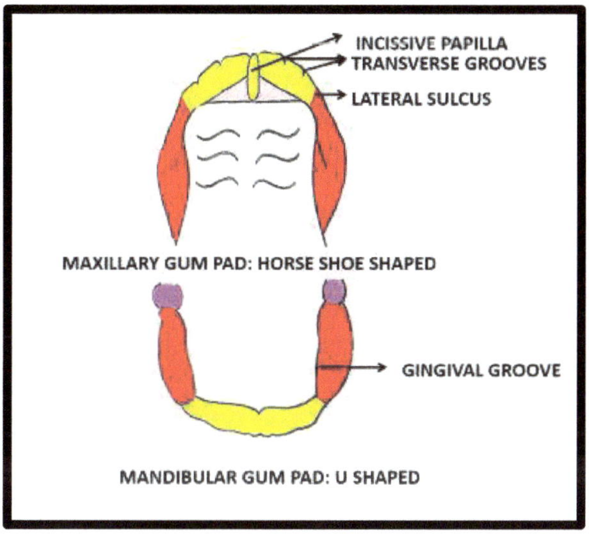

Fig. (6). Upper and Lower Edentulous Gum pads.

b). *Neonatal Jaw Relationship*

The upper & lower gum pads are almost like each other. The upper gum pad is broader and longer than the mandibular gum pad. When the upper and lower gum pads are approximated, there is a complete overjet all around. Contact occurs between the upper and lower gum pads in the first molar region & a space exists between the anterior regions. This infantile open bite is considered normal & it helps in suckling.

At rest, the gum pads are separated by the tongue, which protrudes over the lower gum pad to lie immediately behind the lower lip. At this stage, the upper lip appears short. The upper gum pad is wider than the lower, and when the two are approximated, there is a complete overjet all around. The degree of overjet of the upper gum pad varies considerably, although its significance is still unknown. The lateral sulcus of the lower gum pad is usually posterior to that of the upper, a relation which, if it were to persist, would be abnormal. During the first year of life, the pads grow rapidly, and the growth is most marked in the lateral direction and later in the labiolingual dimensions of the gum pads (Fig. 7).

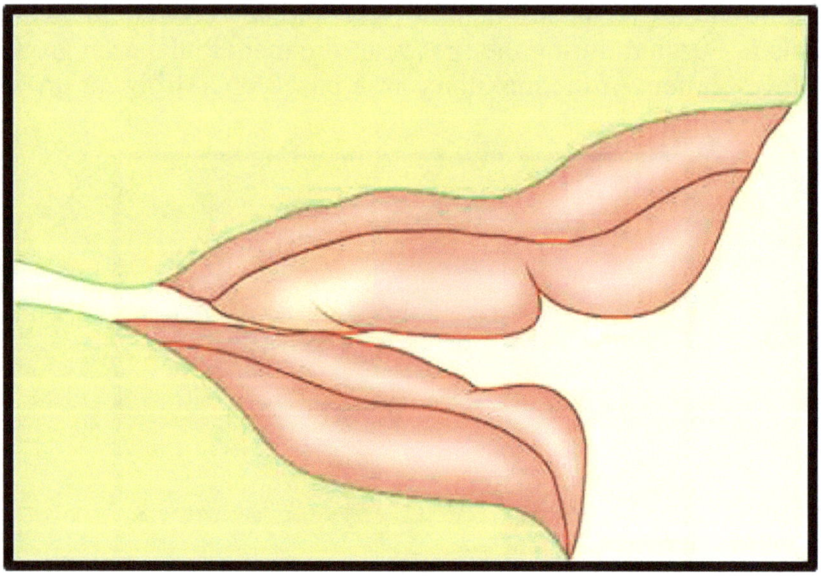

Fig. (7). Contact between Maxillary and Mandibular Gunpad.

c). ***The Status of Dentition***

Usually, there are no teeth present during the pre-dentate period. If any teeth are present in the oral cavity during this period, they are referred to as precociously erupted teeth.

Depending upon the timing of the eruption of teeth, they can be:

- Natal teeth- When infants are born with teeth.
- Neonatal teeth- When teeth erupt during the first month after birth.
- Premature teeth- When teeth erupt in the second or third month after birth.

Synonyms: Congenital teeth, Foetal teeth, Pre deciduous, Dentitia precox.

These teeth are always mandibular incisors, which frequently display enamel hypoplasia. There are familial tendencies for such teeth. Usually, they should not be removed but removed if supernumerary. The most common teeth involved are the mandibular incisors, maxillary incisors, followed by mandibular cuspids and molars. The etiology for precociously erupted teeth is still unclear. Some of the probable aetiologies are shown in Fig. (**8**) [8].

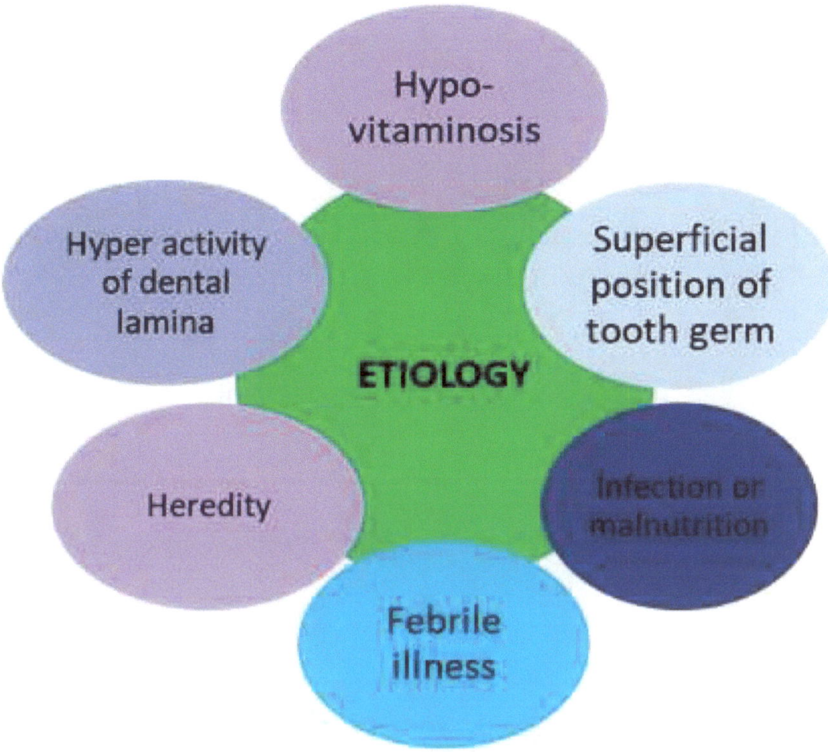

Fig. (8). Aetiology of Precociously Erupted teeth.

2. Deciduous Dentition Period

The deciduous dentition period refers to the period from the eruption of the first primary teeth till the eruption of the first permanent teeth. So primary dentition periods start approximately from the 6th month when the primary mandibular central incisor erupts and lasts till six years when mandibular first permanent molars erupt.

The mandibular central incisors are the first to develop in deciduous dentition, followed by other incisors. They erupt around six months after birth. After 3-4 months, approximately ten months, the mandibular and maxillary first molars erupt, and within 24-30 months, the maxillary & mandibular second molars also erupt. Though all the primary teeth erupt by three years of life, the deciduous dentition period lasts till six years as there are no permanent teeth till that age. From 3-4 years, the dental arch remains stable and changes very slightly [5 - 7].

Favourable Sequence of Eruption of Primary dentition (Fig. **9**).

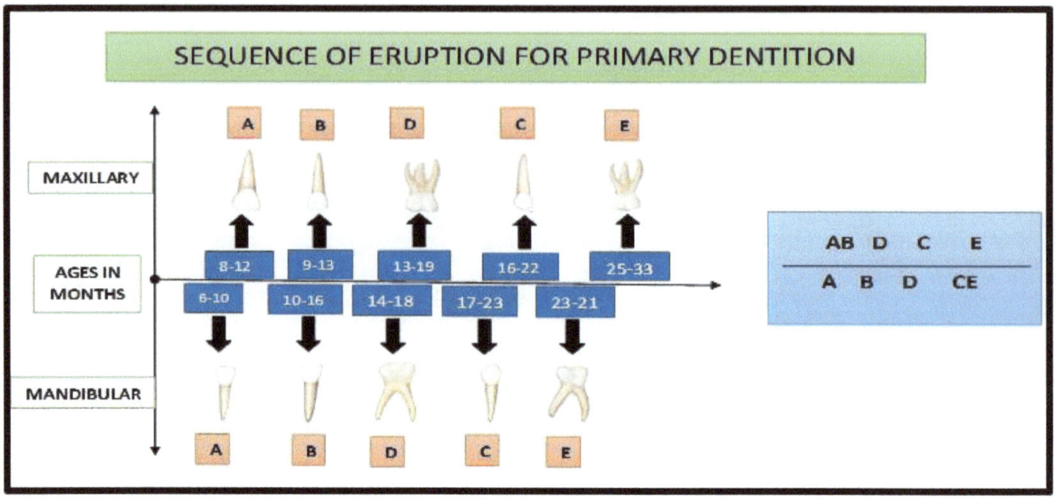

Fig. (9). Sequence of Eruption of Primary teeth.

ABDCE - Maxillary Arch

ABDCE - Mandibular Arch

The deciduous dentition period has the following Ideal characteristic features [9]:

- Ovoid arch form
- Interdental spacing
- Flush terminal plane
- Deep bite more than 4mm
- Upright incisors
- The flat curve of Spee
- Shallow intercuspal interdigitation
- Shallow overbite and overjet

Ovoid Arch Form

Both the arches are half round-shaped or ovoid. The arches are wide enough to accommodate the developing tooth germ of deciduous dentition. The posterior region of both the dental arches keeps growing to accommodate the permanent molars. In developing permanent dentition, the tooth germs are positioned lingually to apices of incisors, just below the apices of canines and between the roots of primary molars for premolars.

Interdental Spacing

- The primary dentition stage may have generalized spacing, no spacing, localized spacing, or crowded dentition.
- These spaces are important and decide the future establishment of occlusion in permanent dentition.
- Spaced dentition is considered good as spaces between the teeth can be utilized to adjust permanent successors, which are always larger than deciduous teeth.
- Generalized spacing occurs in almost 2/3rd of the children, referred to as physiological or developmental spaces. Localized spaces like primate space are also seen.
- The absence of spacing in primary dentition may indicate tooth-size arch-length discrepancy [10] (Table 7).

Table 7. Types of spacing in primary dentition.

Physiological Spaces **Fig. (10)**	**Primate Spaces** **Fig. (11)**	**Non-spaced Dentition** **Fig. (12)**
Spaces between all the primary teeth play an essential role in the normal development of permanent dentition. Total space present may vary from 0 mm to 8 mm with an average of 4mm in maxillary arch and 1 mm to 7 mm with the average of 3 mm in mandibular arch. This space is also referred to as Developmental Space	**Maxillary Arch:** Spaces present between maxillary lateral incisor and the canine (mesial to maxillary canines). Also known as Baume's Space. **Mandibular Arch:** Spaces present between mandibular canine and 1st deciduous molars (distal to mandibular canines). Also known as Anthropoid or Simian spaces.	The dentition is highlighted by the absence of space between primary teeth, either due to small jaw or larger teeth. This type of dentition usually indicates crowding in developing permanent dentition.
Utilized during early mesial shift to settle in Class-I occlusion	Utilized during early mesial shift to settle in Class-I occlusion	Leads to the utilization of Lee Way Space of Nance during Late mesial shift to settle in Class-I occlusion

Spacing in Primary Dentition

Significance of Primate Spaces

- These spaces are essential in the later stage for the alignment of erupting permanent teeth and the establishment of occlusion.
- The absence of these spaces in the primary dentition expresses disproportion between jaw/tooth sizes.
- The establishment and maintenance of normal occlusion constitute one of the

essential objectives of Pedodontics treatment, whether it is preventive, interceptive, or corrective [11, 12].

The early deciduous dentition is of two types as for as the spacing in the primary teeth is concerned.

1. Spaced primary dentition
2. Closed primary dentition (Non-Spaced Primary Dentition)

In the closed type of primary dentition, there is no spacing between the primary teeth. In contrast, spaces are observed in the anterior region between the primary teeth in the spaced primary dentition.

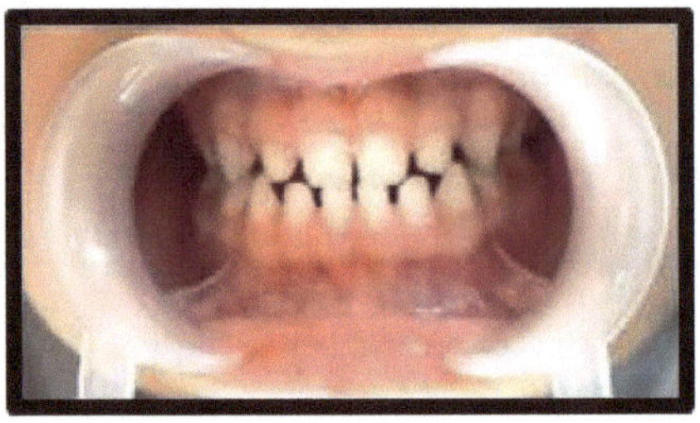

Fig. (10). Physiological.

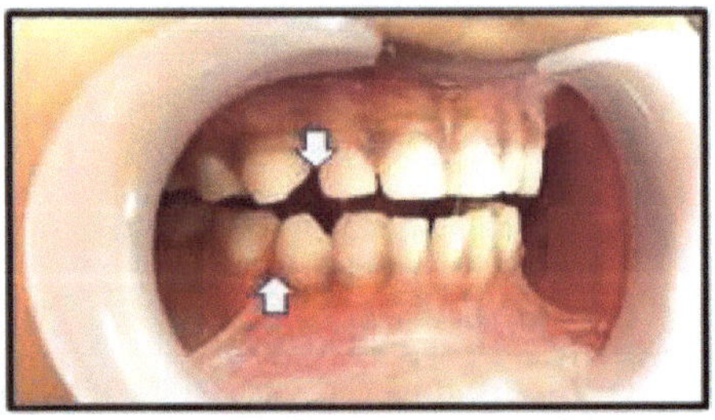

Fig. (11). Primate Space.

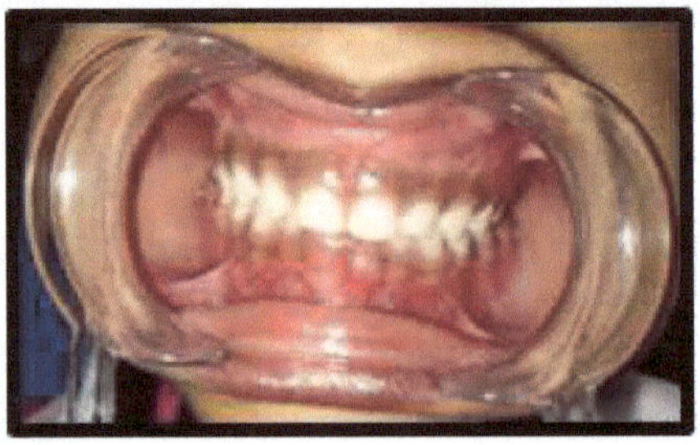

Fig. (12). Non-spaced Space detition.

Molar Relationship in Deciduous Dentition

The mesiodistal relation of the distal surface of the maxillary and mandibular second primary molar is one of the most important factors as it influences the future development of occlusion in permanent dentition and is termed the terminal planes.

Mesio-distal relation between the distal surface of the upper and lower 2nd primary molars when in centric occlusion is called the terminal plane.

As the eruption path of the first permanent molars is guided by the distal surface of the distal root and tooth crown of the second primary molars, the terminal plane determines the interocclusal relationship of the first permanent molars when the upper and lower molars first meet [13, 14].

There are three types of terminal planes (Fig. **13**):

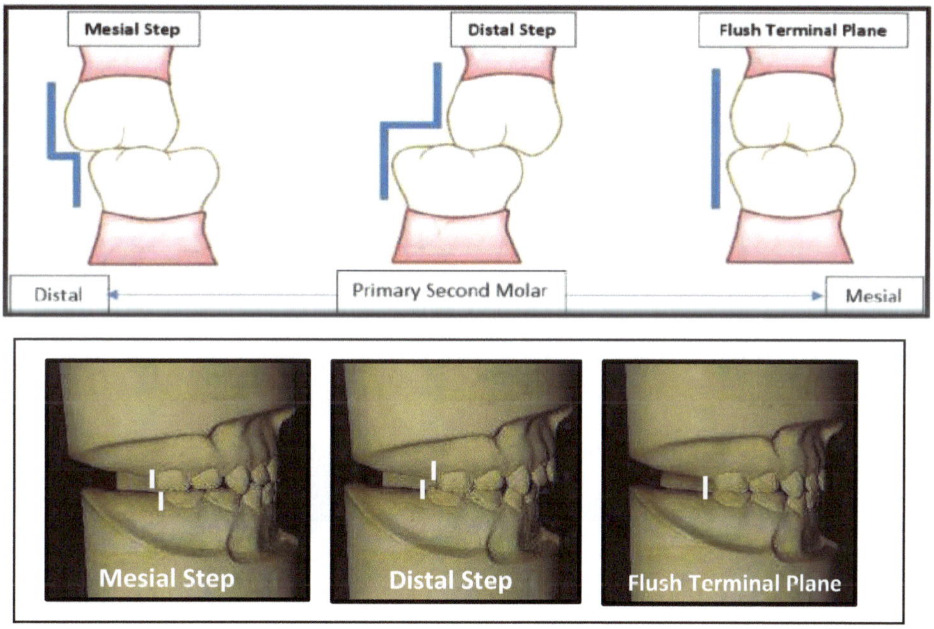

Fig. (13). Terminal planes in primary dentition.

i. **Mesial Step Terminal Plane**- Mandibular terminal plane is more mesial than the maxillary terminal plane. The distal surface of mandibular second molar is more mesial than the distal surface of maxillary second molar. This relation is favourable in guiding permanent molar in Class I molar relationship.

ii. **Distal Step Terminal Plane**- Mandibular terminal plane is more distal to maxillary terminal plane. The distal surface of the mandibular second molar is more distal than the distal surface of maxillary second molar. This relation is favourable in guiding permanent molar in Class II molar relationship.
iii. **Flush Terminal Plane**- Mandibular terminal plane and maxillary terminal plane coincide and are at the same level Antero-posteriorly. The distal surface of mandibular second molar is in the same plane as the distal surface of maxillary second molar. This is the most common molar relationship in deciduous dentition. Primary mandibular molars are wider mesiodistally than maxillary molars. The difference in arch leads to more mesial movement of mandibular permanent 1st molars during the transition. This movement enables the molars to settle in ideal class I relation. Thus, a flush terminal plane is a favourable condition for the development of occlusion.

Upright Incisors

Primary incisors are placed more upright s compared to permanent incisors. Permanent incisors are larger and erupt in the available space. This liability is managed by an increase in labial inclination of permanent incisors.

Shallow Intercuspal Interdigitation (Fig. 14):

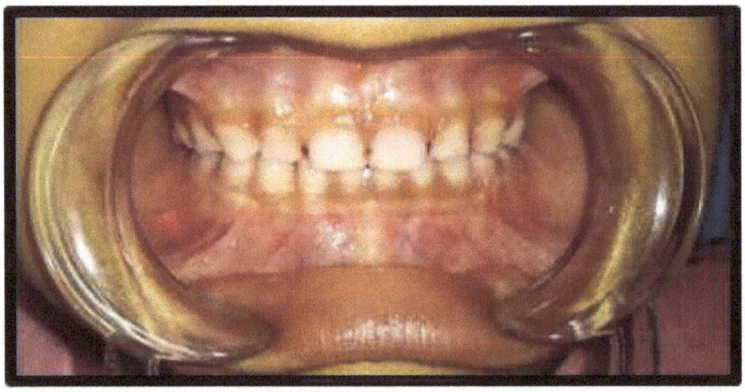

Fig. (14). Primary dentition with of Spee in shallow intercuspation Primary Dentition.

In permanent dentition, the cuspal elevations and deep occlusal fossae are proper. But in primary dentition, as cusps and grooves are less defined, the interdigitations are shallow.

Flat curve of Spee (Fig. 15):

- The curve of Spee is the curvature of the mandibular occlusal plane.
- Acceptable depth is about 2-4 mm.
- In primary dentition, it is flat due to the absence of premolars (Table **8**).

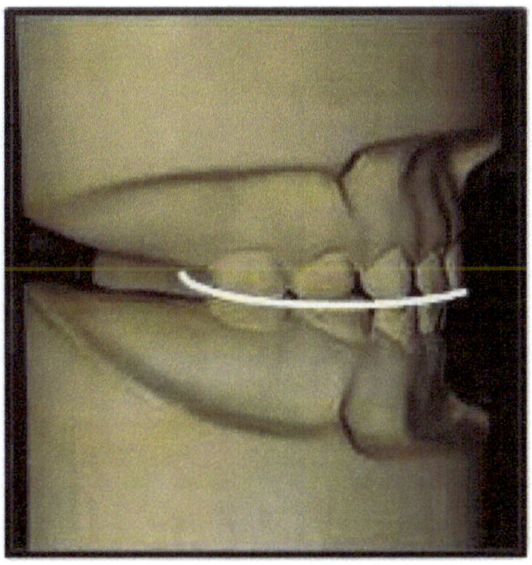

Fig. (15). Flat Curve.

Table 8. Self-Correcting Anomalies in Primary dentition Period.

S. No	Self-Correcting Anomaly	Correction
1	Anterior Deep bite	Eruption of Primary Molars Attrition of incisal edge of primary incisors
2	Flush Terminal Plane	Early mesial shift in the spaced dentition Late mesial Shift in Non-Spaced Dentition Eruption of First Permanent Molar
3	Spacing (Primate and Physiological)	Early Mesial Shift

3. Mixed Dentition Period

- The mixed Dentition period starts with 1st permanent molar eruption by the age of 6 years and lasts till the exfoliation of all deciduous teeth at the age of 12-13 years.
- There may be a temporary open bite in the early part of mixed dentition, usually due to incomplete eruption of incisors or a persistent habit.

- It is a period during which both primary and permanent teeth are in the mouth together, and those permanent teeth that follow into place in the arch once held by a primary tooth are called Successional Teeth (Incisors, Cuspids, and Bicuspids).
- Those teeth that erupt posteriorly to the primary teeth are termed Accessional Teeth (Permanent Molars) (Fig. **16**).

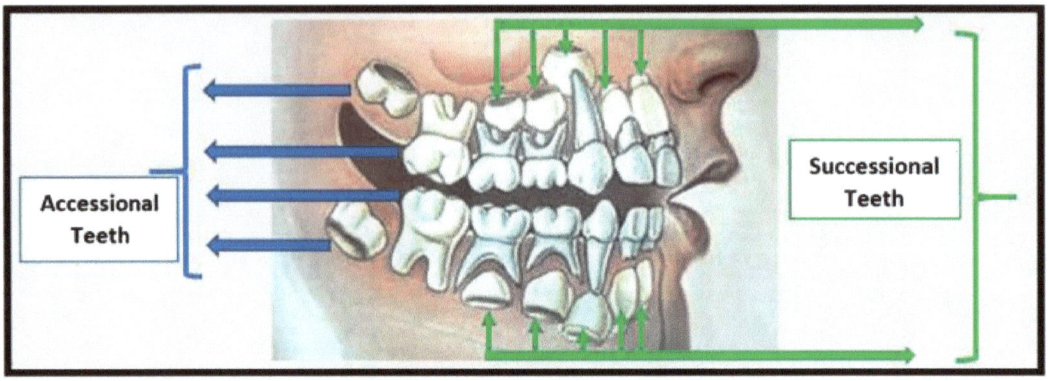

Fig. (16). Successional and accessional teeth.

Phases of Mixed Dentition (Table 9):

First Transition Period:

- Emergence of 1st permanent molar
- Incisor transition
- Establishment of occlusion
    - Inter transition period
    - Second transition period
- Emergence of bicuspids, cuspids & second permanent molar.
- Establishment of occlusion.

First Transition Stage

Emergence of 1st permanent molar:

- Erupts by around the sixth year of life
- Its location & relationship depends upon the distal surface relationship between upper and lower second deciduous molars.
- The distal surface of these deciduous 2nd molars guides the erupting permanent molar into three relations [15] (Fig. **17**).

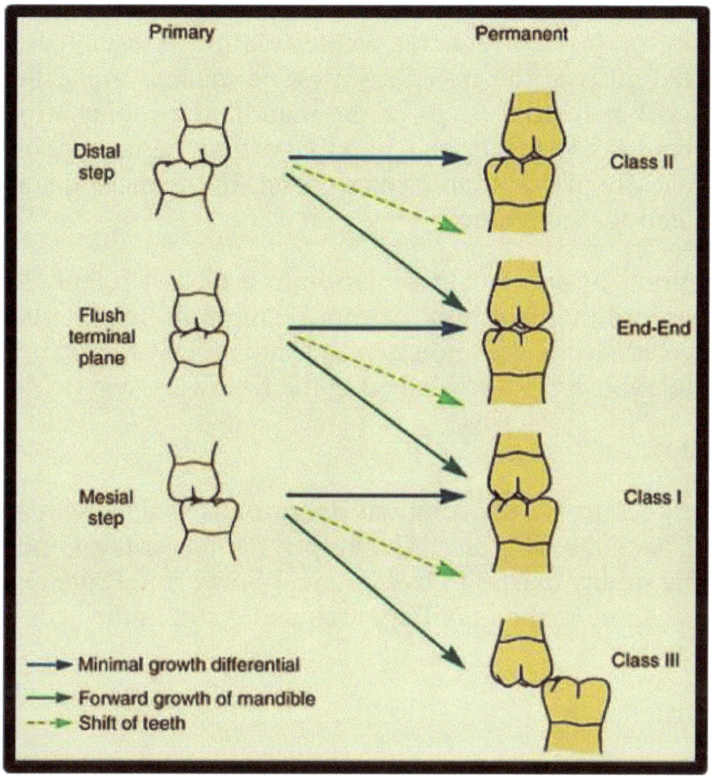

Fig. (17). Progression of terminal planes.

Table 9. List of some important polymers and their roles.

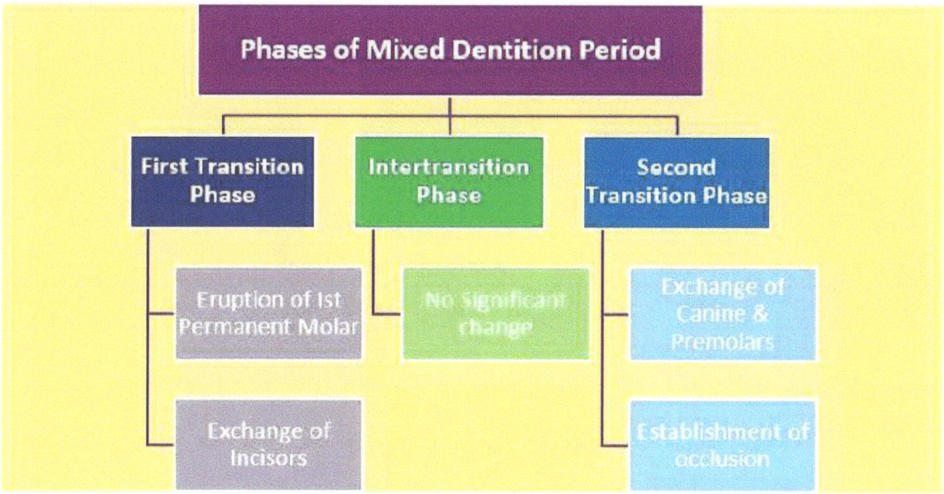

After emergence, the first permanent molars do not attain their maximal contact. However, a more or less correct transverse relation is established because the large mesiopalatal cusp of the maxillary first permanent molar becomes guided between the buccal & lingual cusps of the mandibular molar utilizing the cone-funnel mechanism. As a result, the maxillary first permanent molar becomes slightly more buccally placed than its antagonist. In the mesiodistal direction, the two teeth are in end-to-end relation.

Ideally, the eruption of permanent molars into a class I relationship is desired. Since the flush terminal relation is more common in deciduous dentition, permanent molars are more common to erupt into an end-to-end relationship. The desired Class I relationship is established in the following ways:

Early Mesial Shift

Early mesial shift occurs if the deciduous dentition is spaced with a flush terminal relation of the 2nd deciduous molar. The eruptive force of the 1st permanent molar causes the closure of any existing Physiological Space and Primate Spaces, mesial to the deciduous canine in the maxillary arch and distal to the deciduous canine in the mandibular arch.

Late Mesial Shift

Leeway Space of Nance is the difference between the combined mesiodistal width of primary canine, first molar and second molar (c + d + e) and combined mesiodistal width of their successors, permanent canine, first premolar and second premolar (3 + 4 + 5) (Fig. **18**).

Permanent mandibular first molars migrate mesially utilizing the excess leeway space. This reduces the arch length, converts the flush terminal plane to the mesial step, and provides the class I relationship of permanent molars. This phenomenon is known as ***"late mesial shift."*** (Table **10**).

Table 10. Lee Way space of Nance.

Arch	Leeway Space
Maxillary	1.8 mm (0.9 mm in each arch)
Mandibular	3.4 mm (1.7 mm in each arch)

The Leeway space is utilized for the late mesial shift of the first permanent molars in the non-spaced dentition [16, 17].

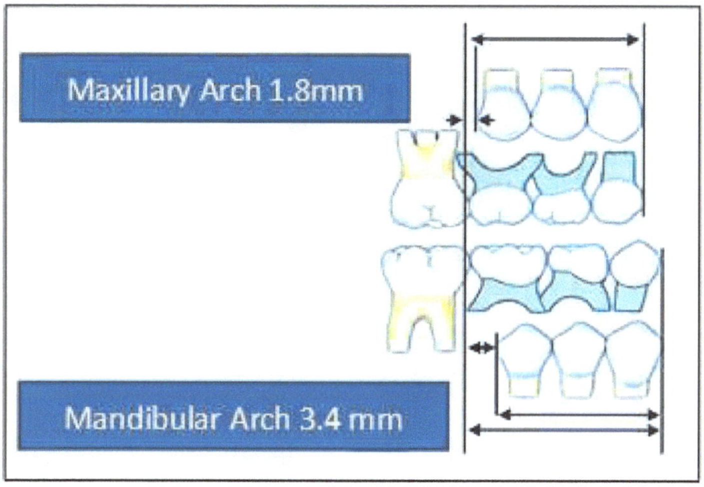

Fig. (18). Lee ways Space of Nance.

Different combination of changes in the deciduous molar relationship to final molar relationship in permanent dentition is because of:

1. Differential growth of the jaws
2. Forward movement of the lower jaws.
3. Shift of teeth.

Incisal Exchange

1. **Incisal Transition-** Interdental spaces are seen in primary dentition, and so its utilization is called incisal translation.
2. **Inter-Canine Width Growth** -Notable growth occurs with the eruption of permanent incisors and canines (Table **11**).

1. **Intercanine Arch Length Increase-** When permanent incisors erupt, they assume a somewhat more anteriorly inclined position than deciduous incisors.

This position of the incisors averages 2.3 mm and results in an increase in

- Inter canine arch length of approximately 3mm without any change in inter canine width (Fig. **19**).
- Inter incisal angle between maxillary and mandibular incisors in primary dentition is 150 degrees. It reduces to 123 degrees in the permanent dentition

due to more proclination and gains space for incisor alignment. This is called ***Incisal Labiality*** (Fig. **20**).

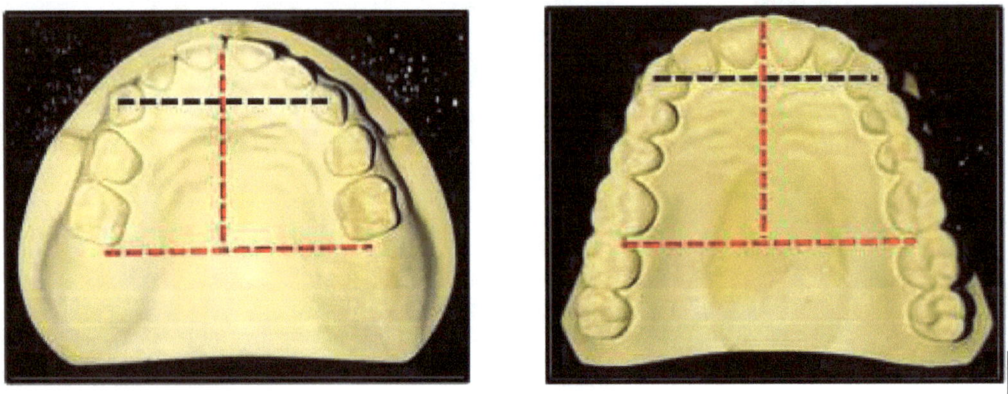

Fig. (19). Arch length (Red) and Intercanine Arch Width (Black).

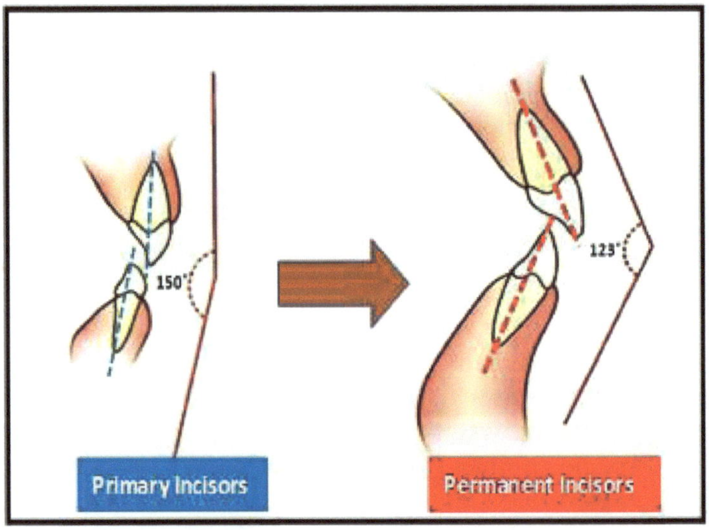

Fig. (20). Incisal labiality.

Table 11. Difference in arch width.

Gender	Dental Arch	Width Increases Between 2-18 Year
Male	Maxilla Mandible	6 mm 4 mm
Female	Maxilla Mandible	4.5 mm 4 mm

Incisal Liability

The unerupted permanent incisors are larger than the deciduous incisors.

The difference between the amount of space needed for accommodation of permanent incisors and the amount of space available is referred to as ***Incisal Liability*** (Table **12**, Fig. **21**).

Table 12. Incisal Liability.

Arch	Incisal liability
Maxillary	7 mm
Mandibular	5 mm

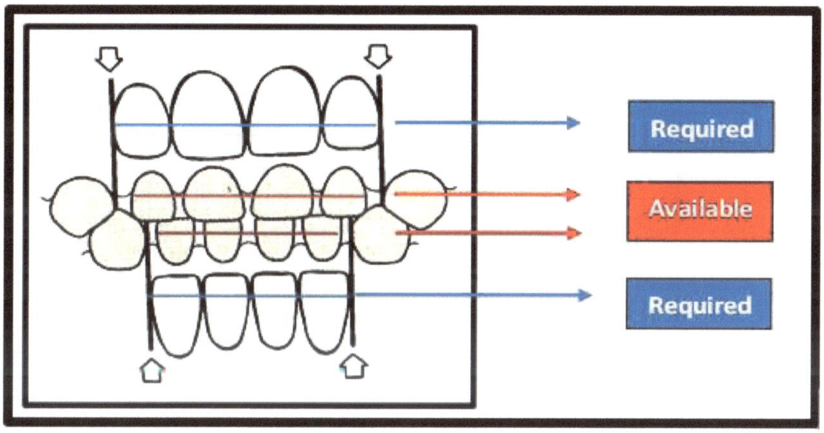

Fig. (21). Incisal Labiality.

The Following Factors Overcome the Incisal Liability

A. Utilization of interdental spaces seen in the deciduous dentition.
B. Increase in inter-canine width
C. Change in interincisal angulation.

Overjet and Overbite (Fig. 22):

OVERJET is the horizontal distance between the lingual aspect of the maxillary incisors and the labial aspect of the mandibular incisors when the teeth are in centric occlusion. The average in primary dentition is 1-2mm.

OVERBITE is the measurement of the incisal edge of the maxillary incisors that overlap vertically past the mandibular incisors' incisal edge. The primary incisors erupt in a deep bite or increased overbite, corrected by the eruption of posterior teeth around five years of age. The average overbite in the primary dentition is 2mm.

Overbite (Vertical overlap) and Overjet (Horizontal overlap) undergo significant changes during the deciduous and mixed dentitions. During the deciduous dentition, the overbite usually decreases slightly, and the overjet is reduced. From the early mixed dentition to the completion of the permanent dentition, the average overbite increases somewhat and then decreases. However, a significant variability can be noticed.

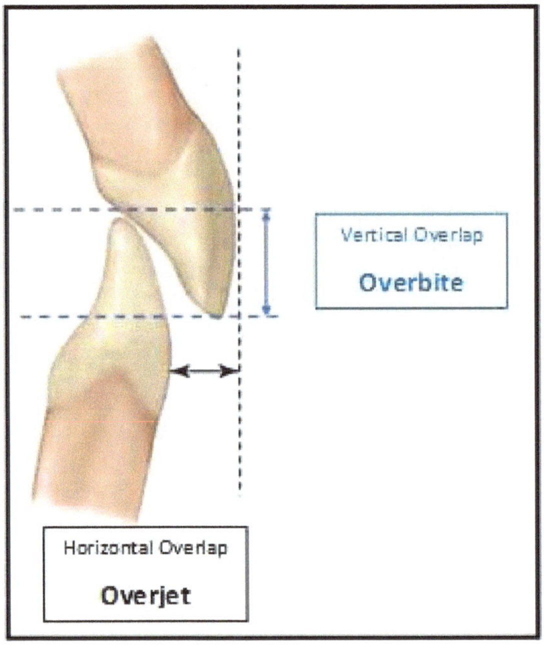

Fig. (22). Overjet and Overbite.

Edge to Edge Bite

When the incisal edges of the two incisors are in the same plane. It is also called ***zero overbite***.

Inter-Transitional Period

- Both sets of teeth present
- 4 permanent incisors & 1st permanent molars present
- Deciduous canines and 1st & 2nd deciduous molars

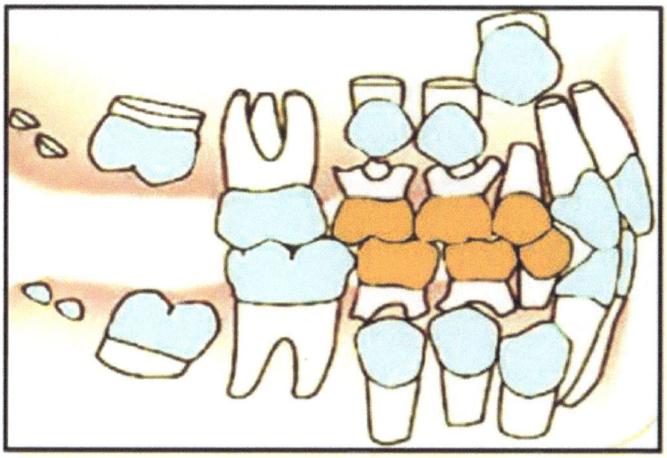

Fig. (23). Inter-transitional Period.

In the Inter-transitional period, the mandibular and maxillary dental arches consist of deciduous and permanent teeth. This phase of the mixed dentition period is relatively stable, and minor change occurs. Deciduous canines and molars are present between the permanent incisors and the first permanent molars.

The maxillary incisors are labially inclined. Mandibular incisors are less labially inclined than in the maxilla. A diastema seldom exists between the mandibular central incisors. All incisor crowns are usually in contact with each other, and the laterals touch the primary canine crowns.

Resorption of the primary roots and reduction in surrounding bone within the jaws occurs. These processes prepare for the second transitional period. The permanent teeth are still to emerge. Their roots increase in length, and the crown of the third molars, if present, starts to calcify. This calcification of a third molar happens at approximately the same time as the furcation of the adjacent second permanent molar is formed. Mandibular third molars start to calcify before their maxillary third molars (Fig. **23**).

Second Transition Period-

This phase is characterized by the exchange of deciduous canines & molars by premolars and permanent cuspids. It occurs at around 9-11 years of age and is very crucial for the alignment of the erupting permanent teeth.

The combined mesiodistal width of permanent canine and premolar is less than that of deciduous canine and molars. This extra space is called the Leeway space of Nance.

To establish Class I occlusion in late mesial shift, it is utilized by the mandibular molars. The mesiodistal dimension of the Deciduous Second Molar (E) is more than that of Permanent Second Premolars (5). This excess space is called ***E-space*** [18] (Fig. **24**).

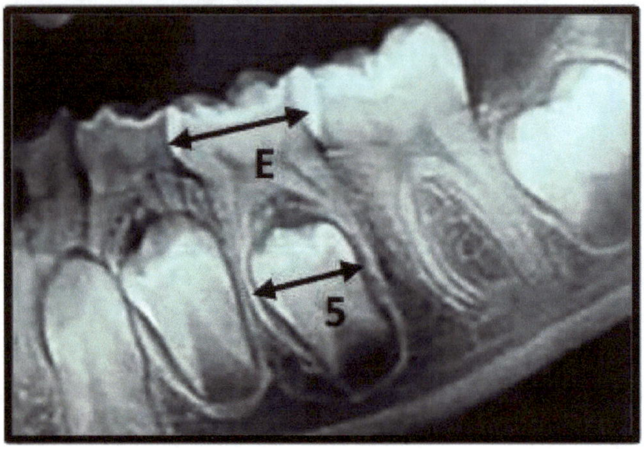

Fig. (24). E Space.

Ugly Duckling Stage

This is also known as the Broadbent phenomenon, as first described by H Broadbent in 1937. He described this situation as the ugly duckling stage.

As the developing permanent canines erupt, they displace the roots of the lateral incisors mesially and, in turn, onto the central incisors. This causes the flaring up of the incisor crowns, thus causing a midline diastema.

This occurs around the age of 9-11 years. This corrects itself when the permanent canine erupts completely.

This stage is called ugly duckling because of the unesthetic appearance of a child during this stage. No orthodontic treatment should be carried out during this stage as there is a danger that the canine can deflect from its path of eruption [19, 20] (Fig. **25**).

PERMANENT DENTITION

This stage begins with the exfoliation of the last primary teeth and eruption of all Permanent teeth except 3rd molar. The normal occlusion in permanent dentition is characterized by correction of anterior deep bite, stabilization of occlusion, reduction in overjet, and shortening of dental arches.

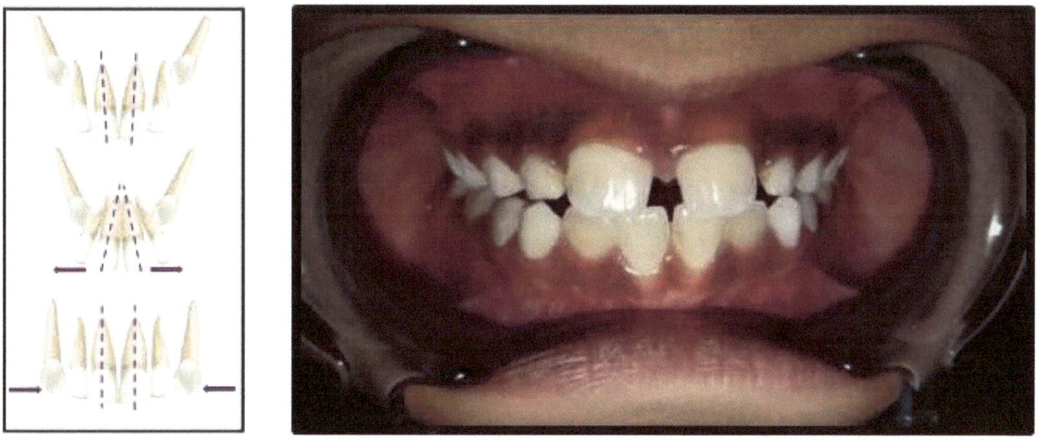

Fig. (25). Ugly Duckling stage.

Favourable Sequence of Eruption of Permanent dentition (Fig. **26**) [7, 8].

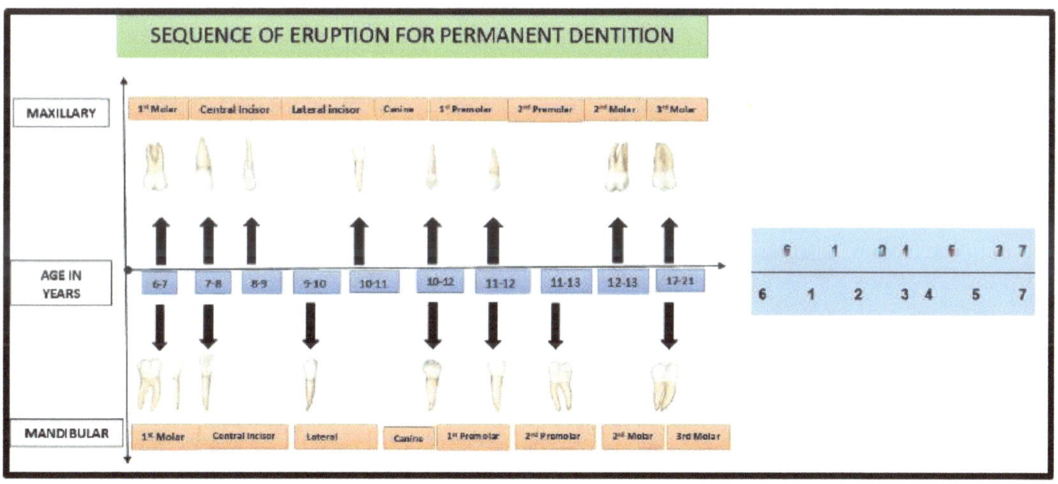

Fig. (26). Sequence of Eruption of Permanent teeth.
6 1 2 4 5 3 7 8 in Maxillary Arch
6 1 2 3 4 5 7 8 in Mandibular Arch

Features of Permanent Dentition

A harmonious relationship exists between the hard structures and soft tissue in the orofacial region, projecting a pleasing profile in normal occlusion. The midline of each dental arch is in line with the other and the face's midline. The lips meet without effort when jaws are at rest. The lips are relatively flush and do not reveal interposed teeth or tongue. The profiles can vary within a range of normal dental occlusion. In normal occlusion, no movement of the lips is seen during deglutition.

Vertical overbite of about one-third the clinical crown height of the mandibular central incisors. Overjet and overbite decrease throughout the second decade of life due to more significant forward growth of the mandible.

Andrew's Keys to Normal Occlusion

Andrew LF in 1972 described Six keys of ideal occlusion. Bolton's Ratio was added later in 1993 by Mc Launghlin.

1. Molar inter-arch relationship
2. Mesio-distal crown angulation
3. Labio-lingual crown angulation
4. Absence of rotation
5. Tight contacts
6. Curve of Spee
7. Bolton's tooth ratio

1) **Molar Inter-Arch Relationship: -** Mesiobuccal cusp of Maxillary first permanent molar occludes in the mesiobuccal groove of Mandibular first permanent molar. Canine and premolars have a cusp embrasure relationship buccally and a cusp fossa relationship lingually (Fig. **27**).

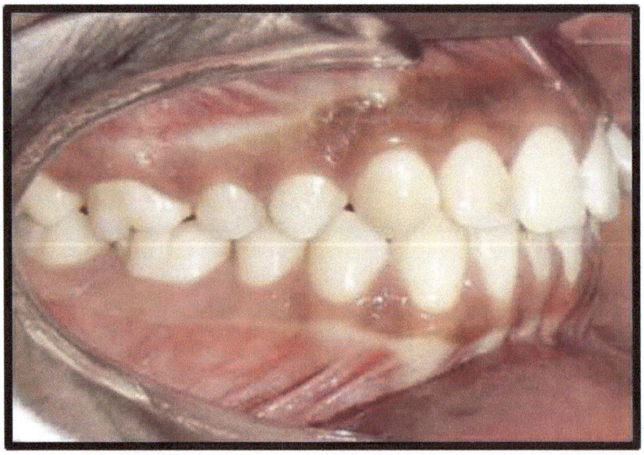

Fig. (27). Molar Inter-arch Relationship.

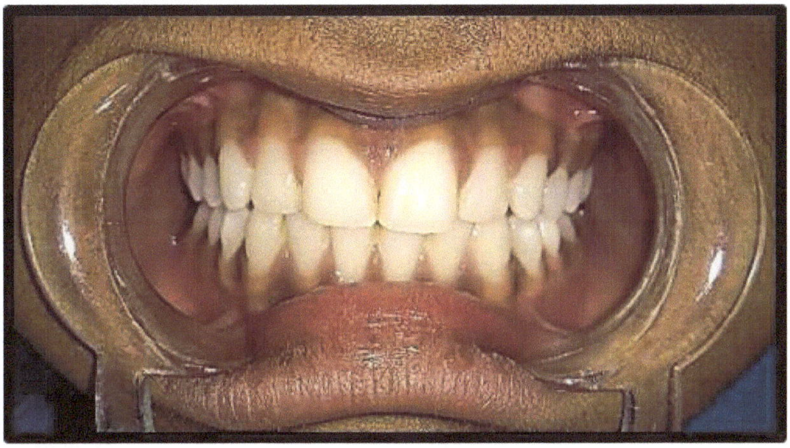

Fig. (28). Crown Angulation.

1. **Mesiodistal Crown Angulation**- Mesiodistal Crown angulation must be positive. Crown angulation refers to angulation of the long axis of the crown, not to angulation of the long axis of the entire tooth. Gingival part of the long axis of all the crown must be distal to that of the Incisal/Occlusal part (Fig. **28**).
2. **Crown Inclination:** Crown Inclination refers to the labiolingual or buccolingual inclination of long axis of the crown, not to the inclination of the long axis of the entire tooth.

   Labio-Lingual Crown Inclination of Maxillary incisors should be Positive, which means the cervical area of the crown is lingually placed. For the rest of all teeth, including Mandibular incisors, crown inclination should be slightly negative, which means the cervical area of the crown is buccally/labially placed (Fig. **29**).
3. **Absence of Rotation-** Normal occlusion consists of teeth free of undesirable rotation. (Fig. **30**).
4. **Tight Contacts-** Permanent teeth should have tight contact to optimize the space. In the absence of abnormalities such as genuine tooth size discrepancies, the contact point should be tight (Fig. **31**).
5. **Curve of Spee-** Curve of Spee should not exceed 1.5cm. The depth of the Curve of Spee ranges from a flat plane to a slightly concave surface. The natural tendency of the Curve of Spee deepens with time. (Fig. **32**).
6. **Bolton's Ratio** (Correct tooth size)- Benett and McLaughlin in 1993 gave the Seventh key to normal occlusion. The upper and lower tooth size should be correct. Roth (1981) adds some functional keys to previous keys given by Andrew:
   a. Centric relationship and centric occlusion should be coincident.
   b. In protrusion, the incisor dis-occludes the posterior teeth, with the guidance

provided by the lower incisal edges passing the palatal contour of the upper incisors.

c. In lateral excursions of the mandible, the canine should guide the working side while all other teeth on that and the other side are dis-occluded.

d. When the teeth are in centric occlusion, there should be even bilateral contacts in the buccal segments.

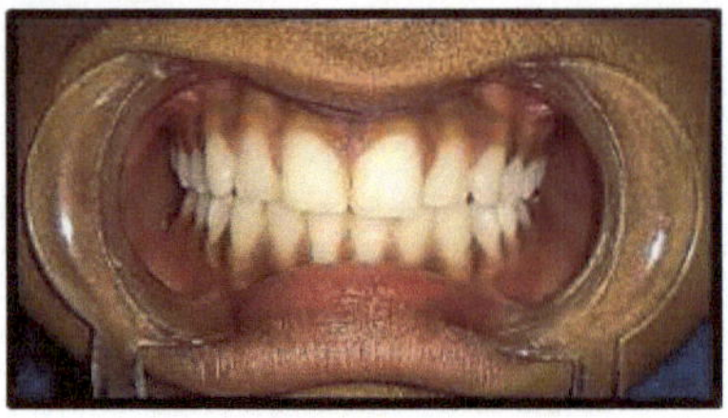

Fig. (29). Crown Inclination.

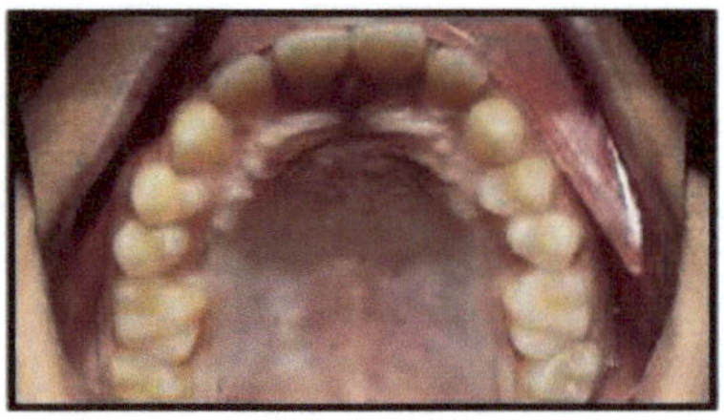

Fig. (30). Absence or rotation.

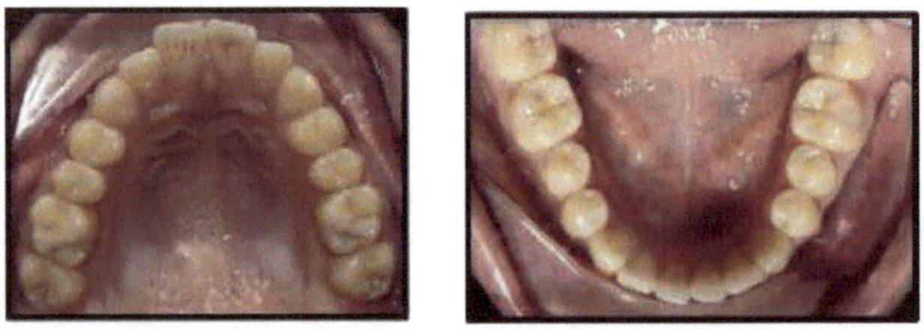

Fig. (31). Tight Contact.

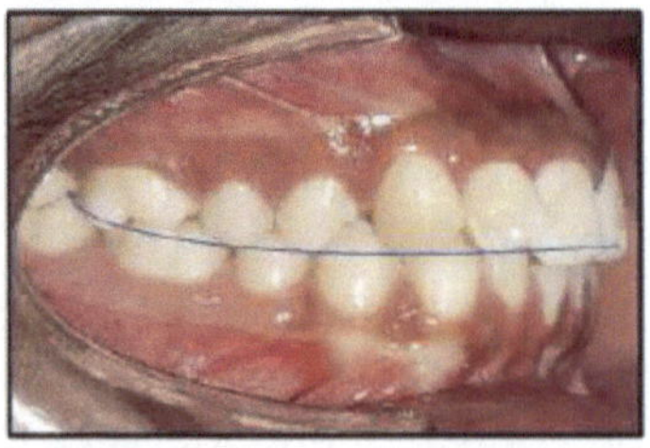

Fig. (32). Curve of Spee.

Self-Correcting Anomalies

During the Development of Occlusion, some Anomalies arise in a child's developing dentition during the transition from pre-dentate to permanent dentition. These anomalies get corrected independently without any dental treatment, referred to as Self-Correcting anomalies. Classification of self-correcting anomalies is based on the period of development of occlusion as in the pre-dentate period (Table **6**), Deciduous Dentition period (Table **8**), and Mixed Dentition period (Tables **13** & **14**).

Table 13. Self-correcting anomalies in mixed dentition period.

S. No	Self-correcting Anomaly	Correction
1	Anterior Deep bite	Super-eruption of Permanent Molars
2	Ugly Duckling Stage	Eruption of Permanent Canine
3	End-On Molar Relation	Super-eruption of Permanent Molars Late Mesial Shift utilizing Lee Way Space of Nance
4	Mandibular Anterior Crowding	Increase in intercanine Width Labial inclination of Mandibular Incisors Tongue Pressure

Table 14. Developmental Anomalies.

Anomaly	Developmental Stage	Etiology	Description	Clinical Features
Number				
Anodontia Hypodontia Oligodontia [21]	Initiation	Hereditary, Systemic Disease, Excess Radiation Exposure, Endocrine Dysfunction.	Hypodontia: Absence of single or multiple teeth. Most common teeth are maxillary lateral incisor and mandibular second premolar. Oligodontia: Absences of six or more teeth. Anodontia: Complete absence of teeth.	May cause disruption of occlusion and aesthetic problems. May need partial or complete dentures, bridges, or implants to replace teeth.

(Table 14) cont.....

Anomaly	Developmental Stage	Etiology	Description	Clinical Features
Hyperdontia Supernumerary teeth	Initiation	Hereditary	Presence of one or more extra teeth. Examples: Mesiodens, Para molars, Distomolar, Supplemental teeth, Odontoma.	Commonly found in maxillary central, distal to 3rd molar, and premolar region may cause crowding, failure of normal occlusion, and disruption of occlusion.
Size				
Microdontia and Macrodontia	Bud stage	Hereditary with partial dysfunction: endocrine dysfunction with complete	Abnormally small or large teeth	It commonly affects the maxillary lateral incisor and 3rd molar with partial microdontia.
Shape				
Dens in Dente and Dens invaginatus	Cap stage	Hereditary	Enamel organ invaginate into dental papilla	It commonly affects the maxillary lateral incisor, has deep lingual pits, and needs endodontic therapy.
Gemination	Cap stage	Hereditary	Splitting to single tooth germ.	Large single-rooted teeth with one pulp cavity twinning in the crown area, a normal number of teeth in dentition, may cause a problem in appearance and spacing.
Fusion [22, 23]	Cap stage	Pressure on area	Union of two adjacent tooth germ	Large teeth with two pulp cavities. and one fewer tooth in dentition may cause a problem in appearance and spacing.
Concrescence	Apposition and maturation stage	Traumatic injury or crowding of teeth.	Union of the root structure of two or teeth by cementum	It commonly affects permanent maxillary molars. Problem with extractions.

(Table 14) cont.....

Anomaly	Developmental Stage	Etiology	Description	Clinical Features
Dens Evaginatus (Leong's premolar, evaginated odontome, occlusal enamel pearl)	Proliferation and evagination of an area of the inner enamel epithelium and subjacent odontogenic mesenchyme into the dental organ during early tooth development.	Local or systemic hereditary.	The condition appears clinically as an accessory cusp or a globule of enamel on the occlusal surface between the buccal and lingual cusp of premolars	It resembles physically. It is an extra cusp that may contribute to the incomplete eruption, displacement of teeth, and or pulp exposure with subsequent infection leads to occlusal wear or fracture.
Talon's cusp	Morpho differentiation	Local or systemic hereditary.	Eagle's talon projects lingually from the cingulum area of the maxillary or mandibular permanent incisor. Maybe prevalent in patients with Rubinstein Taybi syndrome.	Deep developmental groove where the cusp blends with the sloping lingual tooth surface. Problems associated with esthetics, caries control and occlusal accommodation. Treatment can be prophylactically restoring the groove to prevent caries, coronoplasty, endodontic therapy
Taurodontism	Has Primitive pattern It is caused by the failure of Hertwig's epithelial root sheath to invaginate at the proper horizontal level.	Genetic - mendelian recessive trait, Mutation.	Bull-like tooth in which the body of the tooth is enlarged at the expense of the roots.	It affects both primary and permanent dentition. Most commonly, molars can be unilateral and bilateral or in combination .no specific treatment is required.
Dilaceration	Morpho differentiation	Trauma	Sharp angulation, bend or curve in the root or crown of a formed tooth.	Trauma during the period in which the tooth is forming results in the position of the calcified portion of the tooth being changed, and the remaining teeth are formed at an angle.
Tubercle	Cap stage	Trauma pressure or metabolic disease	Extra cusp form effects on enamel organ	Commonly affect permanent molar or cingulum of anterior teeth.

(Table 14) cont.....

Anomaly	Developmental Stage	Etiology	Description	Clinical Features
Enamel pearl	Apposition and maturation stage	Displacement of ameloblast to root	Sphere of enamel on the root.	It may be confused with calculus deposits on the root.
Developmental Disturbance				
Enamel dysplasia Enamel Hypoplasia Turners Hypoplasia	Apposition and maturation stage	Local or systemic hereditary	Faulty development of enamel from interference involving ameloblast	Pitting and extrinsic colour change in enamel with changes in enamel thickness is possible. Problem in function and aesthetics.

CONCLUSION

The masticatory system in a developing child goes through continuous transformation. Therefore, the occlusion of a growing child or teenager should never be considered inactive. The specific situations or positions of the teeth in the dental arch are decided principally by the tongue and by the perioral musculature (the lips and cheeks), normal and abnormal functional characteristics of the face, masticatory forces, shape, and size of the crowns of the teeth, the surrounding supportive tissues and the forces working within the dentition.

Reorganization of eruption timings is more desirable in the present era since dentistry has widened its perspectives towards many specialized fields. Developing norms of the emergence of permanent teeth need to be recognized for diagnosis, treatment planning, preventive dentistry procedures, archaeological, anthropological, paleontological, and may have legal as well as forensic application.

CONSENT FOR PUBLICATION

Not applicable.

CONFLICT OF INTEREST

The author(s) declare no conflict of interest, financial or otherwise.

ACKNOWLEDGEMENT

Declared none.

REFERENCES

[1] Yu T, Klein OD. Molecular and cellular mechanisms of tooth development, homeostasis and repair. Development 2020; 147(2): dev184754. [http://dx.doi.org/10.1242/dev.184754] [PMID: 31980484]

[2] Nolla CM. The development of permanent teeth. ASDC J Dent Child 1960; 27: 254-66.

[3] Nanci A. Ten Cate's oral histology-e-book: Development, Structure, and Function. Missouri. 9th Edition., Elsevier Health Sciences 2017.

[4] Thesleff I. Current understanding of the process of tooth formation: transfer from the laboratory to the clinic. Aust Dent J 2014; 59 (Suppl. 1): 48-54. [http://dx.doi.org/10.1111/adj.12102] [PMID: 24236691]

[5] Kariya P, Tandon S, Singh S, Tewari N. Polymorphism in emergence of deciduous dentition: A cross-sectional study of Indian children. J Investig Clin Dent 2018; 9(1): e12266-83. [http://dx.doi.org/10.1111/jicd.12266] [PMID: 28349669]

[6] Logan WHG, Kronfeld R. Development of the human jaws and surrounding structures from birth to age fifteen. J Am Dent Assoc 1933; 20: 379.

[7] Burgueño Torres L, Mourelle Martínez MR, de Nova García JM. A study on the chronology and sequence of eruption of primary teeth in Spanish children. Eur J Paediatr Dent 2015; 16(4): 301-4. [PMID: 26637254]

[8] Bulut G, Bulut H, Ortac R. A comprehensive survey of natal and neonatal teeth in newborns. Niger J Clin Pract 2019; 22(11): 1489-94. [http://dx.doi.org/10.4103/njcp.njcp_152_19] [PMID: 31719269]

[9] Fernandes S, Gordhanbhai Patel D, Ranadheer E, Kalgudi J, Santokì J, Chaudhary S. Occlusal Traits of Primary Dentition among Pre-School Children of Mehsana District, North Gujarat, India. J Clin Diagn Res 2017; 11(1): ZC92-6. [http://dx.doi.org/10.7860/JCDR/2017/22515.9266] [PMID: 28274054]

[10] Shavi GR, Hiremath NV, Shukla R, Bali PK, Jain SK, Ajagannanavar SL. Prevalence of Spaced and Non-Spaced Dentition and Occlusal Relationship of Primary Dentition and its Relation to Malocclusion in School Children of Davangere. J Int Oral Health 2015; 7(9): 75-8. [PMID: 26435622]

[11] Sun KT, Li YF, Hsu JT, *et al.* Prevalence of primate and interdental spaces for primary dentition in 3- to 6-year-old children in Taiwan. J Formos Med Assoc 2018; 117(7): 598-604. [http://dx.doi.org/10.1016/j.jfma.2017.07.010] [PMID: 28811069]

[12] Srinivasan D, Loganathan D, Kumar SS, Louis CJ, Eagappan S, Natarajan D. An evaluation of occlusal relationship and primate space in deciduous dentition in Kancheepuram District, Tamil Nadu, India. J Pharm Bioallied Sci 2017; 9(5) (Suppl. 1): 45. [http://dx.doi.org/10.4103/jpbs.JPBS_89_17] [PMID: 29284935]

[13] Kumar D, Gurunathan D. Primary Canine and Molar Relationships in Centric Occlusion in 3- to 6-year-old Children: A Cross-sectional Survey. Int J Clin Pediatr Dent 2019; 12(3): 201-4. [http://dx.doi.org/10.5005/jp-journals-10005-1622] [PMID: 31708615]

[14] Anu V, Pavani B, Pavani D, Liana BJX, Lubna FA, Saikrishna YV. Distribution of School Children Based on the Type of Terminal Plane in Primary Dentition: A Study among 3- to 5-year-old Children in Chennai, Tamil Nadu, India. Int J Clin Pediatr Dent 2020; 13(2): 136-7. [http://dx.doi.org/10.5005/jp-journals-10005-1722] [PMID: 32742089]

[15] Dimberg L, Lennartsson B, Arnrup K, Bondemark L. Prevalence and change of malocclusions from primary to early permanent dentition: A longitudinal study. Angle Orthod 2015; 85(5): 728-34. [http://dx.doi.org/10.2319/080414-542.1] [PMID: 25867255]

[16] Vyas M, Hantodkar N. Resolving mandibular arch discrepancy through utilization of leeway space.

Contemp Clin Dent 2011; 2(2): 115-8.
[http://dx.doi.org/10.4103/0976-237X.83077] [PMID: 21957388]

[17] Allen TR, Trojan TM, Harris EF. Evidence favoring a secular reduction in mandibular leeway space. Angle Orthod 2017; 87(4): 576-82.
[http://dx.doi.org/10.2319/091416-688.1] [PMID: 28318312]

[18] Raghav P, Reddy M, Jain S, Mohan S, Wadhawan A. Sequential Utilization of E-space for Correction of Moderate Crowding: A Case Report. Int J Clin Pediatr Dent 2018; 11(6): 519-25.
[http://dx.doi.org/10.5005/jp-journals-10005-1568] [PMID: 31303741]

[19] Tanaka OM, Morino AYK, Machuca OF, Schneider NÁ. When the Midline Diastema Is Not Characteristic of the "Ugly Duckling" Stage. Case Rep Dent 2015; 2015: 1-5.
[http://dx.doi.org/10.1155/2015/924743] [PMID: 26345220]

[20] Masłowska-Kasowicz A, Nowicka-Dudek K, Zadurska M, Shybinsky V, Lesitskiy M, Chukhray N. The incidence of malocclusions in children at the "ugly duckling" stage. Forum Ortodontyczne / Orthodontic Forum 2019; 15(1): 14-26.

[21] Khalaf K, Miskelly J, Voge E, Macfarlane TV. Prevalence of hypodontia and associated factors: a systematic review and meta-analysis. J Orthod 2014; 41(4): 299-316.
[http://dx.doi.org/10.1179/1465313314Y.0000000116] [PMID: 25404667]

[22] Khan R, Kariya PB, Mallikarjuna R, Singh AN. Fusion of permanent maxillary right central incisor and mesiodens in an 8-year-old child. BMJ Case Rep 2015; 2015(jan06 1): bcr2014208541.
[http://dx.doi.org/10.1136/bcr-2014-208541] [PMID: 25564644]

[23] Bernardi S, Bianchi S, Bernardi G, *et al.* Clinical management of fusion in primary mandibular incisors: a systematic literature review. Acta Odontol Scand 2020; 78(6): 417-24.
[http://dx.doi.org/10.1080/00016357.2020.1734233] [PMID: 32125202]

CHAPTER 12

Morphology of Primary Dentition

Parag D. Kasar[1,*], **Dhanashree Sakhare**[2] and **Shailaja Chatterjee**[3]

[1] *Deep Dental Clinic, Nerul, Navi Mumbai, India*

[2] *Lavanika Academy, Melbourne, Australia*

[3] *Department of Oral Pathology, Yamuna College of Dental Sciences and Research, Yamuna Nagar, Haryana, India*

Abstract: Study of dental morphology or characteristics refers to phylogenetic data related to different species. The morphology of a tooth is affected by the genetic constitution, environmental factors, habit of digit sucking, and a variety of parafunctional habits. Tooth development is a long process that involves interactions at molecular and cellular levels, which are influenced by environmental, genetic, and epigenetic factors. Human dentition is undergoing constant evolutionary changes. However, these changes are occurring at different rates in different geographical populations. Knowledge and information about the morphological features of each primary tooth are crucial for pediatric operative dentistry and forensic dentistry. The mesiodistal dimensions of individual teeth provide important information related to human evolution. The differences in tooth eruption, shape, and size can reflect the process of evolution and provide a method of studying evolutionary mechanisms. Measurements of teeth and dental arches have been used for the description and comparison of different populations or racial groups.

Keywords: Crown Size, Mesiodistal Dimensions, Morphology, Primary teeth.

INTRODUCTION

The study of morphological features of the individual primary teeth is very useful for improving the quality of pediatric operative dentistry. The dimensions of the teeth vary according to race and gender [1]. Data regarding the morphological features and dimensions of teeth are valuable in anthropological studies [1, 2]. Genetic and environmental factors influence tooth size. The tooth size estimation is also crucial for determining the abnormal development of dental occlusion.

* **Corresponding author Parag D Kasar:** Deep dental clinic, NL 1 B, 36/7, Shatkarappt owners asson, Sector 10, Nerul Navi Mumbai, Maharashtra 400 706; E-mails: parag.pedodontist@gmail.com

Tooth Numbering System

Commonly used tooth numbering systems for teeth identification in dentistry are:

1. Universal Numbering System (Figs. 1 and 2):

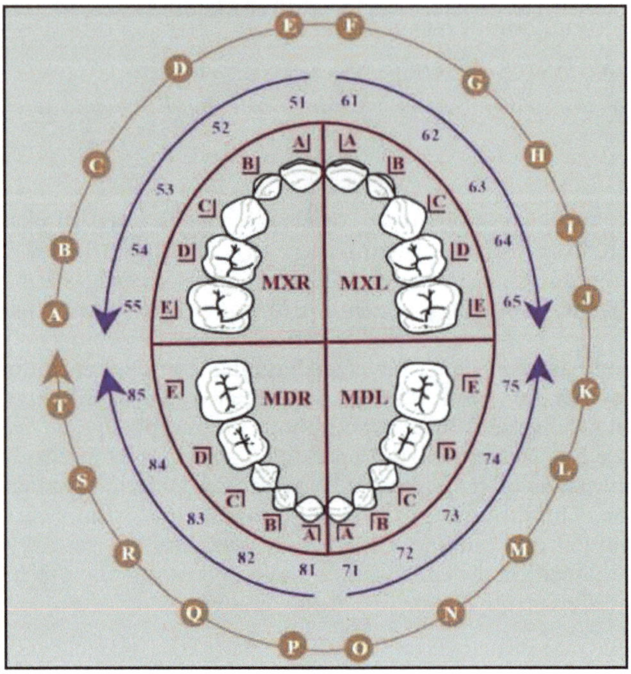

Fig. (1). Primary Dentition Numbering system **Brown: Universal Numbering System; Blue: FDI Numbering System;Red: Palmer Notation System. MXR**: maxillary right quadrant, **MXL**: Maxillary left quadrant, **MDL**: Mandibular left quadrant, MDR: Mandibular right quadrant.

A: The Primary Universal Numbering System (Fig. **1**) was adopted by the ADA in 1968 [3]. The farthest back tooth on the right side of the maxillary jaw is labelled as A. The letters continue along with the maxillary teeth toward the front and across the midline to the farthest back tooth on the left side of the maxillary jaw labelled by the letter J. The letters continue by dropping down to the farthest back tooth on the left side of the mandibular jaw, labelled as K. Letters continue again toward the front and across the midline to the farthest back tooth on the mandibular right side, labelled as T.

B: The Permanent Universal Numbering System (Fig. **2**): The ADA adopted it [3]. The farthest back tooth on the right side of the maxillary jaw is numbered as 1. The numbers continue along with the maxillary teeth toward the front and across the midline to the farthest back tooth on the left side of the maxillary jaw, numbered 16. The numbers continue by dropping down to the farthest back tooth on the left side of the mandibular jaw, numbered 17. Numbers continue again toward the front and across the midline to the farthest back tooth on the mandibular right side, numbered 32.

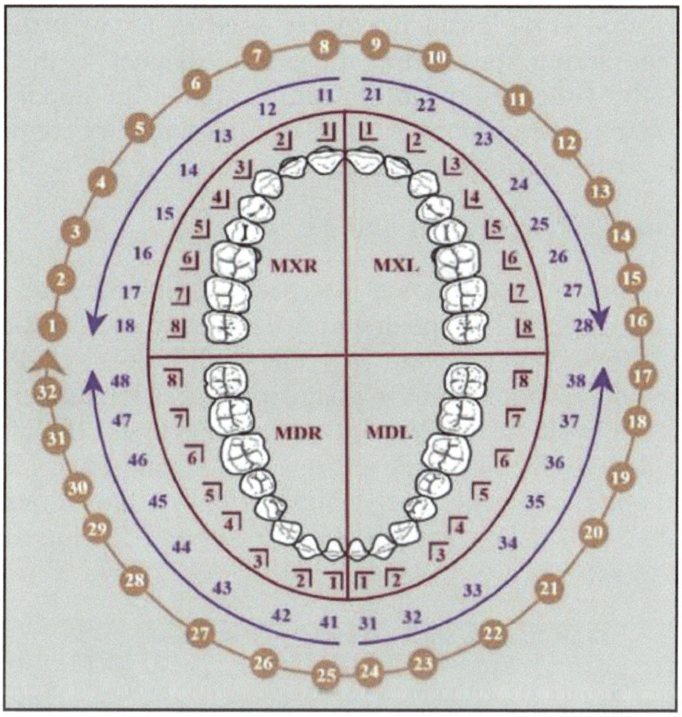

Fig. (2). Permanent Dentition Numbering System. **Brown: Universal Numbering System; Blue: FDI Numbering System;Red: Palmer Notation System. MXR**: maxillary right quadrant, **MXL**: Maxillary left quadrant, **MDL**: Mandibular left quadrant, MDR: Mandibular right quadrant.

2. Palmer Notation System (Figs. 1 and 2):

A: The Primary Palmer Notation Numbering System [3]: The mouth is divided into 4 sections called quadrants. Vertically mouth is divided into right and left halves by a line passing between maxillary and mandibular central incisors while the horizontal line divides the mouth into maxillary and mandibular arches. The letters A through E and a unique symbol (Fig. **1** red lines) is used to identify the teeth in each quadrant. The letters run from the tooth adjacent to the midline to the farthest back tooth of the mouth on the same side. In the upper right quadrant tooth, A denotes the central incisor; the letters continue to the right and back till the second molar, which is denoted by the letter E. Fig. (**1**).

B: The Permanent Palmer Notation Numbering System [3]: This system was originally called Zsigmondy System. The mouth is divided into 4 sections called quadrants. Vertically mouth is divided into right and left halves by a line passing between maxillary and mandibular central incisors, while the horizontal line divides the mouth into maxillary and mandibular arches. The numbers 1 through 8 and a unique symbol (Fig. **2** red lines) are used to identify the teeth in each quadrant. The numbering starts from the tooth adjacent to the midline to the farthest back tooth of the mouth on the same side. In the upper right quadrant, tooth number 1 denotes the central incisor, and the numbers continue to the right and back till the third molar, which is denoted by number 8 (Fig. **2**).

3. FDI Numbering System (Figs. 1 and 2):

A: The Primary Federation Dentaire Internationale Numbering System (FDI). Internationally, Canada and European countries widely use the 2-digit system. In 1996, the ADA adopted this system [3]. The mouth is divided into 4 sections called quadrants, and each quadrant is assigned a specific number. The maxillary right quadrant is assigned the number 5, then in a clockwise direction, numbers 6, 7, and 8 are assigned to the maxillary left quadrant, mandibular left quadrant, and mandibular right quadrant, respectively. The teeth in each quadrant are assigned a number from 1-to 5 with 1 being the central incisor and 5 being the second molar (Fig. **1**).

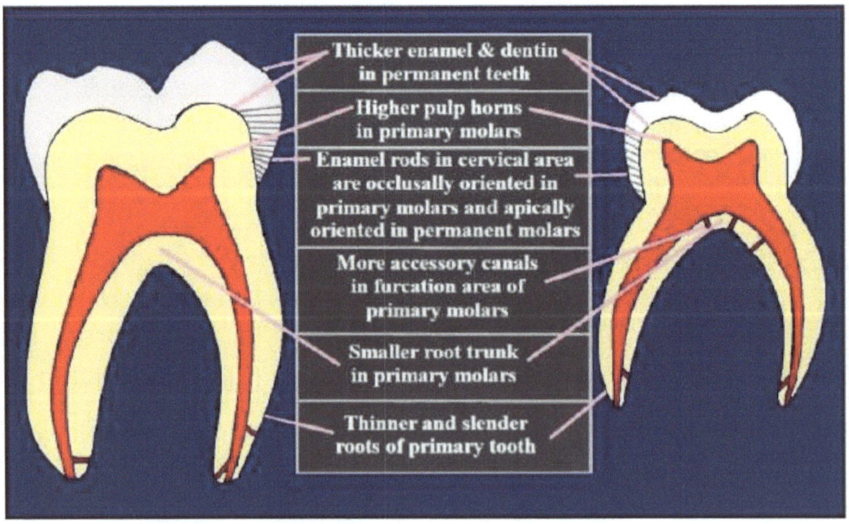

Fig. (3). Differences in Primary and permanent tooth.

B: The Permanent Federation Dentaire Internationale Numbering System (FDI). This system is also called the 2-digit system. Internationally it is the most widely used system worldwide [3]. Each quadrant is assigned a specific number. The maxillary right quadrant is assigned the number 1, then, in a clockwise direction, numbers 2, 3, and 4 are assigned to the maxillary left quadrant, mandibular left quadrant, and mandibular right quadrant, respectively. The teeth within each quadrant are assigned a number from 1 through 8, with 1 being the central incisor and 8 being the third molar (Fig. **2**).

There are 20 primary teeth, 10 teeth in the maxillary arch, and 10 teeth in the mandibular arch [4, 5].. There are four incisors (2 central incisors and 2 lateral incisors), and two canines, and four molars in each jaw [4, 5]. The difference between the primary teeth and the permanent teeth is shown in Table **1** and Fig. (**3**).

Table 1. Differences between primary and permanent teeth.

General Feature			
S. No.	**General Feature**	**Primary Teeth**	**Permanent Teeth**
1	Number	20	32
2	Type of teeth	Incisors (central and lateral), canines and molars (first and second)	Central incisors, lateral incisors, canine, first premolars, secondpremolar,first,second and third molar
3	Dental Formula	2/2,1/1,2/2.	2/2,1/1,2/2,3/3
4	Size	Small	Large
5	Colour	White	Yellowish/white/gray/brown
6	Eruption	In vertical relation to jaw begins at 6th to 10th months after birth and is usually completed by 30th month of age	Oblique relation to the jaw begins at 6 years after birthcompleted by 22 years of age
7	Eruption sequence	Maxillary AB D C E and Mandibular BC D E	Maxillary 6-1-2-4-5-3-7-8 and Mandibular 6-1-2-3-4-5-7-8
8	Root formation	After 1-1$^{1/2}$ years of age	After 2-2$^{1/2}$ years of age
9	Shedding	7-10 of age	Do not undergo shedding
Morphological Features			
S. No	**Morphological features**	**Primary Teeth**	**Permanent Teeth**
1	Shape	More bulbous	Less bulbous
2	Dimensions	Widermesiodistally with short row length	Narrowermesiodistally with long crown length

(Table 1) cont.....

General Feature			
3	Surface	Facial and lingual/palatalurfaceareflat	Facial and lingual, palatal surfaceareconvex
4	Mammelons	Absent	Presentonincisors
5	Cingulum	More prominent	Less prominent
6	Cusps	Short, sharp, pointed	Less sharp
7	Occlusal surface	Narrow Buccolingually	widened Buccolingually
8	Cervical line	Less curved	More curved
9	Cervical ridge	More pronounced	Less pronounced
10	Cervical constriction	More pronounced	Less pronounced
Root Morphology			
S. No.	**Root**	**Primary teeth**	**Permanent teeth**
1	Length of root	Short and slender	Long and plump
2	Crown/root ratio	Longer	No longer
3	Inclination of root	Labial inclination	Do not show any labial Inclination
4	Furcation	Leveloffurcationisnear cervix inmolar	Leveloffurcationis3-4mm fromcervix
5	Root trunk	Not distinct	Longanddistinct
6	Rootflare	Flarebeyondmesiodistaland Buccolingualoutlineofthe crown	. Donotflare either mesiodistally orbuccolinguallyofcrown
7	Anterior root	Narrow mesiodistally	Widened mesiodistally
8	Posterior root	Long	Small
Pulpal Morphology			
Sr. No.	**Pulp**	**Primary teeth**	**Permanent teeth**
1	Pulp chamber	Large	Small
2	Pulp horns	Extendincisally/occlusal	Do notextendedincisally /occlusal
3	Accessory canal	Seeninfurcationarea	As seen in the apical third of the root
Histological Feature			
S. No.	**Histological feature**	**Primary teeth**	**Permanent tooth**
1	Enamelcap	Enamelcapthinnerandmore consistent depth	Thickerand lessprominent depth

(Table 1) cont.....

General Feature			
2	Enamelrods	Enamelrodsinclinedat cervix occlusally	Enamelrodsinclinedatcervix gingivally
3	Dentinthicknessover pulpalwallatocclusalsurface	Greater	Lesser
4	EnamelAnddentin Thickness	Thinner	Thicker
5	Durationoffunctionofpulp	Short period	Long-period
6	Neural development	Less	More
7	Pulp growth and development	Faster	Slower
8	Blood supply	Adequateandinflammatory Response exhibited	Adequate and inflammatory response not exhibited

Morphology of Primary Teeth- The dimension of maxillary primary teeth is shown in Table **2** and of the mandibular primary teeth in Table **3**.

Table 2. Dimension of Maxillary Primary Teeth.

Tooth	Length overall	Length Of Crown	Length Of Root	M-D Diameter of Crown	M-D Diameter of crown at Cervix	La bio/ buccolingual diameter of Crown	La bio/ buccolingual diameter of Cervix
Central Incisor	16.0	6.0	10.0	6.5	4.5	5.0	4.0
Lateral incisor	15.8	5.6	11.4	5.1	3.7	4.0	3.7
Canine	19.0	6.5	13.5	7.0	5.1	7.0	5.5
First Molar	15.2	5.1	10.0	7.3	5.2	8.5	6.9
Second Molar	17.5	5.7	11.7	8.2	6.4	10.0	8.3

Table 3. Dimension of Mandibular Primary Teeth.

Tooth	Length overall	Length Of Crown	Length Of Root	M-D Diameter of Crown	M-D Diameter of crown at Cervix	La bio/ buccolingual diameter of Crown	La bio/ buccolingual diameter of Cervix
Central Incisor	14.0*	5.0	9.0	4.2	3.0	4.0	3.5
Lateral incisor	15.0	5.2	10.0	4.1	3.0	4.0	3.5
Canine	17.5	6.0	11.5	5.0	3.7	4.8	4.0
First Molar	15.8	6.0	9.8	7.7	6.5	7.0	5.3
Second Molar	18.8	5.5	11.3	9.9	7.2	8.7	6.4

Maxillary Central Incisor - The length of the tooth is 16 mm [4, 5].. It is the only tooth in the entire primary dentition set which is broader mesiodistally when compared to cervical-incisal height [4, 5] (Fig. **4**).

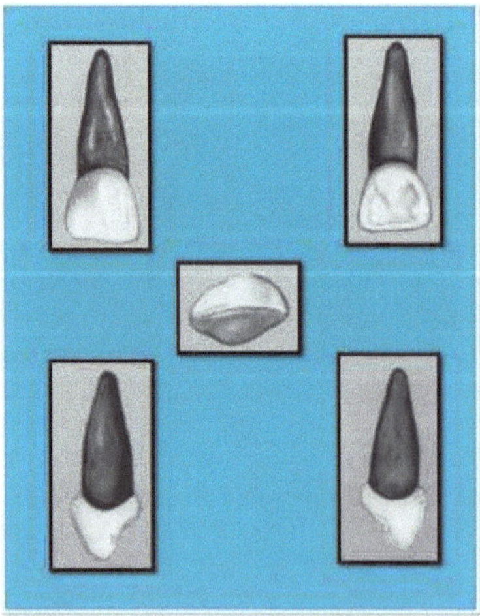

Fig. (4). Primary maxillary central incisor.

a) **Labial surface-** It is smooth without any evidence of developmental lines. The incisal edge meets the mesial surface at an acute angle and the distal surface at an obtuse angle. The crown has mesiodistal width of 6.5 mm, and the incisocervical height is 6 mm. The mesiodistal diameter of the crown at the cervix is 4.5 mm [4, 5].

b) ***Lingual surface-*** This surface shows well-developed marginal ridges with a properly developed cingulum. The mesial and distal fossa is formed by the cingulum extending up to the incisal

c) ***Root-*** The length of the root is 10 mm [4, 5]. It is conical in shape, tapering towards the apex. The mesial surface has developmental grooves. The lingual aspect of the root is narrower than the labial aspect. There is the presence of a ridge on the lingual aspect.

d) ***Mesial and distal surfaces-*** The labiolingual diameter of the crown is 5mm, and at the cervix, it is 4mm. The mesial and distal aspects of the primary maxillary central incisors are similar [4, 5].. The crown appears thicker in the middle third. The curvature of the cervical line is towards the incisal ridge. The cervical curvature on the medial side is more prominent than on the distal side. The shape of the root is conical, having even taper. A developmental groove or concavity may be seen on the mesial surface of the root, whereas the distal surface is convex.

e) ***Incisal Aspect-*** The incisal edge is straight and present in the center of the crown. Labially, the incisal edge is broader and smoother than lingually. This tooth has broad mesial and distal surfaces.

Maxillary Lateral Incisor- The lateral incisor is like the central incisor but smaller in overall dimensions. The crown length is 5.6 mm, and the root length is 11.4mm. The mesiodistal width (5.1mm) of the crown is smaller than the cervicofacial length (5.6 mm). As compared to the central incisor, the distoincisal angles of the crown are more rounded[4, 5]. Although the shape of the roots of the central and lateral incisor is the same, in the lateral incisor the root is much longer in proportion to its crown as compared to the central incisor. The mesiodistal width of the crown is 5.1 mm and at the cervix, it is 3.7 mm. The labiolingual diameter of the crown is 4 mm and at the cervix, it is 3.7 mm.

Maxillary Canine-The length of the maxillary canine is 20 mm. The length of the crown is 6.5mm, and the root is 13.5 mm [4, 5] (Fig. **5**).

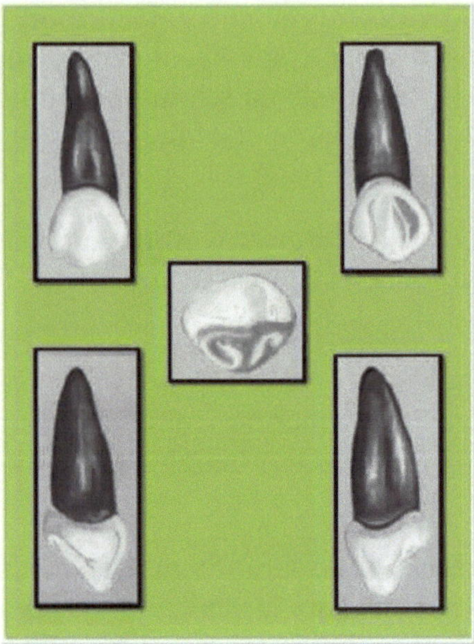

Fig. (5). Primary maxillary canine.

a) ***Labial surface-*** The crown has a cervical constriction with a convex mesial and distal surface [4, 5]. It has a long and well-developed, sharp cusp. The mesial slope of the cusp is longer than the distal slope. The root of the primary canine is long, slender, and tapering and is more than twice the crown length. The mesiodistal width of the crown is 7 mm and at the cervix, it is 5.1 mm.

b) ***Lingual Aspect-*** There are distinct enamel ridges, merging on the lingual aspect [4, 5]. A tubercle is present at the cusp tip. It is the continuation of the lingual ridge connecting the cingulum and the cusp tip. The lingual ridge divides the lingual surface into shallow mesiolingual and distolingual fossae. The root tapers lingually with an inclination towards the distal, above the middle third.

c) ***Mesial Aspect--*** The labiolingual diameter of the crown is 7 mm and at the cervix, it is 5.5 mm. It is conical in shape. On the mesial surface, the curvature of the cervical line toward the cusp ridge is more than that on the distal surface [4, 5].

d) ***Incisal Aspect-*** It appears diamond-shaped from the incisal aspect. When compared to permanent canines, the angles at the cingulum on the lingual surface and the labial surface are more pronounced and less rounded [4, 5]. The cusp remains distally to the Centre of the crown and the distal cusp slope is shorter than the mesial cusp.

Maxillary First Molar

The total length of the tooth is 15.2 mm, with a crown length of 5.1 mm and a root length of 10 mm [5, 10] (Fig. **6**).

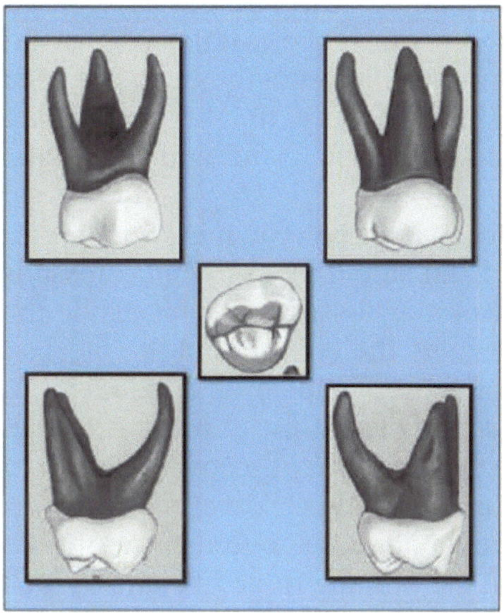

Fig. (6). Primarymaxillary first molar.

a. ***Buccal Aspect***- At the contact areas, the mesiodistal width is 7.3 mm. Apical to the contact areas, the crown converges toward the cervix, and the measurement at the cervix is 2 mm less than the measurement at the contact areas, resulting in a narrow cervical portion of the crown [6, 7]. There is little evidence of developmental grooves on the buccal surface which otherwise is smooth. Three widely spread roots are visible from this aspect. These roots are long and slender, with the mesial root being longer than the distal root. Due to the small length of the root trunk, bifurcation is closer to the cervical line of the crown.
b. ***Lingual Aspect***- The Lingual aspect and the buccal aspect are almost similar. The crown shows convergence lingually. The mesiolingual cusp is the longest, sharpest, and most prominent cusp on this tooth [6, 7]. The distolingual cusp is poorly defined, smaller in shape, and rounded. All three roots may be seen from this aspect with the palatal root being the largest.
c. ***Mesial Aspect***- The mesiolingual cusp is longer and sharper than the mesiobuccal cusp. Mesiodistally, the crown is wider at the cervical third than the occlusal third [7, 8]. The distinguishing feature of this tooth is the presence of a distinct convexity at the cervical third on he buccal outline. The cervical line curves slightly towards the occlusal surface. The palatal and mesiobuccal

roots are visible from this aspect. The palatal root is slender and long with a sharp curvature in a buccal direction above the middle third.

d. ***Distal Aspect***- The crown shows taper towards the distal surface. Well developed, long, and sharp distobuccal cusp is seen, whereas the distolingual cusp is poorly developed [7, 8]. The cervical bulge present on the mesial aspect does not extend towards the distal aspect of the crown. All three roots may be seen from this angle, but mostly the distobuccal and mesiobuccal roots are superimposed, showing only the buccal surface and the apex of the mesiobuccal root. The distobuccal root and the palatal root bifurcate near the cervical line.
e. ***Occlusal Aspect*** – Occlusally the crown is wider on the buccal and mesial side than the lingual and distal side [7, 9]. A central fossa is present on the occlusal surface. A mesial triangular fossa is present inside the mesial marginal ridge. A central groove connects the central and the mesial fossa. The mesiobuccal cusp and the distobuccal cusp are divided by a well-defined buccal developmental groove. A mesial pit is present in the mesial triangular fossa from which many supplementary grooves extend buccally, lingually, and towards the mesial marginal ridge. Sometimes the maxillary first molar shows a well-defined triangular ridge that connects the mesiolingual and distobuccal cusps. It is also called the oblique ridge in some of the teeth; the ridge is poorly developed. This distoocclusal groove, outlining the distolingual cusp, is always seen and may or may not extend through to the lingual mesial marginal ridge.

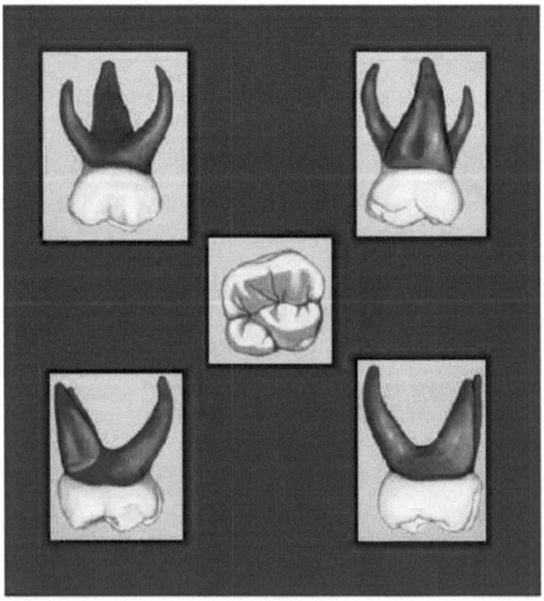

Fig. (7). Primary maxillary second molar.

Maxillary Second Molar

The total length of the tooth is 17.5 mm, with a crown length of 5.7 mm and root length of 11.7 mm. This tooth resembles a permanent maxillary first molar [5] (Fig. 7).

a) ***Buccal Aspect***- The buccal aspect shows two well-defined cusps with a deep buccal developmental groove. The mesiodistal width of the crown is 8.2 mm at the contact areas and 6.4 mm at the cervix resulting in the narrowing of the crown at the cervix [6, 7]. When compared to the first maxillary molar, the roots of the second maxillary molar appear slender, longer, and heavier. The root trunk is short, with the point of bifurcation located close to the cervical line of the crown.

b) ***Palatal Aspect*** - A well-developed and large mesiolingual cusp, a well-developed distolingual cusp, and a supplemental cusp, apical to the mesiolingual cusp, is seen from this aspect [6, 7]. This supplemental cusp is also called the tubercle of Carabelli. Sometimes this cusp is absent. In its place, traces of developmental lines can be seen. All the three roots can be seen from this aspect; the palatal root is larger than the mesiobuccal and distobuccal root.

c) ***Mesial Aspect-*** The mesiolingual cusp, along with the supplementary cusp, appears larger than the mesiobuccal cusp. The mesiobuccal cusp appears short and pointed. The cervical line is almost straight [7, 8]. The mesiobuccal root appears to be broad and flat. The roots are flared. The root trunk is short, and the point of bifurcation between the mesiobuccal root and the palatal root is located 2 or 3 mm apical to the cervical line of the crown. Out of the total width of the root trunk, two-thirds are occupied by the mesial root, and the remaining one-third is occupied by the palatal root. The mesiolingual cusp is seen directly below their bifurcation.

d) ***Distal Aspect-*** The palatal outline of the crown is smooth and rounded. The buccal outline extending from the tip of the buccal cusp to the crest of curvature is almost straight. The distobuccal cusp and the distolingual cusp are of the same length [7, 8]. The cervical line, like on the mesial side, is straight. All three roots are visible from this aspect, with the superimposition of the distobuccal root on the mesiobuccal root. The point of bifurcation between the distobuccal root and the palatal root is more located at the center of the root trunk and usually is in a straight line with the central groove.

e) ***Occlusal Aspect-*** This tooth resembles the permanent first molar from the occlusal aspect. It is rhomboidal in shape with four well-developed cusps and one supplemental cusp: mesiobuccal, distobuccal, mesiolingual, distolingual, and fifth cusp. The buccal surface is flat and the developmental groove between the cusps is less marked as compared to the first permanent molar [7, 9]. The rest of the features like developmental grooves, pits, oblique ridge, and others are almost identical to the permanent first molar. The character of the "mold" is constant. The occlusal surface has a central fossa with a central pit and a well-defined mesial triangular fossa distal to the mesial marginal ridge with a mesial pit at its centre. The 'central groove' located at the bottom of the sulcus is a well-defined developmental groove that connects the mesial triangular fossa with the central fossa. The buccal developmental groove that separates triangular ridges of mesiobuccal and distobuccal cusps extends buccally from the central pit towards the buccal surface. Triangular ridges are the occlusal continuations of the mesiobuccal and distobuccal cusps. Very often supplemental grooves radiate from these developmental grooves.

The oblique ridge is distinct and connects the mesiolingual cusp with the distobuccal cusp. The distal fossa is located distal to the oblique ridge, which harbours the distal developmental groove. The distal developmental groove represents a line of demarcation between the mesiolingual and distolingual cusps and continues to the lingual surface as the lingual developmental groove [7 - 9]. The distal triangular fossa is located mesial to the distal marginal ridge and is indefinitely outlined. The distal developmental groove has branches of supplemental grooves within the distal triangular fossa. The distal marginal ridge is as well developed as the mesial marginal ridge.

Mandibular Central Incisor- The total length of the tooth is 14mm, with the crown length of 5mm and root length of 9mm [4,5] (Fig. **8**).

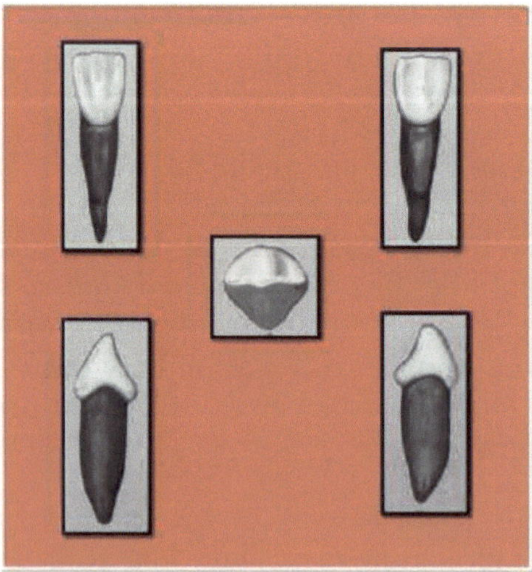

Fig. (8). Primary Mandibular central incisor.

a. ***Labial aspect-*** The mesiodistal width of the crown is 4.2 mm [4, 5, 7]. The labial aspect of the crown is flat. There are no developmental grooves present on this surface. The mesial and distal sides of the crown are tapered evenly from the contact areas, with the measurement being less at the cervix. The mesiodistal width of the crown at the cervix is 3 mm. The root is long and evenly tapered down to the apex. The root is twice the length of the crown.
b. ***Lingual Aspect-*** The marginal ridges and the cingulum are present on the lingual aspect. The lingual surface of the crown at the middle third and the incisal third may have a flattened surface level with the marginal ridges, or it may present a slight concavity, called the lingual fossa [4, 5]. The lingual portion of the crown and root converge so that it is narrower toward the lingual and not the labial surface.
c. ***Mesial Aspect*** - The incisal ridge is centred over the centre of the root and between the crest of curvature of the crown, labially and lingually. The cervical contours are convex at the cervical third with the labiolingual measurement of 4 mm [4, 5]. The mesial surface of the root is evenly tapered and flat; the apex appears blunter when compared to the lingual or labial aspects.
d. ***Distal Aspect-*** This is like the mesial aspect, except that the cervical line of the crown shows less curvature toward the incisal ridge [4, 5]. Usually, a developmental groove is present on the root.
e. ***Incisal Aspect-*** The incisal ridge is straight, bisecting the crown labiolingually. The crown tapers towards the cingulum [4, 5]. There is slight convexity on the labial surface and concavity on the lingual surface.

Mandibular Lateral Incisor- The total length of the tooth is 15 mm, with a crown length of 5.2 mm and root length of 9.8 mm [4, 5]. It is identical to the mandibular central incisor except that the cingulum of the central incisor is a little less distinct than that of the lateral incisor. The lingual surface of the crown between the marginal ridges sometimes is more concave as compared to the central incisor. In addition, the incisal ridge may be sloping downwards towards the distal surface. This results in lowering the distal contact area apically so that proper contact can be established with the mesial surface of the primary mandibular canine.

Mandibular Canine

The total length of the tooth is 17.5mm, with a crown length of 6mm and root length of 11.5 mm (Fig. **9**). It is morphologically like the maxillary canine with some minor exceptions like less pronounced cervical ridges and longer distal cusp slope [4, 5]. The mesiodistal width of the crown is 5 mm, which narrows down to

3.7 mm at the cervix. The labiolingual diameter of the crown is 4.8 mm tapering to 4 mm at the cervix.

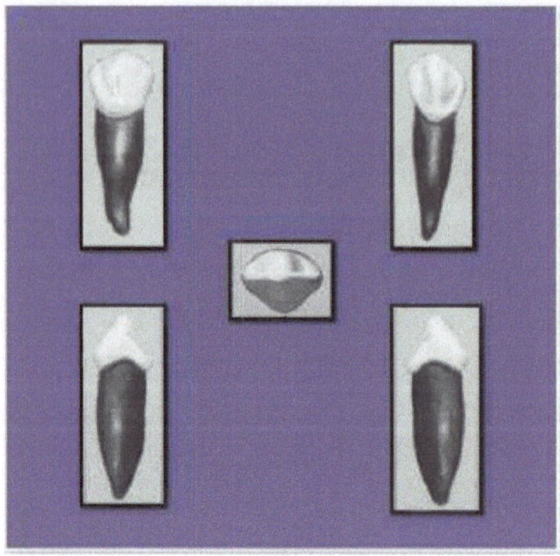

Fig. (9). Primary Mandibular canine.

Mandibular First Molar

During the process of evolution, occlusal groove patterns in mandibular molars have changed from the 'Y' to '+' pattern. The six types of occlusal groove patterns on mandibular molars have been classified as X4, X5, +5, ÷5, Y4, and Y5 [8, 9]. The length of the crown is 6 mm, and the root is 9.8 mm. It is the only primary tooth that does not resemble any other primary or permanent tooth (Fig. **10**).

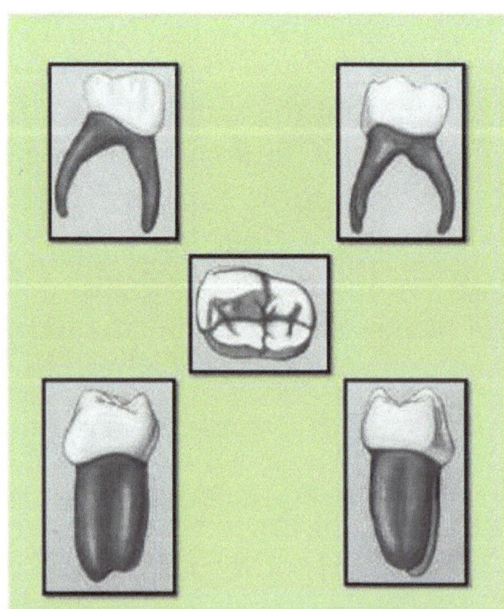

Fig. (10). Primary Mandibular first molar.

a. ***Buccal Aspect***- The mesial outline is straight extending from the contact area to the cervix. The distal outline is comparatively curved with convergence towards the cervix [6, 7]. The crown is short on the distal part than the mesial part. There are two cusps visible, the larger, mesiobuccal cusp and the distobuccal cusp. The roots are long and slender, and they spread at the apical third beyond the outline of the crown.
b. ***Lingual Aspect-*** There is a distinct convergence of crown and root mesially. Two cups are visible, long, and prominent, mesiolingual cusp and rounded distolingual cusp [6, 7]. The cervical line is straight.
c. ***Mesial Aspect-*** The Buccal outline shows a marked curvature at the cervical third. Both the Buccal cusps are placed over the root base. The lingual outline of the crown extends out lingually beyond the confines of the root base [7, 8]. The mesial root has buccal and lingual outlines parallel to each other till two-thirds of the root length and only a slight taper in the apical one-third. The root end is flat and almost square. A developmental depression usually extends the full length of the root on the mesial side.
d. ***Distal Aspect-*** The Buccal and the lingual outline of the crown is uniform. The distobuccal cusp and the distolingual cusp are visible [7, 8]. They are short and rounded. The distal root is round and short with an apical taper.
e. ***Occlusal Aspect-*** Occlusally, the crown is rhomboidal in shape which is due to the prominent mesiobuccal line angle. The mesiolingual cusp is the largest and has a broad, flattened surface lingually. The buccal developmental groove that separates mesiobuccal and distobuccal cusps is short and extends from the central pit to the centre of the crown outline buccally [7, 9]. Two supplemental grooves, one extending buccally and another extending lingually, join the developmental groove in the centre of the mesial triangular fossa. Similar supplemental groves are seen distally mesial to distal triangular fossa [7, 9]. The mesiobuccal cusp shows a well-defined triangular ridge on the occlusal surface, which terminates in the centre of the occlusal surface buccolingually at the central developmental groove.

Mandibular Second Molar

It resembles the permanent mandibular first molar [5, 10] (Fig. **11**).

a. ***Buccal Aspect-*** The mesiodistal dimension of the crown is more at the contact area than at the cervical third. The mesiobuccal and distobuccal developmental grooves divide the buccal surface of the crown occlusally into three cuspal portions almost equal in size [6, 7]. The mesiobuccal, a buccal, and a distobuccal cusp are visible from this aspect. From this aspect, the roots appear slender and long. The point of bifurcation of the roots starts immediately below the CEJ of the crown and root.

b. ***Lingual Aspect*** - Mesiolingual and distolingual cusps of almost equal dimensions can be observed from this aspect. The crown is narrow on the lingual aspect [6, 7]. The mesial portion of the crown seems to be a little higher than the distal portion. The roots are similar in appearance as from the buccal aspect.

c. ***Mesial Aspect-*** A marked cervical constriction can be observed. The marginal ridge is high, a characteristic that makes the mesiobuccal cusp and the mesiolingual cusp appears short [7, 8]. The lingual cusp is longer, or higher than the buccal cusp. The mesial root is unusually broad and flat with a blunt apex that is sometimes serrated.

d. ***Distal Aspect*** – Distally, the crown is narrower than the mesial part. The distolingual cusp appears well developed, and the triangular ridge from the tip of this cusp extending down into the occlusal surface is seen over the distal marginal ridge[7, 8]. The distal marginal ridge dips down more sharply and is shorter buccolingually than the mesial marginal ridge. The distal root is as broad as the mesial root and is flattened on the distal surface.

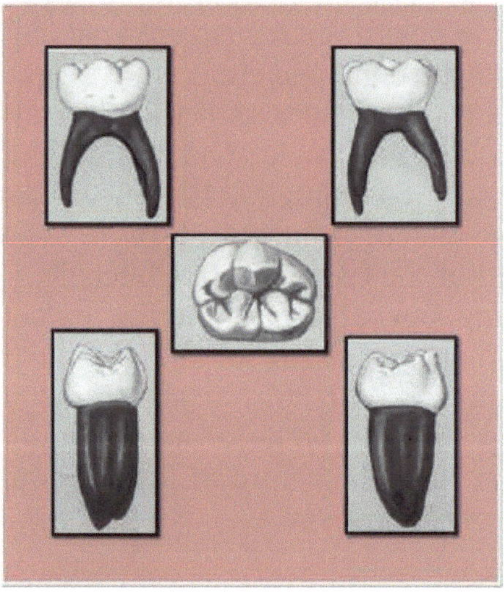

Fig. (11). Primary mandibular second molar.

e. ***Occlusal Aspect-*** It is rectangular in shape. Occlusally total of five cusps are seen: three buccal and two lingual. Each one of these cusp tips has well-defined triangular ridges. The central developmental groove divides the crown buccolingually [7, 9]. The triangular ridges extend from cusp tips to the centre of the crown to the central developmental groove. The central developmental groove follows a staggering course from the mesial triangular fossa, just inside the mesial marginal ridge, to the distal triangular fossa, just mesial to the distal marginal ridge. A well-developed mesial triangular fossa is seen from this aspect, while a distal triangular fossa is not that well developed [7, 9]. Buccal and lingual developmental grooves branch off from the central developmental groove leading to the formation of five cusps. The two buccal grooves, one mesial and one distal are confluent with the buccal developmental grooves of the buccal surface. The single lingual developmental groove is confluent with the lingual groove on the lingual surface of the crown. The mesial marginal ridge is well developed and more pronounced as compared to the distal marginal ridge. The outline of the crown converges distally.

CONCLUSION

It is crucial to comprehend the phases of tooth development to understand the geomorphology of human dentition[2, 4, 5]. These steps give rise to the morphology of a multiplicity of human teeth with dissimilar façades and elevations, which are named using an entomologic scheme, and specified using numbering procedures[3, 5]. This chapter presents a guide to the various phases of tooth development and the tissue composition of teeth at various stages of development and provides an understanding of the terminology and numbering systems used to distinguish and describe human teeth. Subsequently, the anatomy of the crown and root, as well as descriptions of the tooth surfaces and ridges, are also discussed. Thes chapter ended with a discussion of tooth morphology hypotheses that are thought to facilitate/ explain tooth development.

CONSENT FOR PUBLICATION

Not applicable.

CONFLICT OF INTEREST

The author(s) declare no conflict of interest, financial or otherwise.

ACKNOWLEDGEMENT

Declared none.

REFERENCES

[1] Mirzakouchaki B, Shahrbaf S, Talebiyan R. Determining tooth size ratio in an Iranian-Azari population. J Contemp Dent Pract 2007; 8(7): 86-93. [http://dx.doi.org/10.5005/jcdp-8-7-86] [PMID: 17994159]

[2] Kitagawa Y, Manabe Y, Oyamada J, Rokutanda A. Japanese deciduous tooth size: Past and present. Anthropol Sci 2002; 110(4): 335-47. [http://dx.doi.org/10.1537/ase.110.335]

[3] Peck S, Peck L. A time for change of tooth numbering systems. J Dent Educ 1993; 57(8): 643-7. [http://dx.doi.org/10.1002/j.0022-0337.1993.57.8.tb02785.x] [PMID: 8349894]

[4] Savla SN, Gotmare SS, Pereira T, *et al.* Crown Dimensions of Deciduous Teeth: The Tool for Predicting the Physical Height of the Child: A Pilot Study. J Clin Diagn Res 2018; 12: ZC01-3. [http://dx.doi.org/10.7860/JCDR/2018/31369.11659]

[5] Salama FS, Anderson RW, McKnight-Hanes C, Barenie JT, Myers DR. Anatomy of primary incisor and molar root canals. Pediatr Dent 1992; 14(2): 117-8. [PMID: 1502120]

[6] Barbería E, Suárez MC, Villalón G, Maroto M, García-Godoy F. Standards for mesiodistal and buccolingual crown size and height of primary molars in a sample of Spanish children. Eur J Paediatr Dent 2009; 10: 169-75.

[7] Anderson AA. Dentition and occlusion development in African American children: mesiodistal crown diameters and tooth-size ratios of primary teeth. Pediatr Dent 2005; 27(2): 121-8. [PMID: 15926289]

[8] Bravo N, Facal M, Maroto M, Barbería E. Relationship between mesiodistal crown diameters of permanent first molars and deciduous second molars. Eur J Paediatr Dent 2010; 11(3): 115-21. [PMID: 21080750]

[9] Jeevanandan G, Ahsana A, Subramanian E. Evaluation of occlusal groove morphology of primary mandibular second molar in an Indian population. J Forensic Dent Sci 2018; 10(2): 92-5. [http://dx.doi.org/10.4103/jfo.jfds_38_18] [PMID: 30745785]

[10] Avula JSS, Enuganti S, Mallela GM, Margana JSPG, Kakarla P, Eswara K. Deciduous molar sizes and sexual dimorphism: South Indian study. J Paediatr Dent 2014; 2(1): 13-9. [http://dx.doi.org/10.4103/2321-6646.130377]

CHAPTER 13

Teething in Children – Fact and Fiction

Shruti Balasubramanian[1,*] and **Dhanashree Sakhare**[2]

[1] *Department of Pediatric and Preventive Dentistry, Government Dental College and Hospital, Nagpur, India*

[2] *Lavanika Academy, Melbourne, Australia*

Abstract: Teething is a natural process of eruption of the first deciduous teeth. Over the years, teething has been blamed for a wide array of childhood illnesses. Hippocrates (fourth century B.C) and others observed that teething was associated with fever, convulsions, diarrhea, and inflammation of the gums. The association of teething with infant mortality was popular in medieval times. By the twentieth century, the controversy surrounding teething subsided and the morbid conditions initially associated with teeth in infants were found to have other causes. It is assumed that the inflammatory mediators present in the dental follicle are responsible for the local symptoms of teething. The most frequent signs and symptoms associated with teething are irritability, drooling, decreased appetite, sleeping problems, rhinorrhea, fever, diarrhea, rash, and vomiting.

Keywords: Deciduous teeth, Dental Follicle, Eruption, Teething.

INTRODUCTION

In Latin, the term teething was known as "*Dentio difficilis*" which means pathologic dentition or difficult dentition. In medical terminology, it is termed "Odontiasis" which means the eruption of baby teeth through the gums. Teething is considered an index of normal growth and development of children. In the majority of cases, teething does not cause any distress to the infant, but sometimes it may be accompanied by pain and discomfort. The process of primary teeth eruption commences with the eruption of mandibular incisors around the 4th-8th month and is completed with the eruption of deciduous second molars at the age of 30-36 months. However, a variation of as much as 6 months may be observed in the timing of eruption. Disturbances associated with the process of teething are transient but may occur repeatedly for 4-36 months.

* **Corresponding author Shruti Balasubramanian:** Department of Pediatric and Preventive Dentistry, Government Dental College and Hospital, Nagpur, India; E-mail: shruti.310194@gmail.com

Historical Perspective

The effect of teething on the general health of infants has been documented for more than five thousand years. Teething has been associated with morbidity by Hippocrates, Homer, Celsus and Aristotle. Various conditions include fever, diarrhea, convulsions, photophobia, blinking eyes, vomiting, neuralgia, severe headache, loss of weight, cold, inflammation of tonsils, toxemia, para-paresis, cholera, meningeal infections, tetanus, mental illnesses, and sometimes penile discharge have also been associated with teething. Till the nineteenth century, teething was the cause of a substantial number of infant fatalities. It was believed that the link between teething and life-threatening illnesses was the irritation of nerve endings of the 5th cranial nerve in the mucous membrane which led to reflex stimulation of other spinal and cranial nerves. The controversy surrounding teething has subsided in recent decades as morbid conditions initially attributed to teething infants have been associated with other etiologies [1].

Definitions

1. Teething is defined as the process of sequential appearance of an infant's first primary tooth by emerging through the gums.
2. Teething is the process of teeth eruption through the gums.
3. Tooth eruption is a physiologic process wherein the tooth moves from its developmental position within the alveolar bone to its final position in the oral cavity [2].

Signs and Symptoms

There is a window of eight days for the eruption of the tooth. It includes 4 days before the eruption, the day of tooth eruption and the 3 days following it. The signs and symptoms associated with teething are summarized in Table **1** and Fig. (**1**).

Table 1. Signs and symptoms of teething [3, 4].

Mild fever	**Gastrointestinal upset which ranges from constipation to diarrhea**
Lethargy	Lack of sleep/ disturbed sleep/wakefulness
Soreness of gums	Finger sucking
Inflammation of mucous membrane overlying the tooth (with small haemorrhages)	Loss of appetite/alteration in volume of fluid intake
Ear infection	Weight loss
Rubbing of gums/chewing/sucking/biting of objects	Tend to rub ears on the side same as that of erupting tooth

(Table 1) cont.....

Mild fever	**Gastrointestinal upset which ranges from constipation to diarrhea**
General irritability/malaise	Facial flushing /circumoral rash
Gingival pain	Drooling/sialorrhea

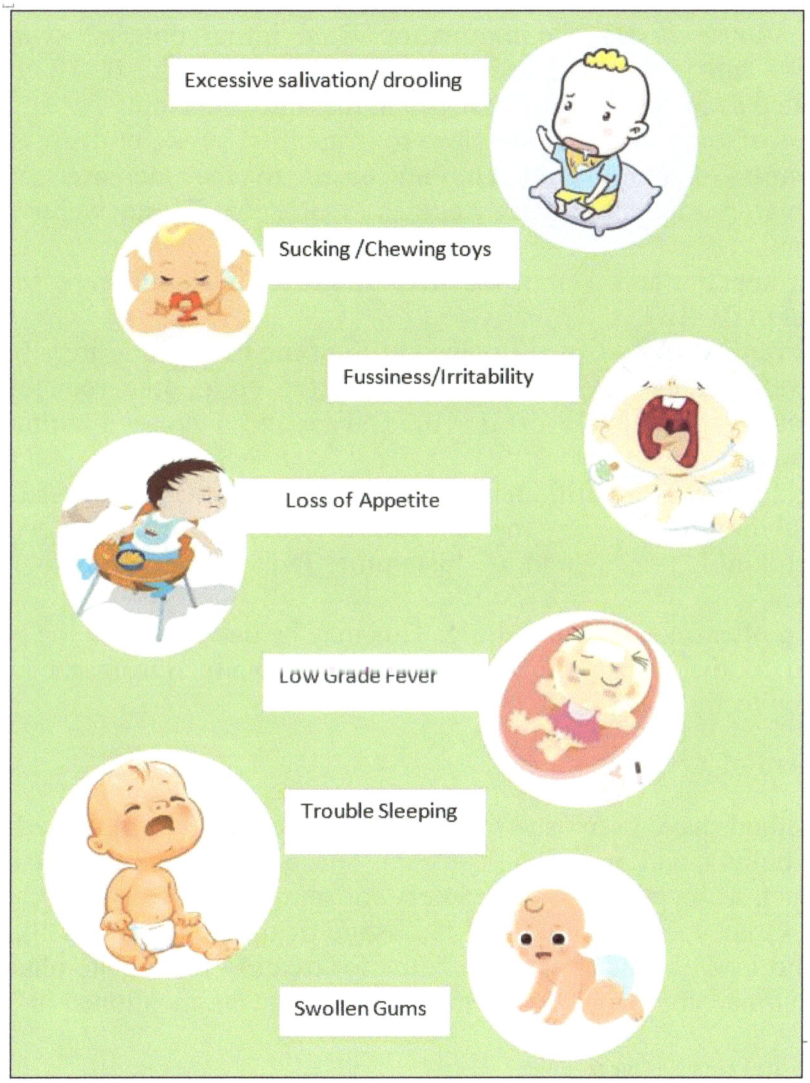

Fig. (1). Signs and symptoms of teething.

1. Drooling - The most common manifestation of teething is drooling. This excessive salivation may be due to increased irritation of the gums. From around three to four months of age, drooling is greater than normal.

2. Coughing - Excess saliva can cause gagging and coughing in infants.
3. Rashes on Chin - Drooling may cause rashes on the chin when saliva comes in contact with the skin around the mouth. It is recommended to regularly wipe the infant's mouth and chin to prevent these rashes.
4. Biting of different objects – Biting of objects creates a counter-pressure which helps to relieve the pressure of the erupting tooth
5. Diarrhea/loose stools- Contamination from biting objects, swallowing of excessive saliva, and increased release of cytokines like IL-1β and IL-8 are implicated as factors causing diarrhea at the time of teething.
6. Soreness of gums and pain may lead to irritability, stress, or distress.
7. Tenderness of gums could be attributed to the increase in levels of inflammatory mediators like cytokines in GCF and the nociceptive receptors are stimulated.
8. Loss of appetite and weight loss can be associated with increased levels of interleukin (IL-1β).
9. Mild fever and disturbance in sleep at the time of teething may be owing to the developmental changes occurring in the child, like reduced maternal immunity, raised levels of IL-1β, TNF-α and increased vulnerability to infections.
10. Itching, local redness, inflammation and sialorrhea may be caused because of degranulation followed by the subsequent release of inflammatory mediators like cytokines, prostaglandins, histamine, leukotrienes, growth factors and proteases.
11. Rubbing of cheeks and ear pulling: This may be due to pain in the gums which radiates to the cheeks as well as ears, especially during the eruption of posterior teeth [1, 2].

Management of Teething [5, 6]

Various methods have been used for the management of teething based on culture, traditional beliefs, and practices (Table **2**). These range from the use of harmful; methods such as local blistering, cautery, or gum lancing to the use of teething necklaces. Other methods involved the usage of opioids, poisons like mercury, bromide and lead acetate or cooling baths for treating fever. The pharmacologic and non-pharmacologic methods to manage to teethe are mentioned in Table **3**.

Table 2. Historical remedies for teething.

Remedies For Teething	Adverse Effects
Salts, purgatives, and emetics	Dehydration
Opioids	Respiratory depression
Mercury	Diarrhea, vomiting, kidney failure

(Table 2) cont.....

Remedies For Teething	Adverse Effects
Lead	Seizures, encephalopathy, paralysis
Bromide	Hallucination, seizures
Honey	Tetanus

Table 3. Management of Teething.

Pharmacological Management	Non-Pharmacological Management (Fig. 2)
Local anesthetics- Lignocaine hydrochloride (0.33%-0.9%), cetylpyridinium chloride (0.02%-0.1%)- Application of 7.5mm of gel onto the tender gums with clean fingertips and rubbed. Twenty minutes should elapse between approaches. It is recommended to use not more than six applications. Products containing lignocaine should be avoided in infants with sensitivity.	Chilled Teething rings – Compared to liquid-filled rings, solid silicone-based teething rings are preferred as there are chances of leakage of the potentially irritant fluid contents in case of damage, which cannot be sterilized. It is advisable to fix the teething rings to the infant's clothing rather than tying them around the neck. This avoids the risk of strangulation.
Minor analgesics- Choline salicylate 8.7%, cetalkonium chloride 0.01% Application of gel onto the tender gums with clean fingertips. It provides analgesic, antipyretic, and anti-inflammatory effects. For children more than 4 months old, it is recommended to use 0.5 inches (7.5 mm) of gel to massage the painful area in less than 3 hourly intervals with a maximum of six daily applications. Frequent use of choline salicylate preparations on oral mucosa should be avoided to prevent chemical burn.	-Hard sugar-free teething rusks/breadsticks/oven-hardened bread. -Frozen items (such as ice cubes to frozen bagels, frozen bananas, sliced fruit, pretzels, and vegetables) -Pacifiers
Paracetamol- 100-120 mg/5ml The recommended dosage of sugar-free paracetamol elixir is: 3–12 months = 60–120 mg 1–5 years = 120–250 mg These doses can be repeated after every 4 to 6 hours with a maximum of 4 times a day. For doses, less than 5 ml, the use of a graduated syringe is recommended and for doses greater than 5 ml, calibrated spoon is recommended. Administering a lesser than recommended dose of paracetamol is ineffective in relieving teething pain, whereas overdosage may cause hepatocellular and renal tubular necrosis.	-Application of mild pressure with a clean finger, preferably with a wet gauze or even a cold spoon, is suitable - Regular wiping of excessive drooling of saliva onto the infant's skin to prevent the development of chin rash.

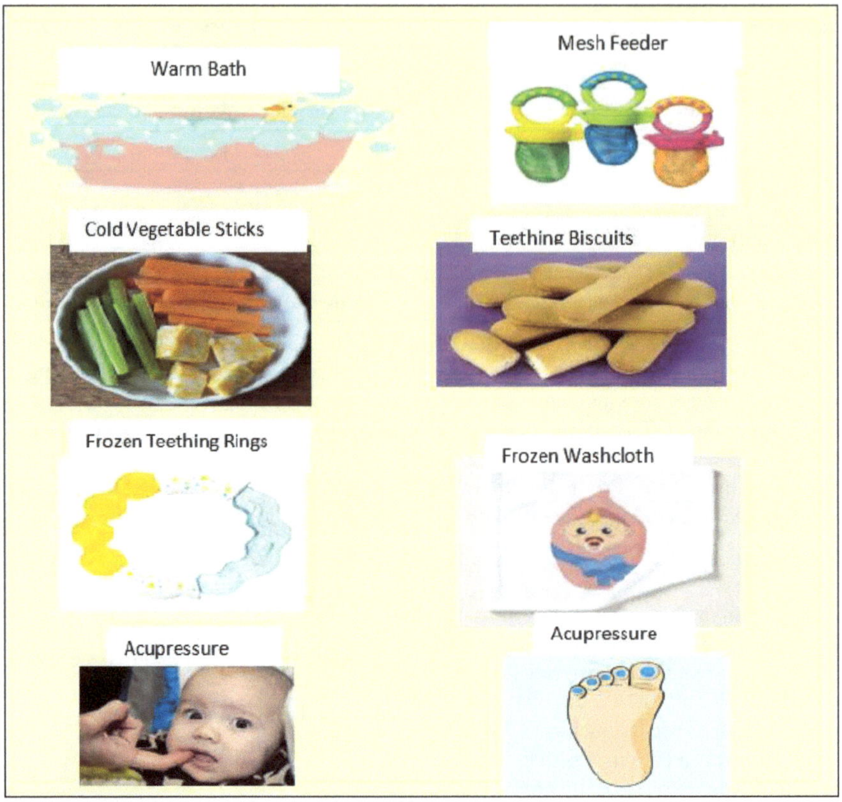

Fig. (2). Teething Remedies.

Practices- Not Recommended [6]

-Parents should avoid adding sugar, jam or honey to the feeding bottles.

- Pacifier should not be dipped in honey or jam.
- Parents should not apply alcohol to the mucous membrane of an infant repeatedly.
- Feeding bottle should not be given while a teething infant is in bed.
- Any medicine, including teething remedies, should not be added to the feeding bottle, as it is difficult to accurately measure the dosage ingested.

-Teething medications should not be kept within reach of children because there is a danger of overdosage due to the added flavorings.

Problems Associated with Teething

a. ***Eruption hematoma (Eruption cyst)***

It presents as an elevated mass of tissue which is bluish-purple. It develops due to trauma of soft tissues during function and is self-limiting. A blood-filled cyst is commonly found in the deciduous or permanent first molar region. They may develop about a few weeks before the eruption of the deciduous or permanent tooth.

Clinical Features – This lesion appears clinically as a fluctuant, translucent, and well-circumscribed swelling present on the alveolar ridge over the site of erupting tooth (Fig. 3). When the cystic cavity consists of blood, it gives a deep blue or purple appearance and is hence termed "Eruption Hematoma."

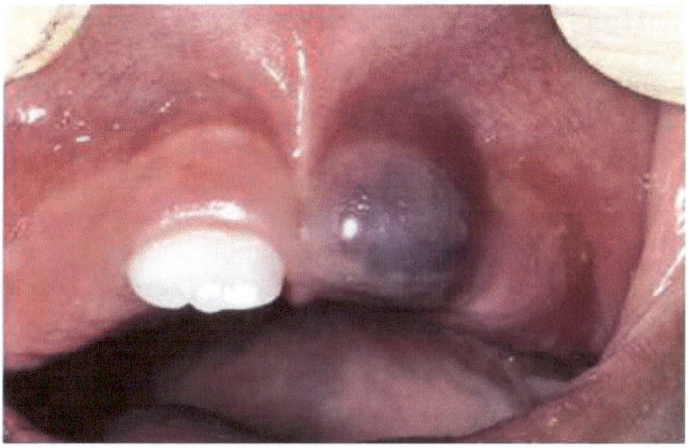

Fig. (3). Eruption hematoma (Eruption cyst).

Differential diagnosis Hemangioma, Pyogenic granuloma, Neonatal alveolar lymphangioma, Amalgam tattoo

Management - Treatment is usually not necessary as it is self-correcting.

-The roof of the cyst may be removed to permit the eruption of tooth although the majority of times they break spontaneously
-Surgical Excision

b. **Eruption Sequestrum**

It is an anomaly associated with erupting teeth in children which were described for the first time by Starkey and Shafer.

Etiology- During the eruption of molar teeth, occasionally there is a separation of a small bony fragment from the surrounding contagious bone. Usually, there is total resorption of this fragment before the eruption. Eruption sequestrum is observed (because of incomplete resorption) if this bony fragment is large or when the eruption occurs earlier.

Clinical Features – This anomaly is a small, irregular piece of bone lying over the crown of erupting permanent molar. It is found either just before or immediately after the cusp tips have emerged. The spicule lies directly over the central fossa of the occlusal region, but it is present inside the soft tissue. This bony fragment undergoes complete sequestration and is lost eventually as the process of eruption continues. For a few days, this bone fragment is visible on the crest of the ridge in a small depression from where it can be removed easily.

Radiographic Features – It appears as a small, irregular opaque area lying over the central fossa however it appears separate from the tooth.

Clinical importance and treatment- The clinical significance of this condition is that occasionally a child may complain of local soreness, mostly due to the compression of soft tissue on the bony spicule during chewing or due to movement of the fragment within soft tissue at the time of mastication. No treatment is necessary as the condition resolves by itself [3 - 7].

c. Natal and Neonatal Teeth

Teeth present during birth are termed as 'natal teeth' whereas the ones erupting within 30 days of birth are known as the 'neonatal teeth' (based on the classification given by Massler and Savara [1950]). They are also known as Dentitia precox, congenital teeth, fetal teeth, infancy teeth, precocious dentition and predeciduous teeth. Natal teeth are three times more common as compared to neonatal teeth. The incidence of this condition ranges from 1:2,000 to 1:3,500. The radiographic evaluation is necessary to differentiate between the supernumerary tooth and prematurely erupted primary tooth. Among the cases of natal and neonatal teeth, 90% prematurely erupt primary teeth and only <10% are supernumerary teeth. The supernumerary tooth needs to be extracted, but this decision should be based on the possibility of local and general complications as well as on the parent/caregiver's consent. They are commonly found in the lower central incisor region. Apart from this, the most common to least commonly affected teeth are maxillary incisors, mandibular canines/molars, and lastly, maxillary canine/molar. Natal or neonatal cuspids are extremely rare.

Etiology-Specific etiology is not known.

- Previously, neonatal teeth were merely considered to be dental laminal cysts. Usually, they appear white, corniform, consisting of compact keratin and projected above the ridge of alveoli. Some suggested it to be a result of inheritance as an autosomal dominant trait.

- Endocrine dysfunction of the pituitary gland, thyroid or gonads may also be the contributing factor.
- Excessive or increased resorption of the overlying bone may lead to the early eruption of the natal or neonatal teeth.
- Pregnancy-related complications and congenital syphilis are also considered predisposing factors for natal and neonatal teeth.
- Natal teeth may also be associated with the primary tooth agenesis
- Associated Syndromes- Ellis-Van Creveld, Pachyonychia Congenital, Rubinstein-Taybi, Hallermann-Streiff, Steatocystoma Multiplex, Pierre-Robin, Cyclopia, Cleft lip and palate, Pfeiffer syndrome, Pallister-Hall, Wiedemann-Rautenstrauch syndrome, Craniofacial dysostosis, Van der Woude syndrome, Walker-Warburg, Epidermolysis-Bullosa and Adrenogenital syndrome.

Classification

1. Massler and Savara (1950)-Natal and Neonatal tooth(Depending upon the time of eruption)
2. Spouge and Feasby (1966)- Mature – when the natal tooth is fully developed and its shape and morphology resemble that of the primary tooth; Immature – represents incomplete development of natal teeth. The term mature suggests that the tooth is well developed in comparison to the remaining primary teeth and has a relatively good prognosis, whereas the term immature denotes an incomplete structure which shows a poor prognosis.
3. Hebling (1997) classified natal teeth clinically into 4 categories [8]:

1. Shell-shaped crown without any root and is fixed poorly to the alveolus with the help of gingival tissue.

2. Solid crown structure with little or no root, which is fixed poorly to alveolus with gingival tissue.

3. Eruption of the crown's incisal edge through the gingival tissue.

4. Tooth is unerupted but is palpable along with oedema of the gingival tissue.

Histological Characteristics-Hypoplastic Enamel

- No root formation,
- Vascularization of pulp,
- Irregular formation of dentine,
- Absence of cementum

Complications and treatment- The decision regarding whether these teeth have to be retained in the oral cavity or not depends on the following:

- Degree of mobility
- Inconvenience during breastfeeding
- Inconvenience experienced during suckling
- Possibility of trauma
- Whether the tooth is supernumerary or is part of the normal dentition

The preferred treatment is to maintain these teeth in the mouth; if it is

-Part of the normal dentition
-Well implanted

Their Removal is Indicated

- When they interfere with feeding
- When they are mobile
- When there is an increased risk of aspiration.
- Sharp incisal edge causing trauma to the infant's tongue or the mother's breast

Riga-Fede Disease- Ulceration observed on the ventral surface of the tongue due to the impinging sharp incisal edge of the tooth

The precautions to be taken during extraction of natal and/or neonatal teeth [9]:

1) Avoid extracting at least for the first 10 days of life to reduce the risk of haemorrhage,
    1. Considering the general health of a newborn, vitamin K is administered before the extraction.
2) Precautions to prevent injury to the gingiva, and
    1. Alertness to prevent aspiration during removal.

It is imperative to wait for the first 10 days for extraction to allow the establishment of intestinal flora and commence production of vitamin K (necessary for forming prothrombin). If the extraction has to be done urgently, it is recommended to assess the need for administering vitamin K along with an opinion from his/her pediatrician. Vitamin K is administered intramuscularly at a dose of 0.5-1 mg/to prevent hemorrhage.

CONCLUSION

Several ancient misapprehensions and related perilous medications regarding teething persist to date. In the rural areas of eastern Africa, the swelling of gums that precedes eruption was believed to be the cause of fever, vomiting and diarrhoea. Treatment of these symptoms includes removing the tooth (ebinyo), cutting or lancing the gums and hot nails pressed into the gums. These remedies were believed to have relieved the tension on gums hence alleviating vomiting and diarrhoea. The complications of such procedures are often deadly. Traditionally, villagers used unsterile equipment, which led to infections. Lancing or removal of teeth may lead to defects in enamel, malformation of teeth and alteration in the size of the mandible. The current treatment regimen for teething includes teething rings, topical anaesthetics, homoeopathic oils. Although the majority of treatments pose no threat but, few of them may be risky. Pediatric dentists should work towards increasing the awareness of parents regarding teething myths and must answer their queries and alleviate their concerns.

CONSENT FOR PUBLICATION

Not applicable.

CONFLICT OF INTEREST

The author(s) declare no conflict of interest, financial or otherwise.

ACKNOWLEDGEMENT

Declared none.

REFERENCES

[1] Getaneh A, Derseh F, Abreha M, Yirtaw T. Misconceptions and traditional practices towards infant teething symptoms among mothers in Southwest Ethiopia. BMC Oral Health 2018; 18(1): 159. [http://dx.doi.org/10.1186/s12903-018-0619-y] [PMID: 30241521]

[2] Markman L. Teething. Pediatr Rev 2009; 30(8): e59-64. [http://dx.doi.org/10.1542/pir.30.8.e59] [PMID: 19648257]

[3] Memarpour M, Soltanimehr E, Eskandarian T. Signs and symptoms associated with primary tooth eruption: a clinical trial of nonpharmacological remedies. BMC Oral Health 2015; 15(1): 88. [http://dx.doi.org/10.1186/s12903-015-0070-2] [PMID: 26215351]

[4] Massignan C, Cardoso M, Porporatti AL, *et al.* Signs and Symptoms of Primary Tooth Eruption: A Meta-analysis. Pediatrics 2016; 137(3): e20153501. [http://dx.doi.org/10.1542/peds.2015-3501] [PMID: 26908659]

[5] Nemezio MA, De Oliveira KMH, Romualdo PC, *et al.* Association between Fever and Primary Tooth Eruption: A Systematic Review and Meta-analysis. Int J Clin Pediatr Dent 2017; 10(3): 293-8. [http://dx.doi.org/10.5005/jp-journals-10005-1453] [PMID: 29104392]

[6] Ispas RS, Mahoney EK, Whyman RA. Teething signs and symptoms: persisting misconceptions

among health professionals in New Zealand. N Z Dent J 2013; 109(1): 2-5.
[PMID: 23923149]

[7] Gugwad S, Bommanavar S, Garud S. Teething: a relook. Int J Dent Case Reports 2012; 2: 115-20.

[8] Noor-Mohammed R, Basha S. Teething disturbances; prevalence of objective manifestations in children under age 4 months to 36 months. Med Oral Patol Oral Cir Bucal 2012; 17(3): e491-4.
[http://dx.doi.org/10.4317/medoral.17487] [PMID: 22143712]

[9] Wake M, Hesketh K, Lucas J. Teething and tooth eruption in infants: A cohort study. Pediatrics 2000; 106(6): 1374-9.
[http://dx.doi.org/10.1542/peds.106.6.1374] [PMID: 11099591]

CHAPTER 14

Developmental Disturbances of Oral Structure

Jay Gopal Ray[1,*], **Deepika Bablani Popli**[2], **Aman Chowdhry**[3] and **Priyanka Bhaje**[4]

[1] *Burdwan Dental College and Hospital, West Bengal, India*

[2] *Department of Oral Pathology and Microbiology, Faculty of Dentistry, Jamia Millia Islamia, New Delhi, India*

[3] *Faculty of dentistry, Jamia Milia Islamia (A Central University) New Delhi, India*

[4] *Senior lecturer, Rungata college of Dental sciences and research center, Bhilai, Chhattisgarh, India*

Abstract: Childhood developmental disorders have serious adverse impacts on the psychological and social well-being of children and their families. Despite the burden that developmental disorders impose on children and adolescents, most countries do not provide satisfactory care to those in need. These developmental disorders can either be present as a single finding or as a part of syndrome. This chapter focuses on the developmental disorders affecting the teeth, tongue, and lip. The spectrum of these developmental disorders varies widely. In each case, the anomaly is first described, followed by diagnostic information, including the availability of various treatment options. Early diagnosis is often crucial for the effective treatment of functional and developmental aspects. This will improve the prognosis for better functional and aesthetic outcome for these patients and lead to a better quality of life, not only for the patients themselves but also for their families.

Keywords: Developmental disorders, Early diagnosis, Quality of life.

INTRODUCTION

Developmental disorders of teeth, tongue and mucosa are of prime importance in children because of their unsightly appearance and even the loss of functioning sometimes (Fig. **1**). Identification of these defects and managing them effectively is the primary task of a Pediatric Dentist. Thus, the knowledge of these conditions can help the Pediatric Dental Surgeon to identify the problem accurately and diagnose & treat it effectively.

* **Corresponding author Jay Gopal Ray:** Professor and Head, Burdwan Dental College and Hospital, West Bengal, India; E-mail: sharathchandrah2012@gmail.com

Satyawan Damle, Ritesh Kalaskar, Dhanashree Sakhare & Abdulkadeer Jetpurwala (Eds.)

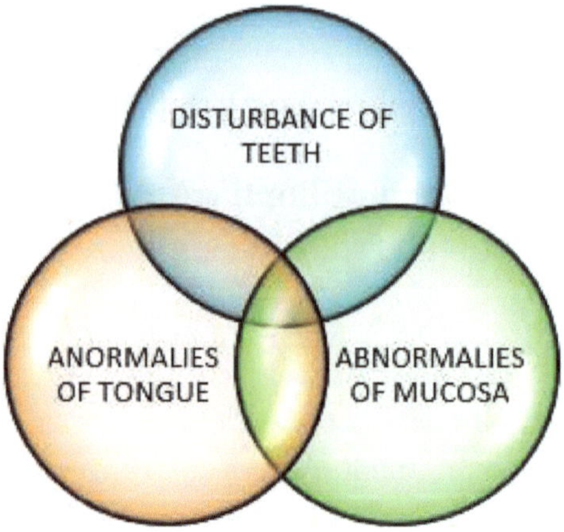

Fig. (1). Developmental disturbances of teeth, tongue, and mucosa.

DISTURBANCES OF TEETH (FIG. 2)

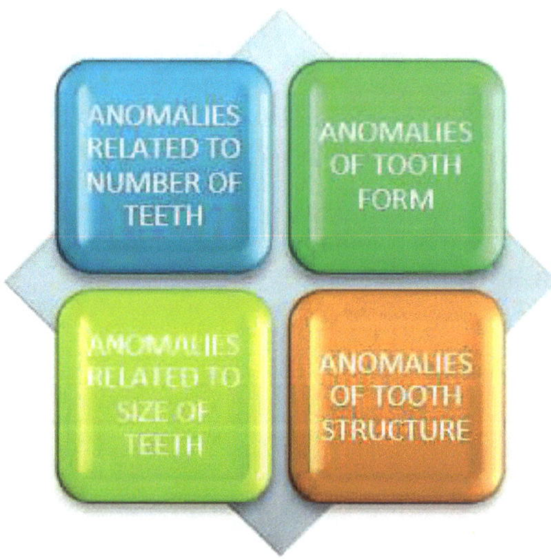

Fig. (2). Disturbances of teeth.

Anomalies related to number of teeth (Fig. 3)

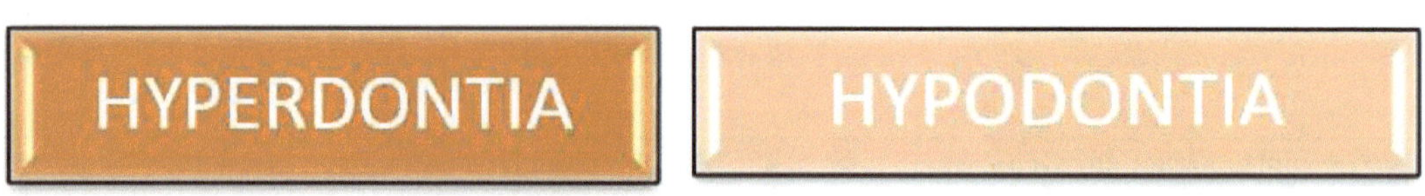

Fig. (3). Anomalies related to number of teeth.

Alterations in the number of teeth result due to interruptions in the normal developmental stages.

Hyperdontia

- In this condition, teeth are more than normal in number and these extra teeth are known as 'supernumerary teeth'.
- Associated syndromes include Apert's syndrome, Gardner syndrome Cleidocranial dysplasia and Sturge Weber syndrome.
- Different theories have been mentioned in the formation of the supernumerary tooth which include:
  - Hyperactivity theory suggests that supernumeraries are formed as the result of hyperactivity of dental lamina.
  - Dichotomy of tooth bud.
- Hyperdontia more frequently occurs in the upper arch compared to the lower arch (Fig. **4**). Most found supernumerary tooth is Mesiodens. Males are more commonly affected, with a male to female ratio of 2:1.
- Horizontal proliferation or hyperactivity of the permanent or deciduous dental lamina are the reasons for the development of the majority of supernumerary teeth.
  - i. Supplemental supernumerary teeth duplicate the typical position and structure of anterior and posterior teeth.
  - ii. Rudimentary supernumerary teeth are dysmorphic & may assume conical forms. This condition is generally found in some syndromes, such as Cleidocranial dysplasia, Gardner's syndrome, Orofacial digital syndrome, *etc*.

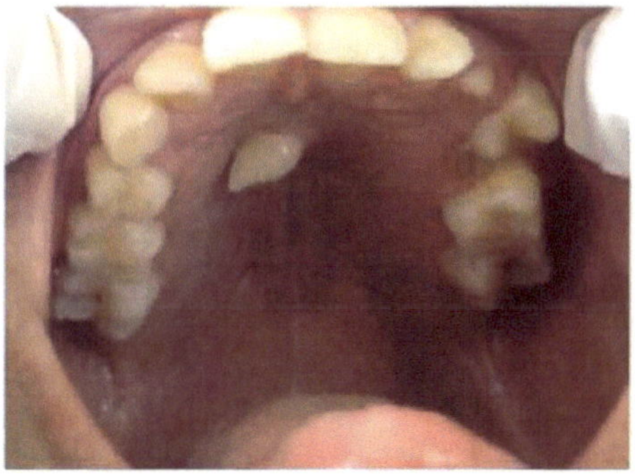

Fig. (4). Hyperdontia: ectopically erupted rudimentary supernumerary seen on the palate.

Treatment

- Management is based on the type and position of the supernumerary tooth and its potential effects on the adjacent tooth. Hypodontia in a young child.

- If a delay or inhibition of eruption of permanent teeth is found, removal of supernumerary teeth is advised.
- Associated pathology with supernumerary teeth compromises secondary alveolar bone grafting in cleft lip and palate patients. Treatment is decided based on clinical status and may include cosmetic crown placement.
- If the prognosis of the tooth is poor due to caries or there is a tooth displacement, extraction followed by management for space closure is recommended. Results of the study carried out by Omer *et al.* stated that if the impacted supernumerary tooth is removed surgically at stage C of Demirjian (aged 4 to 5 years), it poses minimal complications. The arrest of root development can occur if the supernumerary teeth are removed at stage D of Demirjian, at 5 to 6 years of age. Delayed removal at stage H, until the permanent tooth has been achieved, may lead to more defects like root resorption [1, 2].

Hypodontia (Figs. 5 and 6)

In this condition teeth are present in less than the normal number. Maxillary lateral incisors, third molars and mandibular second premolars (Fig. **5**) are the commonly missing permanent teeth at birth (congenitally). 'Anodontia' is a complete absence of teeth in the oral cavity (Fig. **6**). In anodontia, the growth of the alveolar process is restricted. Hypodontia, more commonly occurs in permanent dentition compared to primary dentition. A subtype of hypodontia characterized by the lack of development of six or more teeth is known as 'oligodontia', which may be true or false (Fig. **5**) [3].

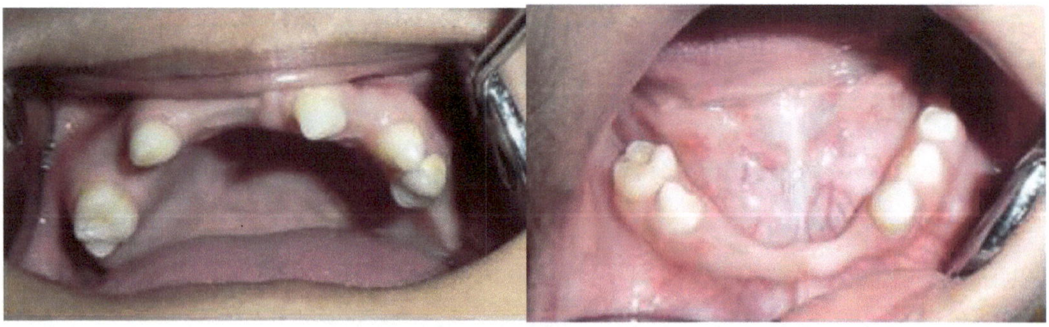

Fig. (5). Oligodontia: Multiple developmentally missing permanent teeth in maxillary and mandibular arch.

Hypodontia is often associated with several syndromes (Table **1**) and has a strong genetic basis. The associated syndromes include hereditary Down's syndrome, ectodermal dysplasia, Crouzon syndrome, Focal Dermal Hypoplasia, Ehlers-Danlos syndrome, Turner syndrome, *etc.*

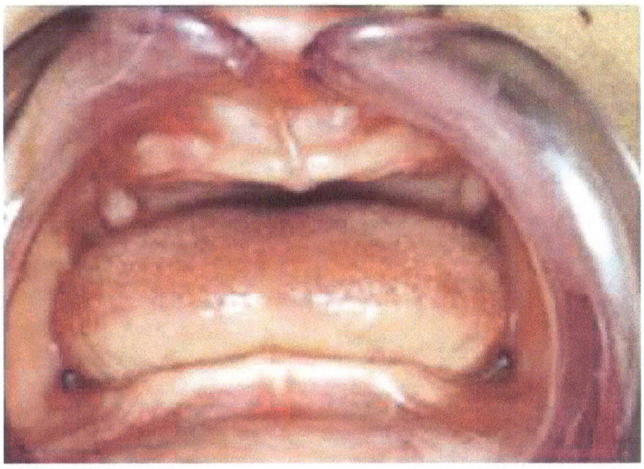

Fig. (6). Anodontia.

Table 1. Syndromes associated with Hypodontia.

Ectodermal dysplasia
Bilateral cleft lip and palate
Dubowitz syndrome
Fucosidosis
Hypoglossal-hypodactylia
Down syndrome
Ellis-van Crevald syndrome
Down syndrome
Marfan syndrome
Goldenhar
Gorlin
Sturge-Weber
Monilethrix-anodontia
Focal dermal hypoplasia
Coffin-Lowry
Tooth-and-nail
Turner
Progeria

Treatment

- Treatment depends upon the clinical involvement and include maintenance of oral hygiene, use of fluoride, pit & fissure sealants, and endodontic therapy.

- Prosthetic replacement of missing teeth is indicated in some cases with the use of dentures, bridges, and crowns. Orthodontic intervention can also be required.
- In the long term, implants can be an important treatment option.

Abnormalities Related to the Size of Teeth

Microdontia (Fig. 7)

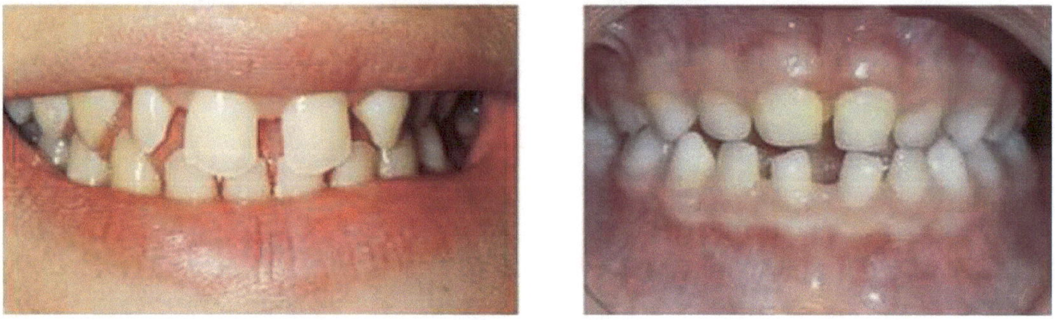

Fig. (7). Microdontia.

- The term is used to describe teeth that are smaller than normal.
- It can be of three types-
    1. True generalized microdontia-all the teeth are smaller than normal. It is exceedingly rare.
    2. Relative generalized microdontia- normal or slightly smaller than normal teeth are present in jaws that are somewhat larger than normal; there is an illusion of true microdontia. Hereditary factors play an important role.
    3. Microdontia involving only a single tooth is a rather common condition. It affects most often the maxillary lateral incisor and third molar. One of the common forms of localized microdontia is that which affects the maxillary lateral incisor, a condition known as *peg lateral* [*4*].

Treatment:

- Management includes esthetic restoration or prosthetic replacement.
- Orthodontic intervention can also be required.
- In older patients, implant placement can be a suitable treatment option.

Macrodontia (Fig. 8)

- Teeth are larger than normal in this case. It can be of three types-
    1. True generalized macrodontia-The condition in which all the teeth are larger than normal, has been associated with pituitary gigantism but is extremely rare.

2. Relative generalized macrodontia- is somewhat more common and is a result of the presence of normal or slightly larger than normal teeth in small jaws. Hereditary factors are responsible.
3. Macrodontia of single teeth- is relatively uncommon but occasionally seen. The etiology is unknown. A variant of localized macrodontia is seen in hemihypertrophy of face [5].

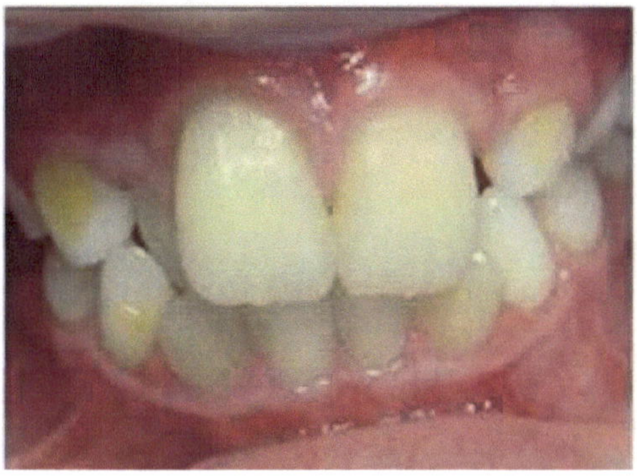
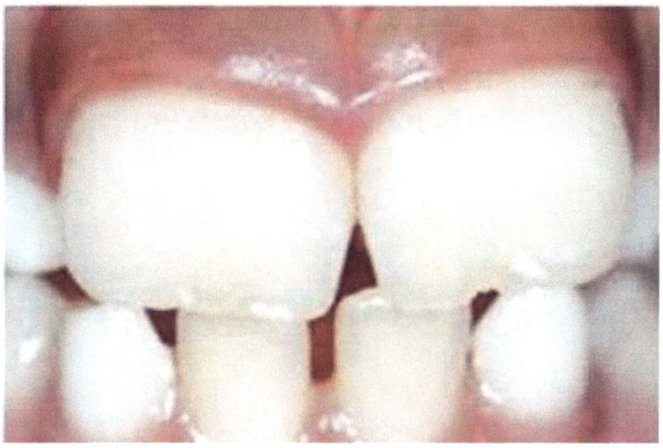

Fig. (8). Macrodontia.

Treatment

- Management may consist of esthetic restoration like double veneer indirect composite restoration.

Abnormalities of Tooth Form

Fusion (Fig. 9)

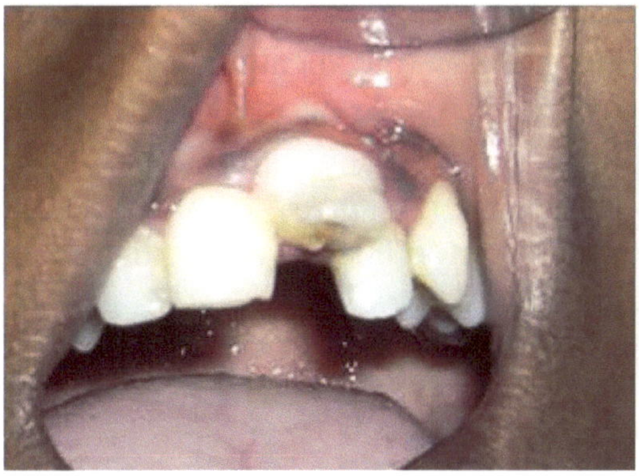
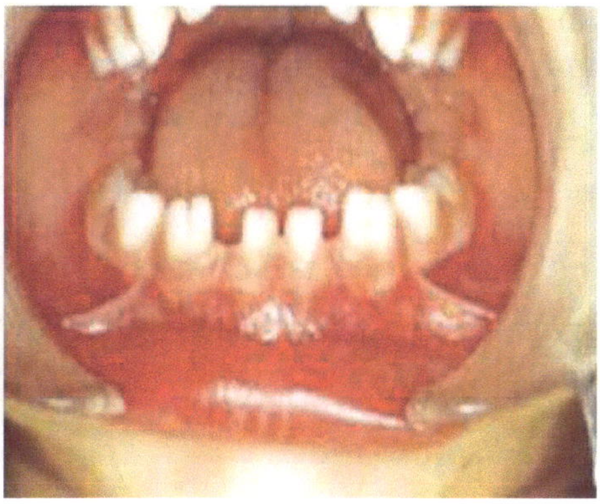

Fig. (9). Macrodontia.

- Fused teeth arise through union of two normally separated tooth germs.
- Depending upon the stage of development of teeth, at the time of union, fusion may be complete or incomplete. It has been thought that some physical force or pressure produces contact of the developing teeth and their subsequent fusion. If this contact occurs early, at least before calcification begins, the two teeth may be completely united to form a single large tooth.
- If the contact of teeth occurs later, when a portion of the tooth crown has been completed, there may be a union of roots only [6].
- In addition to affecting two normal teeth, fusion may also occur between a normal tooth and a supernumerary tooth such as Mesiodens or distomolar.

<u>Treatment</u>

Treatment of choice is mostly based on the patient's periodontal, functional, and esthetic needs. A multidisciplinary approach is usually required for successful results.

- A most preferred treatment option is a 'two-step surgical separation technique'.
- Endodontic therapy requires special consideration due to separate pulp chambers and root canals. Composite restoration of the teeth can then be the next step done.
- Orthodontic treatment may also be needed.

Concrescence

- Concrescence of teeth is a form of fusion which occurs after root formation has been completed. In this condition teeth are united by cementum only.
- It is thought to arise because of traumatic injury or crowding of teeth with resorption of the interdental bone so that the two roots are in contact approximately and become fused by the deposition of cementum between them.
- Concrescence may occur before or after the teeth have erupted [7].

<u>Treatment</u>

- Treatment varies as per the morphology of the tooth. Endodontic therapy, *i.e.*, non-surgical endodontic therapy, may be advised.
- Periodontal intervention is indicated in some cases.
- Surgical extraction is advised when needed. However, this may result in considerable loss of alveolar bone and can cause sinus perforation.

Gemination (Fig. 10)

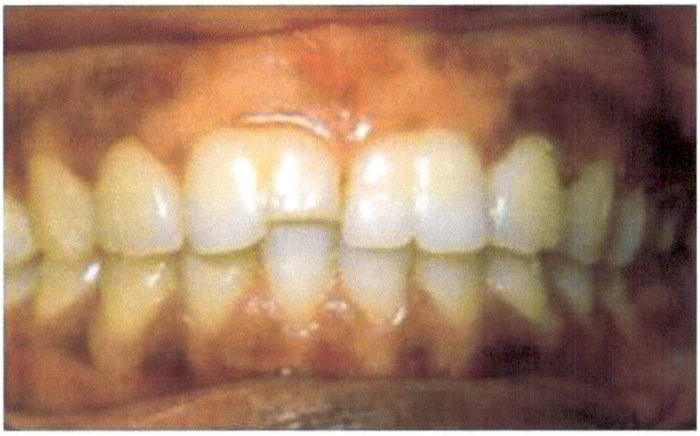

Fig. (10). Gemination.

• Gemination is the division of a single tooth germ during the proliferation stage of tooth development.

• It appears as a bifid crown on a single root. It is seen both in primary and permanent dentition. The affected tooth has two pulp chambers and a single root canal.

Treatment

• Periodontal surgical separation of tooth germs and esthetic restoration using a crown.

• Endodontic treatment required, because of two pulp chambers and a single root canal system.

This condition may have comorbidities like achondrodysplasia and chondroectodermal dysplasia. If found, this should prompt further detailed systemic evaluation [8].

Dens in Dente (Dens Invaginatus/tooth within a Tooth/ Invaginatedodontome/ Dilated Gestantodontome/dilated Composite Odontome/ Dentinoid in Dente) (Fig. 11)

- It is a developmental variation thought to arise because of an invagination in the surface of the tooth crown before calcification has occurred. The causes can include an increased localized external pressure, focal growth retardation and focal growth stimulation in certain areas of tooth bud.

- The permanent maxillary lateral incisors are the most frequently involved. Radiologically, it is recognized as a pear-shaped invagination of enamel and dentin with a narrow constriction at the opening on the surface of the tooth, and closely approximating the pulp in its depth.
- To prevent caries, pulp infection and premature loss of teeth, the condition must be recognized early, and the tooth prophylactically restored [9].

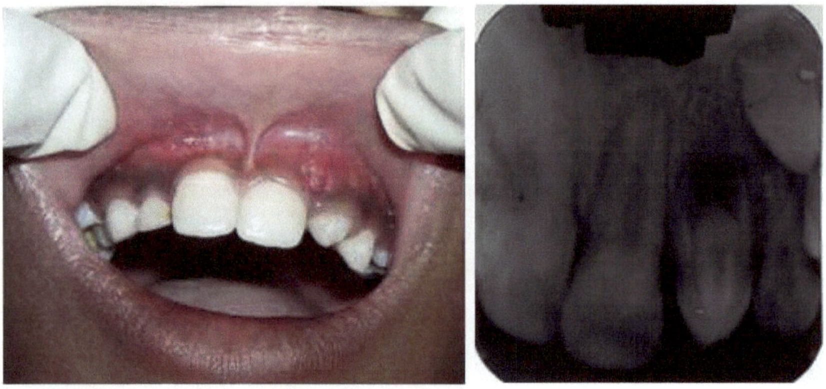

Fig. (11). Dens in dente.

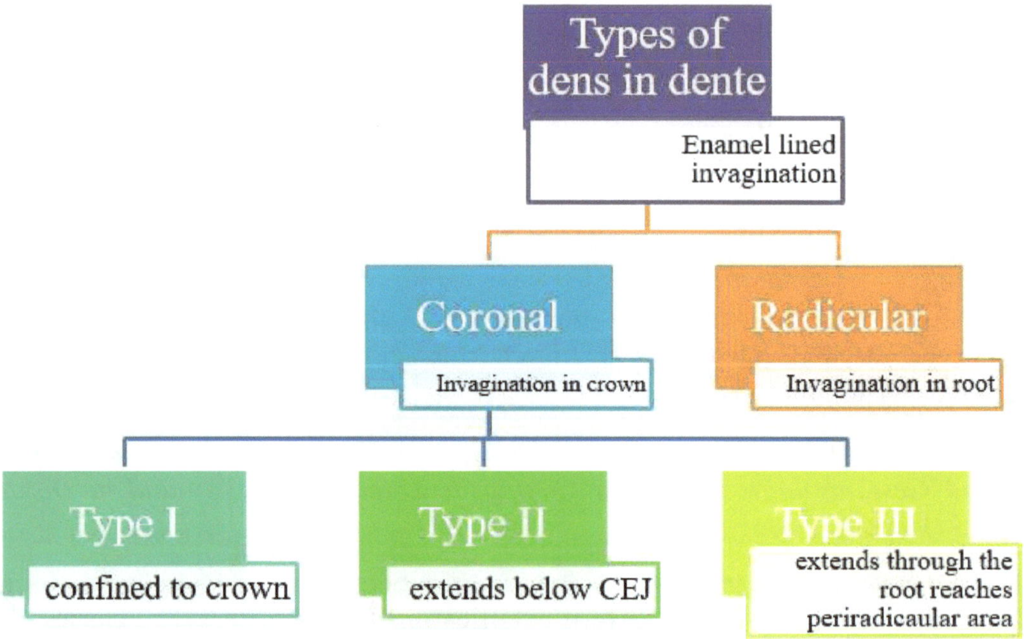

Etiological theories for Dens invaginatus

- Growth pressure of dental arch resulting in buckling of enamel organ.
- Invagination resulting from focal failure of inner enamel epithelial growth while the normal epithelium proliferates (Kronfeld, 1939).
- Invagination is the result of rapid proliferation of inner enamel epithelium infiltrating dental papilla (Rushton, 1937).
- Oehlers (1957) considered distortion of enamel organ and protrusion of enamel organ leading to formation of an enamel lined channel.
- 'Twin-theorie' proposed by Buiszt (1950) suggests fusion of two tooth germs.
- Fischer (1936) and Spranson (1937) suggested inflammation as a probable cause.
- Gustafson and Sundberg (1950) described trauma as a causative factor.

Treatment

The invagination can serve as a site for food lodgment resulting in the development of caries which then requires endodontic intervention. Endodontic non-surgical management in affected teeth with open apex using Mineral trioxide aggregate can be done.

Dens Evaginatus

- It is a developmental condition which appears clinically as an accessory cusp or a globule of enamel on the occlusal surface between the buccal and lingual cusps of the premolars, unilaterally or bilaterally, although it is mainly reported rarely in molars, cuspids and incisors. It is usually seen in people of the Mongoloid ancestry- Chinese, Japanese, Filipinos and Eskimos.
- The pathogenesis of the lesion is associated with the proliferation and evagination of an area of the inner enamel epithelium and subjacent odontogenic mesenchyme into the dental organ during early tooth development. It can lead to displacement of teeth or pulp exposure [10].

Talon Cusp (Fig. 12)

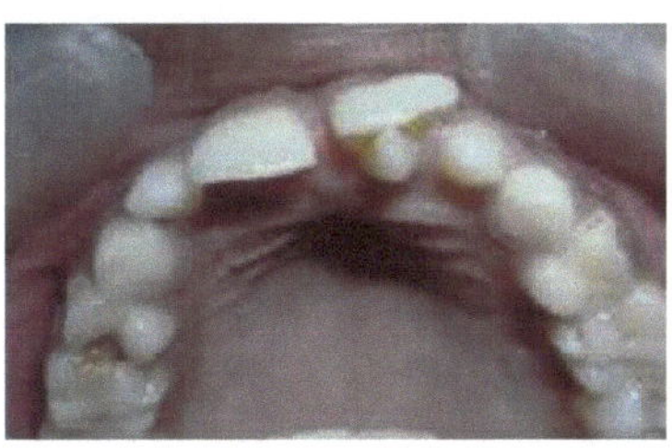

Fig. (12). Talon cusp.

- It is an anomalous structure resembling the talon of an eagle and projects lingually from the cingulum areas of a maxillary or mandibular permanent incisor. The cusp blends smoothly with the tooth, except that there is a deep developmental groove where the cusp blends with the sloping lingual tooth surface. It is composed of normal enamel and dentin and contains a horn of pulp tissue.
- It is associated with Rubinstein Taybi syndrome [11].

Treatment

- Caries may develop in the affected tooth, which then requires endodontic therapy followed by esthetic restoration or full crown coverage.
- Occlusal interference, if present, can be corrected by occlusal grinding.
- Complete removal of the anomaly followed by endodontic therapy and crown restoration can be required for esthetics and function.
- Orthodontic correction and realignment may also be needed.

Taurodontism (Fig. 13)

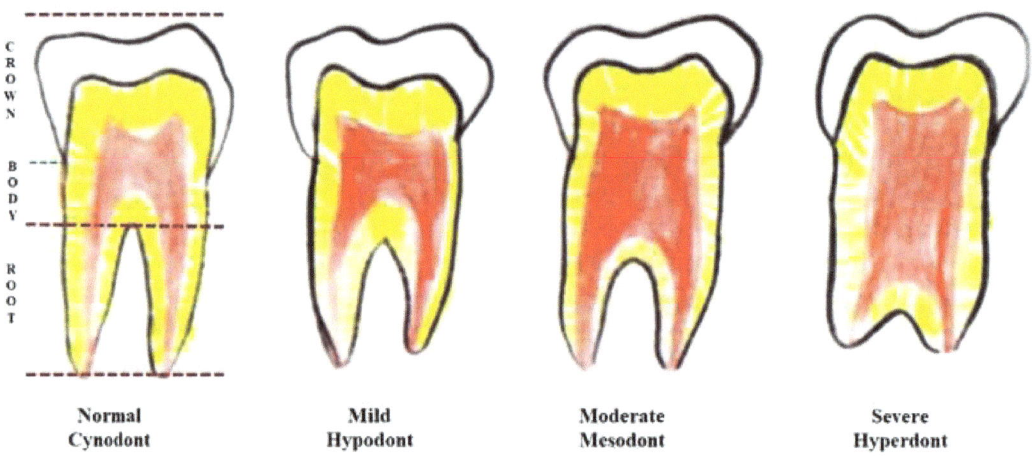

Fig. (13). Taurodontism- Diagrammatic representation of increasing grades of taurodontism.

- The term Taurodontism was originated by Sir Arthur Keith to denote a particular dental anomaly in which the body of a tooth is enlarged at the expense of the roots. Shaw classified taurodont tooth into mesotaurodont, hypotaurodont and hypertaurodont forms. The tooth involved is usually molars.
- The pulp chamber is extremely large with a much greater apico occlusal height than normal (Fig. **14**).

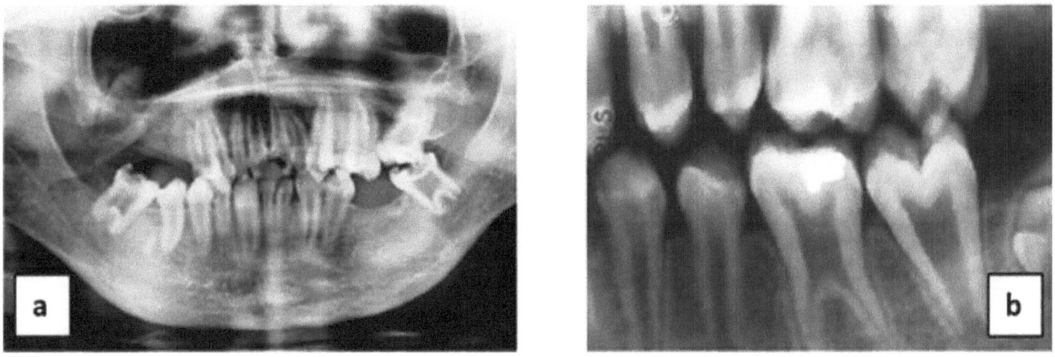

Fig. (14). Taurodontism: A and B- Large sized pulp chambers can be observed in molars.

Classification	Crown-Body: Root Ratio (CB: R)
Cynodont (Normal tooth)	<1.10
Hypodont	1.10–1.29
Mesodont	1.30–2.0
Hyperdont	>2.0

Treatment

- Assessment and evaluation of the complexity of the canal, obliteration and configuration of the canal, potential for an additional root canal, *etc*., are needed while performing root canal treatment on such teeth.
- The endodontic therapy may need modification depending on the length of the root canals and the diameter of the apical foramen. If it is wide, it can restrict the use of sodium hypochlorite during the irrigation process.
- Modified obturation technique consists of a combination of lateral compaction in the apical region and vertical compaction of the enlarged pulp chamber.
- A taurodont cannot be used for post-placement or as an abutment, or for orthodontic purposes because of lack of surface area.
- Apart from the dental treatment, clinicians should also help to uncover the systemic comorbidities associated with the condition [12].

Dilaceration (Fig. 15)

- Dilaceration is an angulation, curve, or a sharp bend in either the root or crown of a formed tooth.
- It is hypothesized to be caused by a trauma during the period of tooth formation, which results in the change in position of a calcified portion of the tooth. This also causes the remainder of the tooth to be formed at an angle.

- The bend or curve can occur anywhere across the length of the root, at the cervical portion, midway or at the apical portion of the tooth. The preoperative radiographic investigation is important in this regard [13].
- It occurs in relation to the permanent tooth where trauma has occurred in the corresponding deciduous tooth *i.e* when the roots of the permanent teeth are not formed completely (Fig. **14A**).

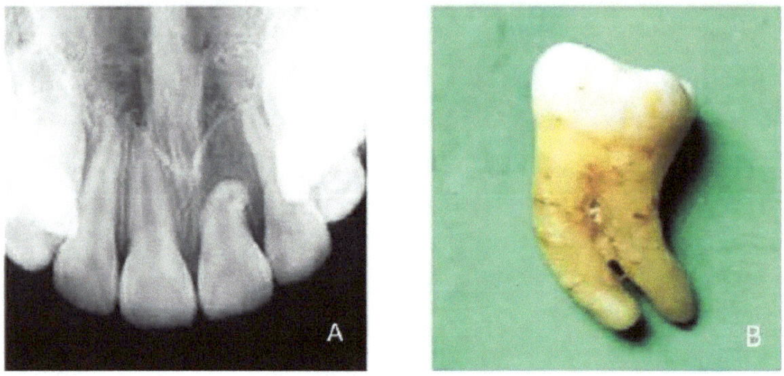

Fig. (15). Dilaceration seen in roots of permanent molar.

Treatment: A

- No treatment is needed in cases of mild dilaceration.
- This condition may result in problems during the extraction of carious teeth. Therefore, in cases of the severely dilacerated tooth, surgical exposure of the tooth with an apically repositioned flap along with orthodontic retraction may be required.

Abnormalities of tooth structure (Fig. 16)

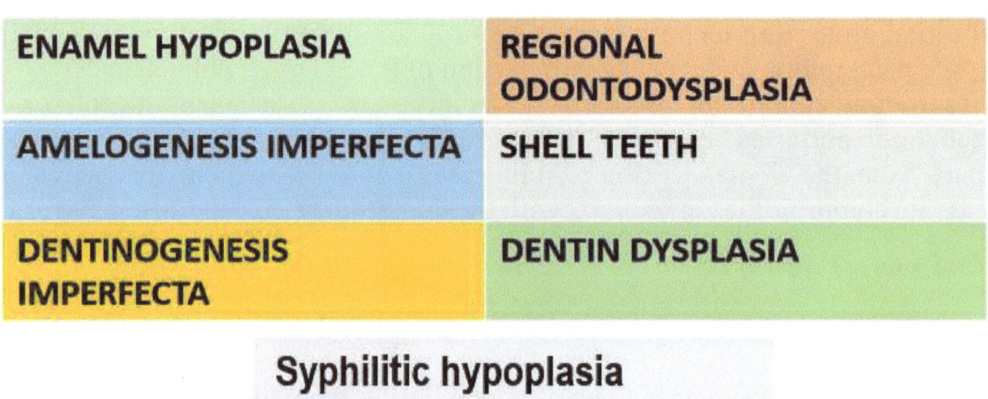

Fig. (16). Anomalies related to Tooth Structure.

Enamel Hypoplasia (Figs. 17 and 18)

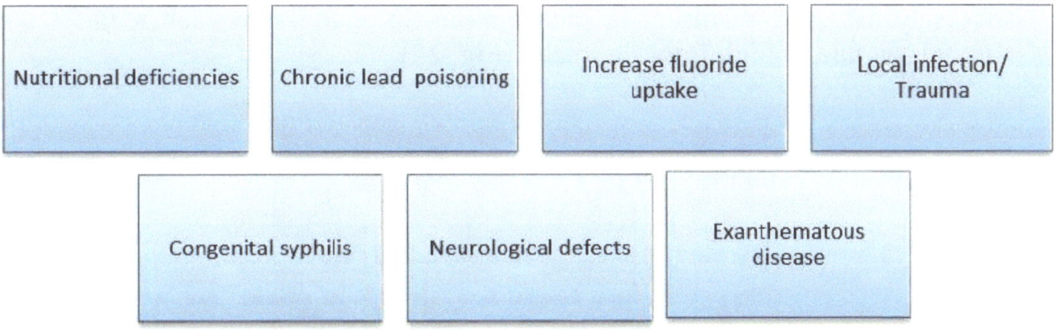

Fig. (17). Causes of Eamel hypoplasia.

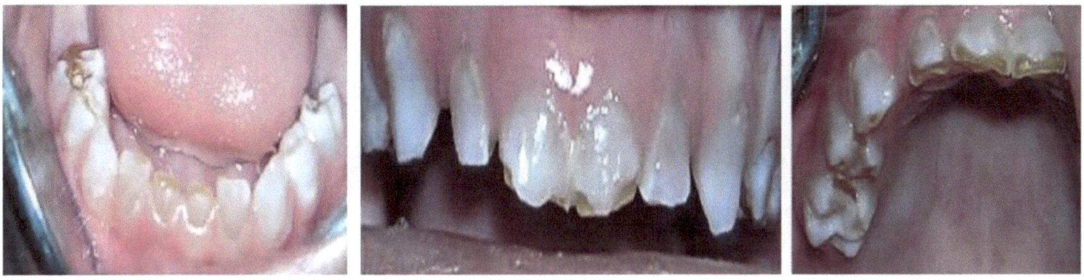

Fig. (18). Enamel hypoplasia.

Enamel hypoplasia is caused due to interference in the formation of the enamel matrix. Based on the severity, it is graded as mild, moderate, and severe. The primary dentition is usually associated with the mild form, while the severe form is commonly found in permanent dentition.

Classification

i. Hypoplasia secondary to local infection or trauma (Fig. **19**): Hypoplastic areas are commonly seen on the crowns of primary teeth due to the infection or trauma. The term used for the hypoplasia resulting from the local infection is 'Turner's tooth' or 'Turner's hypoplasia'. Trauma to the primary teeth may interfere the calcification or matrix formation of the developing permanent teeth, resulting in hypoplasia.
ii. Hypoplasia due to nutritional deficiencies: Hypoplasia is mostly seen in children having deficiency of vitamin A, C, D, calcium and phosphorous.
iii. Hypoplasia associated with allergies: Rattner and Myers first discovered the correlation between hypoplasia and allergic reactions. This type of hypoplasia is commonly found in children with severe allergic reactions.

iv. Hypoplasia due to radiation: In children undergoing radiation therapy for malignancy, it is found that, the process of enamel matrix formation is adversely affected, resulting in the hypoplastic changes in such teeth.
v. Hypoplasia due to high fluoride intake (Fig. **20**):

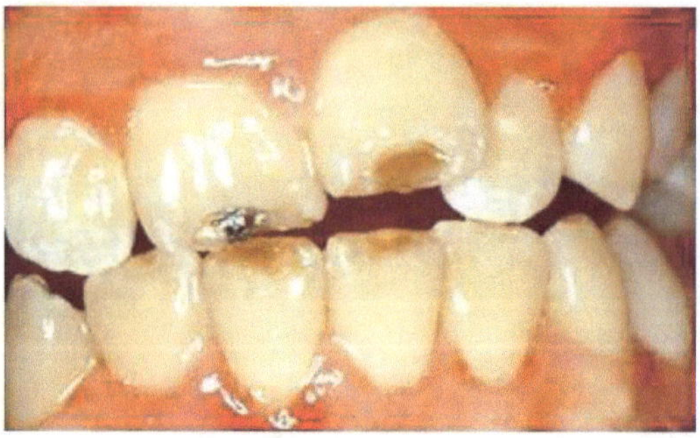

Fig. (19). Turner's hypoplasia.

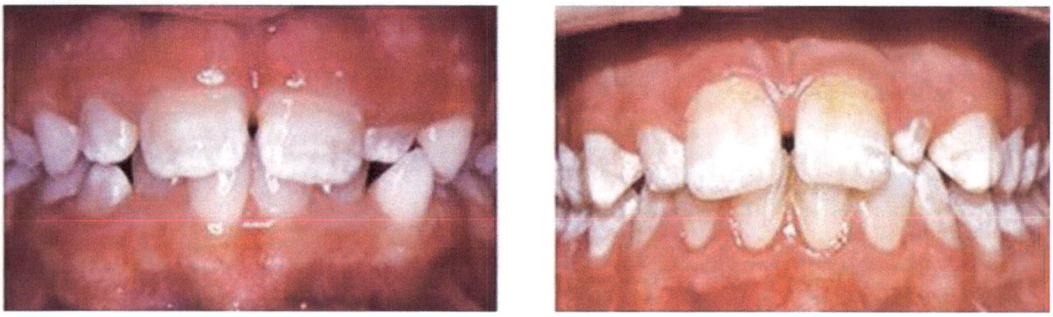

Fig. (20). Fluorosis.

Excess consumption of fluoride can result in enamel hypoplasia.

The enamel shows white opaque or pitted areas that vary in extent and severity as per the degree of fluorosis.

i. Hypoplasia in association with neurological defects: Hypoplasia is commonly found in children having low Intelligence scores (IQ) and neurological defects. There is a direct relationship between the time of brain injury and the defect. Thus, children who have suffered brain damage may also show hypoplastic changes in the enamel.
ii. Hypoplasia due to chronic lead poisoning: Children of mothers having a history of lead poisoning during pregnancy can be affected, as lead can readily cross the placental barrier. Pitting enamel hypoplasia is seen in these children.

iii. Hypoplasia associated with congenital syphilis: Hutchinson's triad has been found in patients with this disorder. The triad consists of eighth nerve deafness, keratomalacia and enamel hypoplasia.
iv. Hypoplasia is associated with exanthematous diseases like scarlet fever [14].

Treatment

- Hypoplastic teeth are susceptible to caries. In patients with mild enamel hypoplasia, the small carious lesions can be restored with amalgam, resin, or glass ionomer cement. Composite resin restorations may be required for anterior tooth restorations.
- Sensitivity of teeth, a common complaint, can be relieved with topical fluoride application.
- Severe enamel hypoplasia is associated with large areas of defective enamel and exposed dentin. In cases of severe crown destruction, stainless steel crowns can be placed on posterior teeth. Restorative rehabilitation can help to reproduce the natural tooth appearance by means of microabrasion, composite resin restoration and bleaching.

Amelogenesis Imperfecta (Fig. 21)

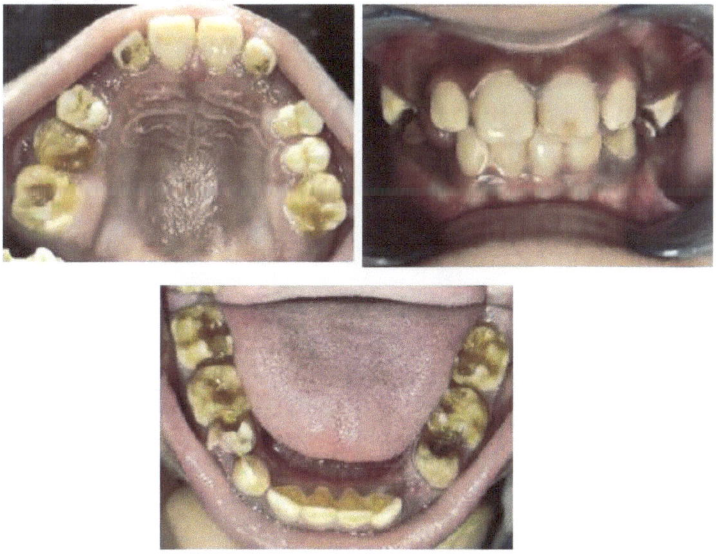

Fig. (21). Amelogenesis imperfect.

- This is a rare hereditary ectodermal disorder in which the mesodermal components of the teeth are not altered. Etiology is genetic and related to the alteration of genes that are associated with the process of formation and maturation of the enamel.

Classification:

i. Hypocalcified type
ii. Hypomaturation type
iii. Hypoplastic type.

- The defect in tooth structure is limited to the enamel. On radiographic examination of the pulpal outline, the morphology of the root usually appears normal.
- Hypocalcified type: The enamel matrix formation is normal, but the calcification is deficient, which results in soft enamel. This defect is clinically manifested by the softened, pigmented enamel that is easily detachable.
- Hypomaturation type: The enamel matrix is improperly formed through calcification does occur. The enamel is hard but deficient in the proportion, which can be expressed clinically as thin enamel. It has grooves and pits on its surface.
- Hypoplastic type: The enamel matrix is improperly formed, calcification in the matrix occurs, and enamel is hard but deficient in amount. Clinically it is expressed as thin enamel with grooves and pits on the surface [15].

Treatment

- Multidisciplinary approach is generally needed for management of such teeth.
- Periodontal surgery (for example, crown lengthening procedures) is recommended in cases of excessively shortened crowns.
- Esthetic restoration on discolored teeth and endodontic intervention in cases of pulpal involvement are mandatory.

Dentinogenesis imperfecta (Fig. 22)

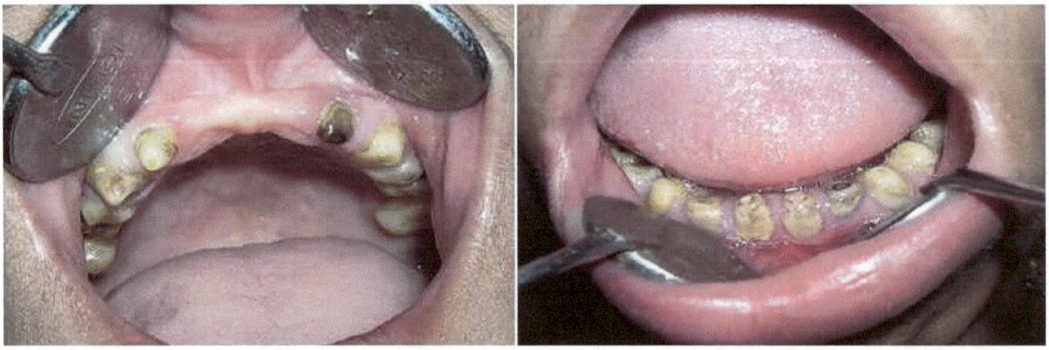

Fig. (22). Dentinogenesis imperfecta.

It is inherited as an autosomal dominant trait.

Classification:

i. Type I Dentinogenesis imperfecta is a dentin defect occurring in association with osteogenesis imperfecta.
ii. Type II Dentinogenesis imperfecta is an isolated trait.
iii. Type III (Brandy wine type) with multiple pulpal exposures in deciduous dentition. This condition affects both the dentitions and is characterized by reddish-brown to grey opalescent discoloration of the teeth.

The enamel is extremely brittle and easily chips off, resulting in the exposure of underlying dentin. Dentin is soft and abrades easily, which gives it a smooth polished appearance. The pulp chamber and canals appear diminutive on the radiograph or may be completely absent.

Roots can be slender with ribbon-like canals and root fractures are common. Permanent teeth show relatively less destruction. Enamel and dentin show normal histologic structures.

The fracturing of the enamel has been attributed to the lack of scalloping at the junction of dentin and enamel [16 - 18].

Treatment

- Basic preventive measures like maintenance of oral hygiene and use of fluoridated toothpastes are advised.
- To avoid tooth abrasion in primary dentition, stainless steel crowns and Polycarbonate crowns can be fabricated.
- Cast crowns are the treatment of choice in permanent molars.
- Anterior teeth can be restored with strip crowns, polycarbonate crowns and metal ceramic restorations.
- Extraction is needed for teeth with root fractures.
- For esthetic purpose, composite veneers can be placed over maxillary and mandibular anteriors.
- The treatment of this condition continues up to adulthood, with placement of crown placement, over-dentures, and dental implants.
- In cases of periapical abscess, an endodontic intervention may be needed.
- Psychological and genetic counseling of the parents and child is important in these cases.

Shell Teeth (Fig. 23)

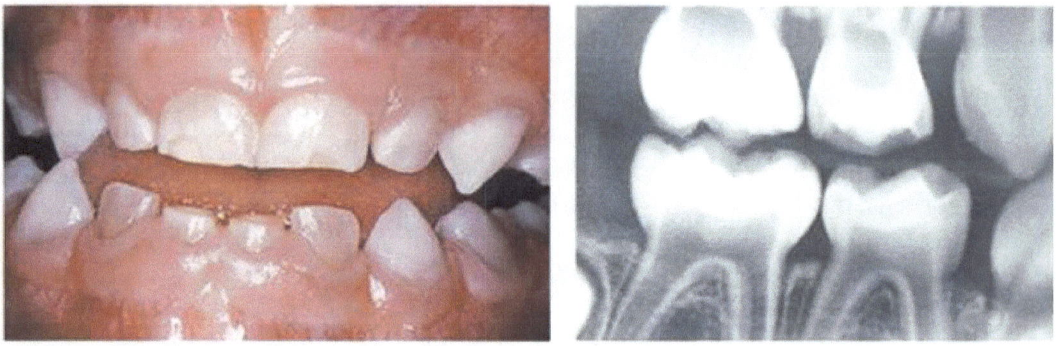

Fig. (23). Shell teeth.

• Shell teeth were first described by Rushton, as a form of dentinal dysplasia.

• The shape and color of the teeth are generally normal, though the teeth may darken with age. Both primary and permanent dentitions are affected, but different teeth within the arch are not affected equally.

• Enamel thickness is usually normal, but the dentin is thin, giving it the appearance of a thin shell of a hard tissue surrounding a large pulp chamber and canals.

• The roots appear short and have closed apices. Histopathologically, normal dentin is seen subjacent to dentinoenamel junction for 1 to 2 mm, followed by abrupt changes *i.e.*, alteration in the tubule directions & morphology and an apparent arrest in further dentin deposition.

Treatment:

- These teeth carry the risk of pulpal exposure during restorative procedures and increase the susceptibility of the teeth to fracture.
- Preserving the teeth by orthodontic, restorative, surgical and endodontic procedures, if possible, ensures adequate alveolar support for future prosthodontic treatment.

Dentin Dysplasia (Fig. 24)

- This condition is a hereditary, autosomal dominant disorder resulting in atypical dentin formation. (Fig. **24**)
- Dentine dysplasia (a) Type I; (b) Type II abnormal pulpal morphology.

- It is of two types (Type I- radicular and Type II- coronal). Since the teeth have short roots, exfoliation occurs prematurely.
- Radiographically, type-II dentin dysplasia shows a 'thistle tube appearance'. Microscopically, type I dentin dysplasia shows 'lava flowing around boulders' appearance [19].

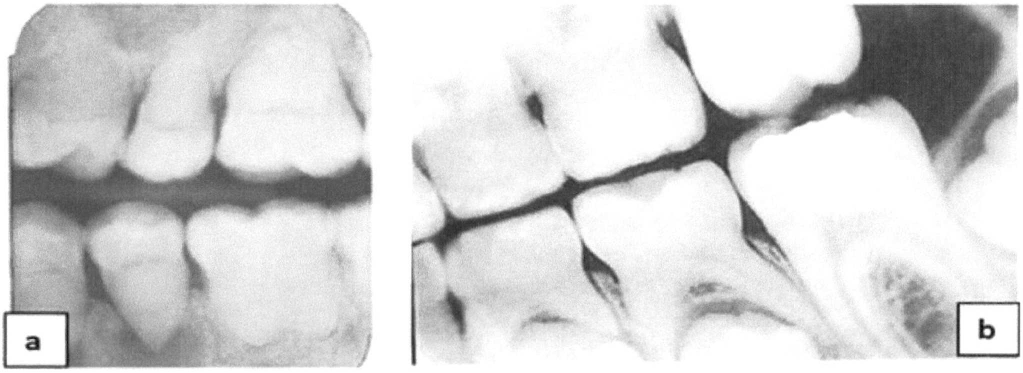

Fig. (24). Dentine dysplasia **(a)** Type I; **(b)** Type II.

Treatment:

- Prosthetic replacement using dentures and over-dentures is recommended.
- Composite facings or strip crowns can be used to ensure the esthetic restorations.
- Dental implants can be considered on growth completion, for which ridge augmentation can be performed.
- Routine endodontic treatment for teeth with pulpal necrosis and a periapical abscess is done.
- As early tooth exfoliation occurs, bone grafting and sinus lift procedure can be performed to enable implant placement once the growth completion occurs.

Regional Odontodysplasia

• This is an unusual anomaly of unknown etiology, characterized by the presence of several teeth, in a localized area, radiographically exhibiting thin enamel and dentin surrounding an enlarged radiolucent pulp (ghost tooth appearance). Maxillary central, lateral incisors and cuspids are the most common teeth involved [20].

Treatment

- The affected tooth needs extraction followed by prosthetic replacement with a denture or a crown along with a bridge preparation.

Syphilitic Hypoplasia (Fig. 25)

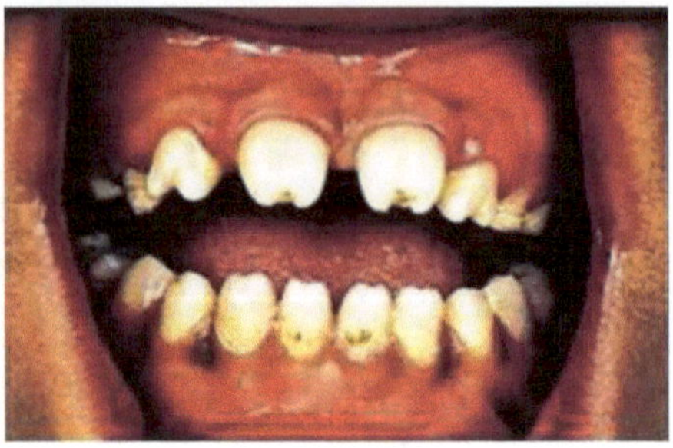

Fig. (25). Hutchinson's teeth.

- It is a characteristic of congenital syphilis.
- In this condition, the shape of the center incisors is peg shaped or screwdriver shaped which are widely spaced.
- The incisors are notched at the end with crescent shaped deformity.
- It is seen along with Hutchinson triad which consists of deafness, Hutcinson's incisor and neurosyphilics.
- Another condition seen in congenital syphilis is the presence of multiple rudimentary enamel cusps on 1st molar giving the appearance of mulberry, called as Mulberry molar.

Treatment

- It includes cosmetic corrections such as composite resin, veneers, or full crown.

Anomalies of tongue (Fig. 26)

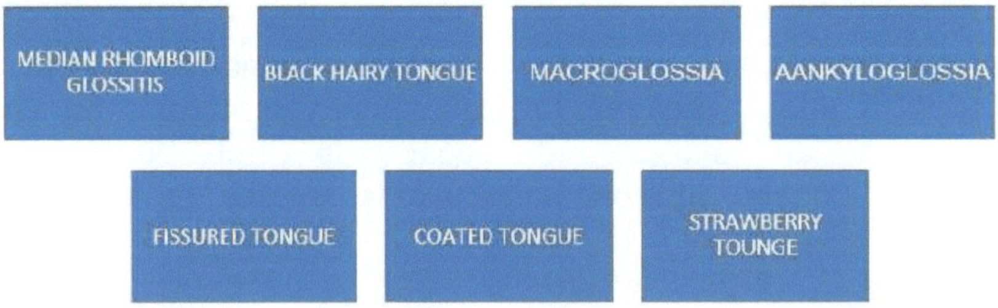

Fig. (26). Anomalies of Tongue.

The tongue should be thoroughly examined during the examination procedure.

Macroglossia (Fig. 27)

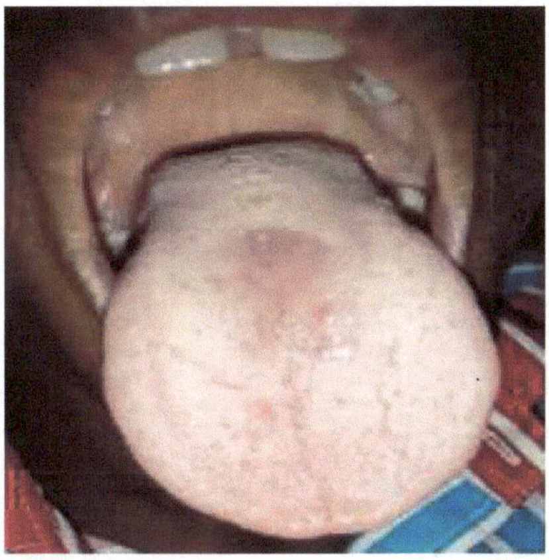

Fig. (27). Macroglossia.

- It is an abnormally enlarged tongue which can be congenital or acquired. Congenital macroglossia results from the overdevelopment of associated musculatures, which may or may not involve other parts of the body. Acquired or secondary macro glossia can occur because of a tumor (lymphangioma, hemangioma, neurofibroma), acromegaly, cretinism, or amyloidosis.
- Macroglossia is a prominent feature of Beckwith-Widermann syndrome. The components include macroglossia, postnatal somatic gigantism, microcephaly, umbilical hernia, visceromegaly and neonatal hypoglycemia.

Treatment

- Management includes the identification of the exact underlying cause, and accordingly treatment must be done. In cases of Congenital macroglossia surgical debulking of excess tongue tissue may be done.
- Glossectomy can be performed for the treatment of macroglossia.
- When the underlying etiology is neoplastic or due to endocrinal disturbance, primary management should be the treatment of the cause.
- When a syndromic comorbidity or genetic condition is present, surgery needs to be performed for functional and esthetic reasons.

Microglossia and Aglossia

- A small or rudimentary tongue is a rare congenital anomaly which is known as microglossia. Complete absence of the tongue, *i.e.*, Aglossia has been reported.

- Because of the lack of muscular stimulus between the alveolar arches, these do not develop transversely, and the mandible does not grow in an anterior direction.
- The problems encountered are obvious and include severe difficulties with speech, mastication, deglutition, and phonation.

Ankyloglossia (Fig. 28)

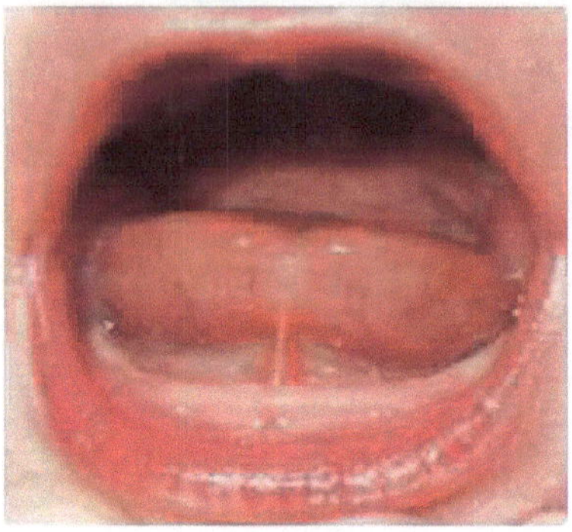

Fig. (28). Ankyloglossia.

- Ankyloglossia or tongue-tie is said to exist when the inferior frenulum attaches to the bottom of the tongue and subsequently restricts the free movement of the tongue.
- The criteria for diagnosis are based on observation of lingual mobility. Tongue-tie can cause feeding problems in infants.
- Speech defects, especially articulation of the sounds l, r, t, d, n, th, sh and z, can take place. The Ankyloglossum superium syndrome or oral-facial digital syndrome, the cleft lip or palate, and congenital lip pits syndrome should be considered when ankyloglossia occurs.

Treatment

Frenulectomy is recommended.

Cleft Tongue

- A complete cleft or bifid tongue is a rare condition that is apparently due to lack of merging of the lateral lingual swellings of this organ. A partially cleft tongue is considered more common and is manifested simply as a deep groove in the midline of the dorsal surface.
- The partial cleft results because of incomplete merging and failure of groove obliteration by underlying mesenchyme proliferation.

- It is part of an oral-facial-digital syndrome in association with thick fibrous bands in the lower anterior mucobuccal fold, eliminating the sulcus.
- It is of little clinical significance except that food debris and microbes may collect in the base of the cleft and cause irritation.

Fissured tongue (Fig. 29)

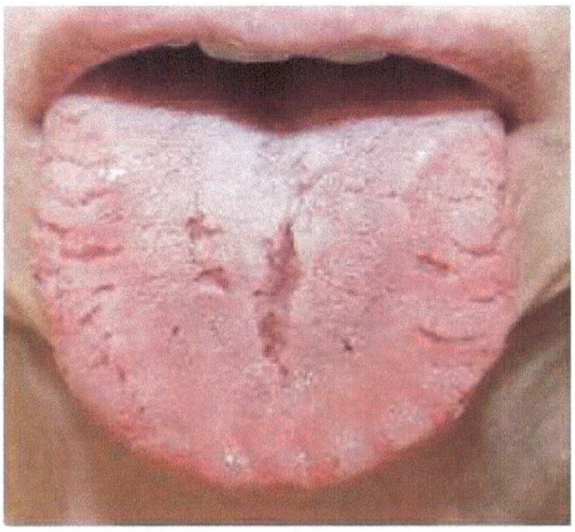

Fig. (29). Fissure tongue.

- Fissured tongue manifests itself as numerous small furrows or grooves often radiating out from a central groove along the midline of the dorsal surface of the tongue. It is usually part of a syndrome such as Melkersson Rosenthal syndrome or Down syndrome.
- The components of MR syndrome include the fissured tongue, 7th cranial nerve paralysis and cheilitis granulomatosa. The grooves and fissures may be upto 6 mm deep. A polygenic mode of inheritance and deficiency of Vit B12 may be associated with fissured tongue. There may be an accumulation of food debris in these fissures and grooves, causing discomfort and irritation. Keeping the grooves and fissures clean helps eliminate clinical problems associated with irritation in this condition.

Treatment

No treatment is indicated as maintaining oral hygiene can resolve most secondary symptoms.

Coated Tongue (Fig. 30)

- The tongue appears to be coated with a white layer when dead and degenerated epithelial cells, food debris and microorganisms become lodged between enlarged papillae.

- The condition is normally harmless, despite the odd appearance. But a coated tongue can be a symptom of a serious health condition.

Causes of the coated tongue are myriad-

- Oral thrush-thick, white cottage cheese-like appearance
- Poor oral hygiene
- Mouth breathing
- Leukoplakia
- Dry mouth
- Alcohol consumption and tobacco usage
- Fever and congenital heart disease

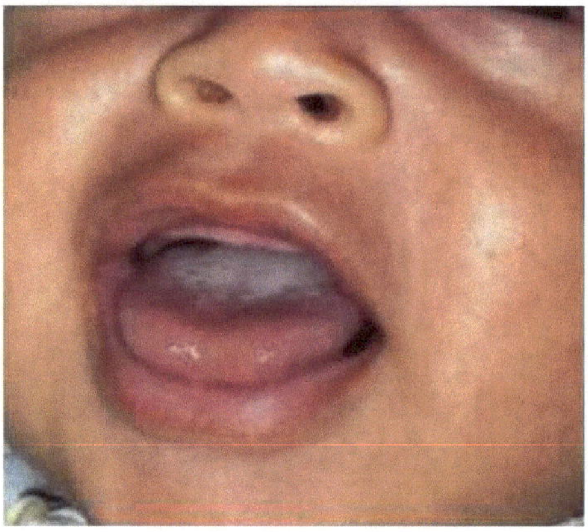

Fig. (30). Coated tongue.

Important causes are-

- Antibiotic and corticosteroid use
- Diabetes
- Poorly fitted dentures
- HIV and cancer
- Pregnancy

Treatment

- Maintaining oral hygiene along with regular tongue scraping should be done as a preventive method.
- Systemic therapy using Vitamins can resolve this problem. Nowadays, oil pulling is being recommended as a line of treatment.

Strawberry Tongue (Fig. 31)

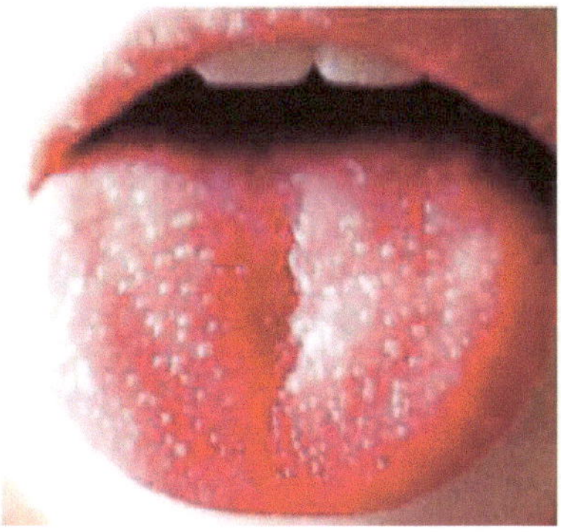

Fig. (31). Strawberry tongue.

- It is a result of the enlargement of fungiform papillae above the level of filiform papillae. The term refers to a tongue that is swollen, bumpy and bright red.
- It generally occurs in children and is a symptom of medical conditions, like Kawasaki disease and scarlet fever. It can also occur due to Vit B12 and folate deficiencies and allergies.

Treatment

The underlying systemic condition should be corrected, and antihistaminics can control allergic conditions. Proper diet and Vit B12 supplements can correct vitamin deficiencies. Antibiotic treatment can resolve the problem as it is merely a benign manifestation of scarlet fever.

Geographic Tongue (Benign Migratory Glossitis)

- Patchy, multifocal, circinate, sharply demarcated and irregular areas of surface erosion, characterized by the loss of filiform papillae, constitute the lesions of the geographic tongue. At the periphery, whitish serpiginous lines at least partially surround the lesions. The fungiform papillae remain. They may show evidence of swelling and erythema. Most of the cases are asymptomatic. Some patients complain of glossodynia.
- The lesions wax and wane. Remissions occur, and during recurrences, the lesions appear in different locations. The apparent movement of the lesions and the geographical appearance of the lesion have led to the descriptive terminology. Psychological stress is associated with the condition and is also seen in people with psoriasis [21].
- Microscopically there is a loss of the filiform papillae with a spongiotic abscess (Monroe's abscess) appearing in the epithelium. This appearance, including the

presence of neutrophils, is like that seen in Reiter syndrome and psoriasis. A mild chronic inflammatory infiltrate is generally seen in underlying connective tissue.

- No treatment is necessary. We can only administer topical steroids like prednisolone and antifungals in severe cases.

Median Rhomboid Glossitis (Fig. 32)

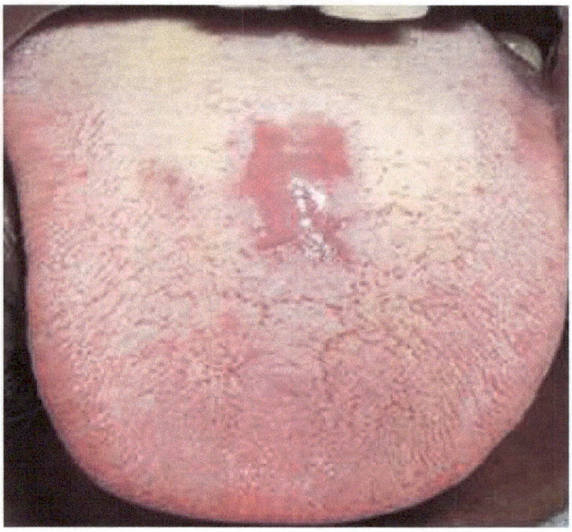

Fig. (32). Median rhomboidal glossitis.

- MRG presents as a smooth surfaced, rhomboid-shaped, pink, nodular elevation of the tongue located immediately anterior to the foramen caecum and the circumvallate papillae in the midline of the dorsum of the tongue.
- It likely represents a developmental defect, presumably arising because of the persistence of the tuberculum impar and its failure to retract during embryogenesis. However, several investigators have suggested that Candida organisms play a causative role in the development of MRG. In patients with central papillary atrophy, Candida could be demonstrated.
- Microscopically the epithelial rete ridges extend well into the mucosal connective tissue. Candida organisms are often demonstrated in the parakeratin layer, while the underlying CT shows a mild inflammatory infiltrate.

Treatment

- The lesions normally regress spontaneously. Sometimes antifungal therapy like nystatin and clotrimazole lozenges must be instituted.

Black Hairy Tongue

- A hairy tongue is characterized by a marked accumulation of keratin on the filiform papilla of the dorsal surface of tongue, resulting in a hair-like appearance. The condition apparently represents an increase in keratin production or a decrease in the normal keratin desquamation. The elongated papillae are usually brown, yellow, or black because of the growth of pigment-producing bacteria or staining from tobacco or food
- The tongue should be thoroughly examined during the intraoral examination for any anomalous presentation.

Treatment

- No treatment is indicated as good oral hygiene can prevent this condition. Maintenance of good oral hygiene, including cleaning of the tongue, should be followed.

DEVELOPMENTAL LESIONS OF ORAL MUCOSA (FIG. 33)

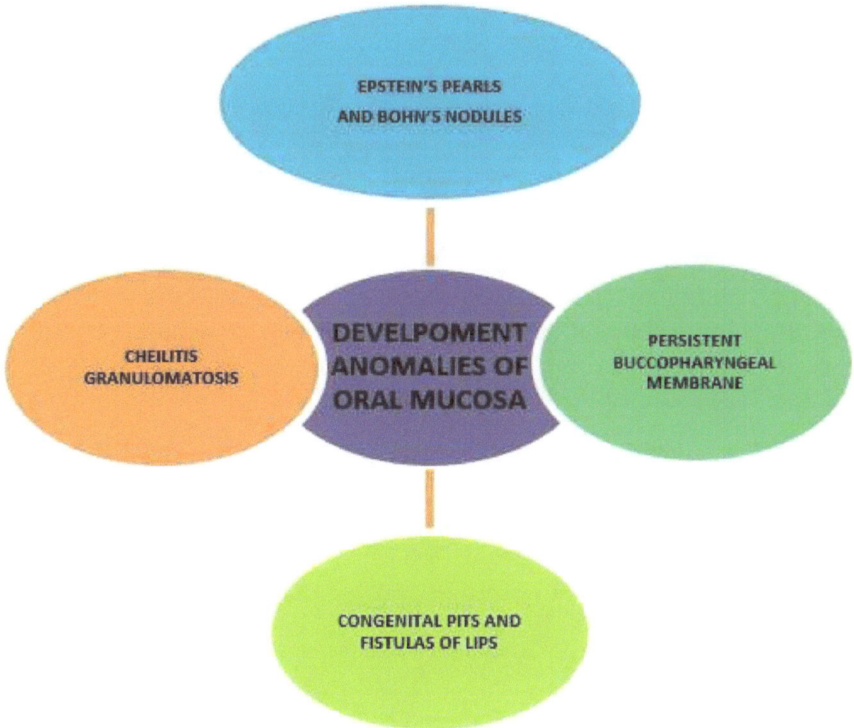

Fig. (33). Developmental lesions of the oral mucosa.

Fordyce's Granules

- It is a developmental anomaly caused by a heterotopic collection of sebaceous glands at various sites in the oral cavity. It may arise from inclusion in the oral cavity of ectoderm having some of the potentialities of skin during the development of maxillary and mandibular processes during embryonic life. It appears as multiple discreetly dispersible or focally condensed yellowish papular spots frequently bilaterally in the buccal mucosa along with the molar teeth. Histologically heterotopic lobular aggregations of sebaceous glands will be evident.

Focal epithelial hyperplasia or Heck disease (Fig. 34)

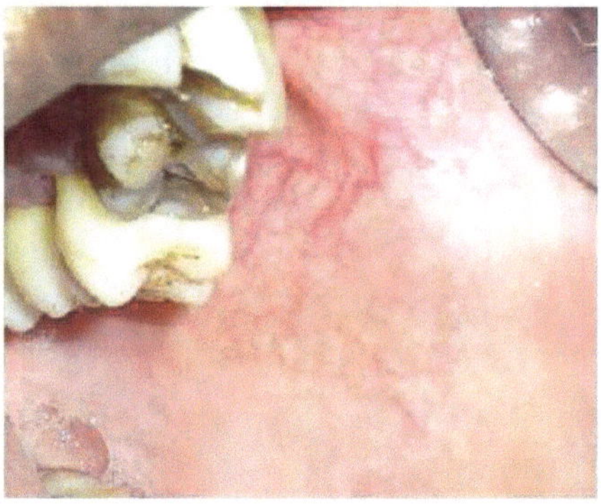

Fig. (34). Fordyce's granules – Yellow dots on the buccal mucosa representing ectopic sebaceous glands.

- It is caused by HPV 13 AND 32. Children and young adults are commonly affected. Well demarcated, smooth-surfaced and flat-topped papular lesions involving the labial, buccal and lingual mucosa are usually present. If they coalesce together, they can produce a *cobblestone* appearance. It might represent as an oral manifestation of AIDS.

Epstein's pearls and Bohn's nodules (Fig. 35)

- Multiple or single white raised nodules are seen on the alveolar ridges in nearly 80% of newborn infants. These are called 'Epstein's pearls' or 'Bohn's nodules' depending on the location. Epstein's pearls are commonly seen in the mid palatal raphe area.
- They occur because of trapped epithelial remnants along the line of fusion of the palatal halves. Bohn's nodules are remnants of salivary gland epithelium and are usually present on the buccal and lingual aspects of the ridge, away from the midline.

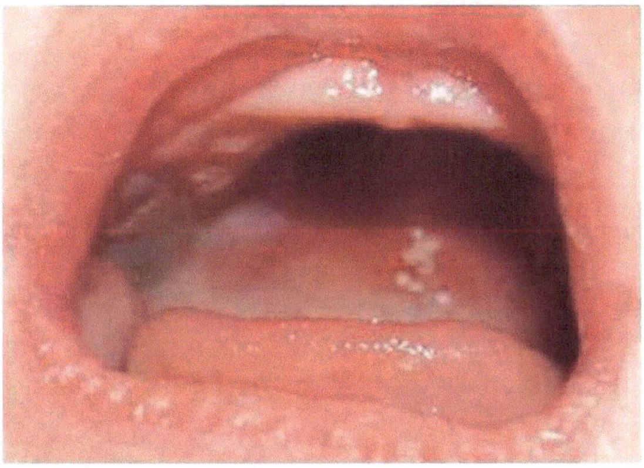

Fig. (35). Bohn's nodules.

Treatment

- These lesions do not increase in size and do not require any treatment as they regress on their own, leading to complete disappearance. Parent should be counseled about the harmlessness of these entities.

Persistent Buccopharyngeal Membrane

- The primitive oral cavity or stomodeum is lined by stratified squamous epithelium called the oral ectoderm. The oral ectoderm contacts the endoderm of the foregut to form the buccopharyngeal membrane.
- On twenty-seventh day of gestation, this double-layered epithelial membrane ruptures and the primitive oral cavity establishes a connection with the foregut and the development of the oropharynx occurs. Sometimes, the membrane does not rupture completely, and part of it persists in the oral cavity. This can obstruct swallowing [22].

Treatment

- Management using custom-made polyurethane stent has been used as a prosthetic treatment to facilitate swallowing.

Congenital Pits and Fistulas of the Lip (Fig. 36)

- These are usually seen on the lower lip and often show some secretion. Sometimes these become infected and show signs of inflammation. Congenital lip pits (Van der Woude Syndrome) are seen as small mucosal invaginations that occur at the corners of the mouth on the vermillion border [23].

Treatment

- Pits are treated by surgical excision. Superimposed Candidiasis can be treated by application of antifungal agents topically.

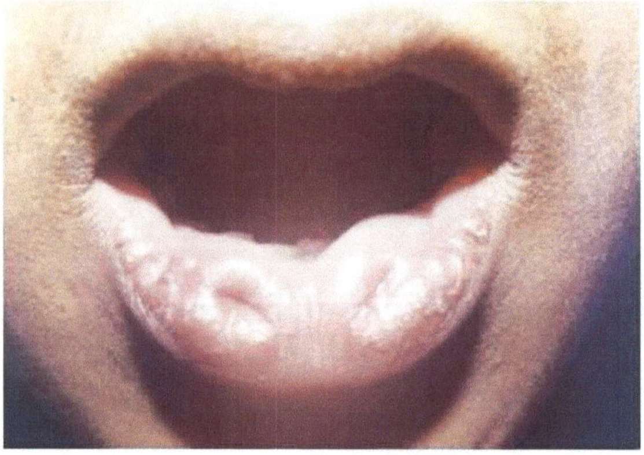

Fig. (36). Congenital lip pits.

Cheilitis Granulomatosa

This is an autosomal dominant condition where the affected lip appears diffusely swollen. Histopathology reveals macrophages and lymphocytes within granulomatous clusters separated by fibrous septa. The differential diagnosis of this condition includes angioedema, allergic reaction, and soft tissue trauma [24].

Treatment

Management includes steroid (Triamcinolone) injections along with surgical intervention to resolve the swelling (Fig. **37**).

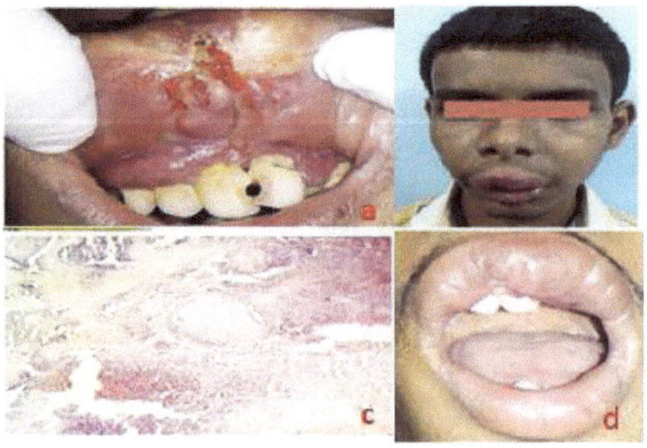

Fig. (37). A, b- Intraoral and extraoral photograph of diffuse swelling of upper lip, c- Histopathology shows granulomatous lesion. d- After treatment with steroids.

CONCLUSION

Childhood developmental disorders globally account for significant health and societal burden. As the evidence presented in this chapter indicates, key treatment protocols have the potential to reduce developmental disorders in childhood. Evidence suggests that these can be feasibly delivered in both clinical and hospital setups. The screening of children for developmental disorders is possible; however, the evidence for intervention once identified is limited. The systems required for reducing these development disorders require intersectoral collaboration and significant parent and child cooperation. The widespread implementation and evaluation of parenting skills training in all countries is recommended to achieve a meaningful reduction in the global prevalence and burden of childhood developmental disorders.

CONSENT FOR PUBLICATION

Not applicable.

CONFLICT OF INTEREST

The author(s) declare no conflict of interest, financial or otherwise.

ACKNOWLEDGEMENT

Declared none.

REFERENCES

[1] Application of the International Classification of Diseases to Dentistry and Stomatology. 2011.

[2] Pereira MN, de Almeida LE, Martins MT, da Silva Campos MJ, Fraga MR, Vitral RWF. Multiple hyperdontia: Report of an unusual case. Am J Orthod Dentofacial Orthop 2011; 140(4): 580-4. [http://dx.doi.org/10.1016/j.ajodo.2010.02.038] [PMID: 21967947]

[3] Villa A, Albonico A, Villa F. Hypodontia and microdontia: clinical features of a rare syndrome. J Can Dent Assoc 2011; 77: b115. [PMID: 21846459]

[4] Bargale SD, Kiran SDP. Non syndromic occurrence of true generalized microdontia with mandibular mesiodens - a rare case. Head Face Med 2011; 7(1): 19-29. [http://dx.doi.org/10.1186/1746-160X-7-19] [PMID: 22035324]

[5] Fuentes R, Borie E. Bilateral macrodontia of mandibular second premolars: a case report. J MorpholSci 2011; 28(3): 212-5.

[6] Tewari N, Pandey RK. Bilateral fusion in primary mandibular teeth: A report of two cases. J Indian Soc Pedod Prev Dent 2011; 29(1): 50-2. [http://dx.doi.org/10.4103/0970-4388.79936] [PMID: 21521919]

[7] Foran D, Komabayashi T, Lin LM. Concrescence of permanent maxillary second and third molars: case report of non-surgical root canal treatment. J Oral Sci 2012; 54(1): 133-6. [http://dx.doi.org/10.2334/josnusd.54.133] [PMID: 22466898]

[8] Oelgiesser D, Zyc R, Evron D, Kaplansky G, Levin L. Treatment of a fused/geminated tooth: a multidisciplinary conservative approach. Quintessence Int 2013; 44(7): 531-3. [PMID: 23534048]

[9] Mupparapu M, Singer SR. A review of dens invaginatus (dens in dente) in permanent and primary teeth: report of a case in a microdontic maxillary lateral incisor. Quintessence Int 2006; 37(2): 125-9. [PMID: 16475374]

[10] Borie E E, Oporto V G, Aracena R D. Dens evaginatusin haemophiliac patient. Int J Morphol 2010; 28(2): 375-8. [http://dx.doi.org/10.4067/S0717-95022010000200006]

[11] Hattab FN, Yassin OM, al-Nimri KS. Talon cusp--clinical significance and management: case reports. Quintessence Int 1995; 26(2): 115-20. [PMID: 7568721]

[12] Jafarzadeh H. azarpazhooh A, Mayhall JT. Taurodontism: a review of the condition and endodontism treatment challenge. Int Endod J 2008; 41: 375-88. [http://dx.doi.org/10.1111/j.1365-2591.2008.01388.x] [PMID: 18363703]

[13] Chew MT, Ong MMA, Perio C. Orthodontic-surgical management of an impacted dilacerated maxillary central incisor: a clinical case report. Pediatr Dent 2004; 26(4): 341-4. [PMID: 15344628]

[14] Arrow P. Enamel hypoplasia of the primary dentition in a 4-year-old with intestinal lymphangiectasia. Int J Paediatr Dent 2005; 15(5): 380-4. [http://dx.doi.org/10.1111/j.1365-263X.2005.00662.x] [PMID: 16129004]

[15] Aldred MJ, Savarirayan R, Lamand SR, Crawford PJM. Clinical and radiographic features of a family with autosomal dominant amelogenesis imperfecta with taurodontism. Oral Dis 2002; 8(1): 62-8. [http://dx.doi.org/10.1034/j.1601-0825.2002.1c766.x] [PMID: 11936459]

[16] Kantaputra PN. Dentinogenesis imperfecta-associated syndromes. Am J Med Genet 2001; 104(1): 75-8. [http://dx.doi.org/10.1002/ajmg.10031] [PMID: 11746032]

[17] Stephen L, Beighton P. Dental management of severe dentinogenesis imperfecta in a mild form of osteogenesis imperfecta. J Clin Pediatr Dent 2003; 26(2): 131-6. [http://dx.doi.org/10.17796/jcpd.26.2.r852g46052604266] [PMID: 11878277]

[18] Abukabbos H, Al-Sineedi F. Clinical manifestations and dental management of dentinogenesis imperfecta associated with osteogenesis imperfecta: Case report. Saudi Dent J 2013; 25(4): 159-65. [http://dx.doi.org/10.1016/j.sdentj.2013.10.004] [PMID: 24371383]

[19] Toomarian L. mashhadiabbas F, MirkarimiM, Mehrclad L. Denti dysplasia type I: a case report and review of literature. J Med Case Reports 2010; 4: 1-6. [http://dx.doi.org/10.1186/1752-1947-4-1]

[20] Fulari S, Tambake D. Rootless teeth: Dentin dysplasia type I. Contemp Clin Dent 2013; 4(4): 520-2. [http://dx.doi.org/10.4103/0976-237X.123063] [PMID: 24403801]

[21] Ishibashi M, Tojo G, Watanabe M, Tamabuchi T, Masu T, Aiba S. Geographic tongue treated with topical tacrolimus. J Dermatol Case Rep 2010; 4(4): 57-9. [PMID: 21886753]

[22] Tan SSW, Tan HKK, Lim CS, Chiang WM. A novel stent for the treatment of persistent buccopharyngeal membrane. Int J Pediatr Otorhinolaryngol 2006; 70(9): 1645-9. [http://dx.doi.org/10.1016/j.ijporl.2006.04.009] [PMID: 16797730]

[23] Ziai MN, Benson AG, Djalilian HR. Congenital lip pits and van der Woude syndrome. J Craniofac Surg 2005; 16(5): 930-2. [http://dx.doi.org/10.1097/01.SCS.0000164335.27171.B1] [PMID: 16192885]

[24] Krutchkoff D, James R. Cheilitis Granulomatosa. Arch Dermatol 1978; 114(8): 1203-6. [http://dx.doi.org/10.1001/archderm.1978.01640200057015] [PMID: 677920]

CHAPTER 15

Lesions of Oral Mucosa

Jay Gopal Ray[1] and **Priyanka Bhaje**[2,*]

[1] *Burdawan Dental College and Hospital, West Bengal, India*

[2] *Rungata College of Dental Sciences and Research Centre, Bhilai, Chhattisgarh, India*

Abstract: In children, lesions of the oral mucosa are common, and they can have various clinical signs such as ulceration, changes in the colour of mucosa or the presence of nodular lesions. Some lesions are asymptomatic, whereas others are symptomatic and sometimes even can disturb the routine activities of a child. It is important that, while evaluating the soft tissue lesions, dentists should be able to distinguish between normal, pathological conditions and normal anatomical variations. Sometimes children can present with oral mucosal lesions like those present in adults with a predisposition for some lesions. It was also observed that most of the common oral diseases were dental caries and mucosal diseases associated with cancer treatment. In literature, ere is a scarcity of information about oral lesions in children. This chapter explains various oral mucosal lesions in children along with their clinical presentation and management.

Keywords: Children, Color Change, Oral Lesions, Soft Tissue Nodules.

INTRODUCTION

Oral mucosal lesions always appear frightening to patients, especially in the pediatric age group. The clinical features of oral mucosal lesions can show variation and differ from common oral pathologies seen in adults.As substantial literature is found in the oral cavity of a child (Fig. **1**), it becomes important to make an accurate diagnosis and the right treatment plan. Thus, a Pediatric dentist should be knowledgeable in identifying these conditions to alleviate the fear of the parents, and in counselling for treatment, as per the need.

* **Corresponding author Priyanka Bhaje:** Rungata College of Dental Sciences and Research Centre, Bhilai, Chhattisgarh, India; Email: priyanka22bhaje@gmail.com

WHITE LESIONS
Geographic tongue
Geographic tongue
Candidiasis
White sponge nevus

VESICULAR ERYTHMATOUS AND ULCERATIVE LESIONS
Primary herpetic gingivostomatitis
Herpengina

AUTOIMMUNE DISORDERS
Pemphigus/pemphigoid
Systemic Lupus erythematous
Ectodermal dysplasia
Papillon-lefevre syndrome
Apthous stomatitis

LESIONS OF BACTERIAL ORIGIN
Impetigo
Scarlet fever
Syphilis
Tuberculos gingivitis
Actinomycosis
Noma

PIGMENTED LESIONS
Hereditary hemorrhagic telangiectasis
Hemangioma
Sturge Weber Syndrome
Black hairy tongue

SOFT TISSUE ENLARGEMENTS
Reactive tumors/ neoplasms

IDIOPATHIC LESIONS
Pterygoid ulcer/ Bednar ulcer

Fig. (1). Different oral mucosa lesions in children.

White lesions of the Oral Cavity (Fig. 2)

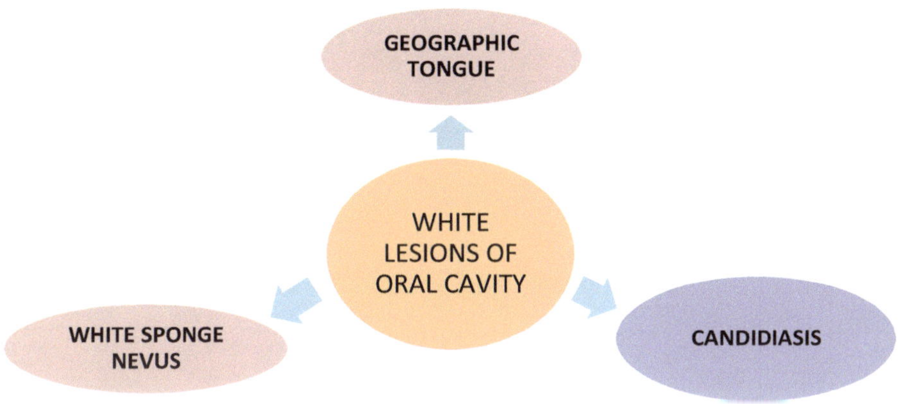

Fig. (2). White lesions of Oral Cavity (Representative diagram).

Benign Migratory Glossitis (Geographic Tongue)

- Patchy, multifocal, circinate, sharply demarcated and irregular areas of surface erosion, characterized by the loss of filiform papillae constitute the lesions of the geographic tongue. At the periphery, whitish serpiginous lines at least partially surround the lesions. The fungiform papillae remain. They may show evidence of swelling and erythema. Most of the cases are asymptomatic. Some patients complain of glossodynia (Fig. **3**).
- The lesions wax and wane. Remissions occur, and during recurrence, the lesions appear in various locations. The apparent movement of the lesions and the geographical appearance of the lesion have led to the descriptive terminology. Psychological stress is associated with this condition and is also seen in people with psoriasis.
- Microscopically, filiform papillae are lost with a spongiotic abscess (Monroe's abscess) appearing in the epithelium. This appearance, including the presence of

neutrophils, is like that seen in Reiter syndrome and psoriasis. A mild chronic inflammatory infiltrate is seen in underlying connective tissue [1].

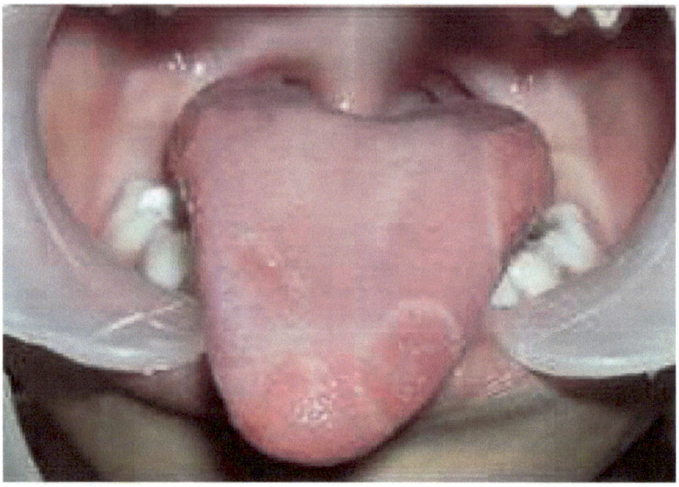

Fig. (3). Benign migratory glossitis.

Treatment

- Usually, no treatment is required.
- In severe cases, topical steroids like prednisolone and antifungals can be prescribed.

Candidiasis/Moniliasis

- Candidiasis or Oral thrush is a common opportunistic fungal infection in infants and neonates. The spectrum of infections caused by species of Candida includes infections of the nails, skin, mucous membrane, and internal organs. Candida albicans is the commonest causative agent.
- The factors which predispose to Candidiasis include infancy, pregnancy, immunosuppression, prolonged use of wide-spectrum antibiotics and malnourished state.
- Candidiasis which affects neonates, is known as acute pseudomembranous candidiasis. It is characterized by multiple white, curdy, loosely attached patches on any part of the oral mucosa. Preferred sites are the buccal mucosa and tongue. The patches can be easily wiped off with a wet gauze piece leaving a denuded, erythematous surface (Fig. **4**).
- Diagnosis by PAS stain is of importance. It shows thread-like magenta-coloured hyphae and budding spores [1].

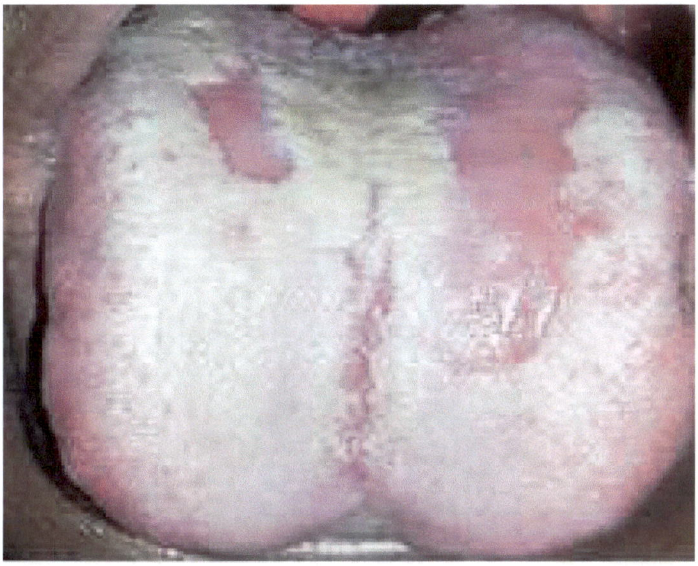

Fig. (4). Candidiasis on tongue.

Treatment

- Systemic antifungal agents are prescribed such as Fluconazole or Itraconazole
- In severe or azole-resistant candidiasis, amphotericin B is also advised.
- For local therapy, nystatin is given.
- Ethanolic propolis extract has also been reported to be equally curative as Nystatin.

White Spongy Nevus

- It is a rare autosomal dominant disorder which is due to a defect in the normal keratinization of the oral mucosa. The lesions of White spongy nevus usually appear at birth or in early childhood. Symmetrical, diffuse, thickened, white and corrugated plaques bilaterally involving the buccal mucosa are usually found. Other sites of involvement are the ventral tongue, labial mucosa, soft palate, alvcolar mucosa, and floor of the mouth.
- Histopathologically, prominent hyperparakeratosis, marked acanthoses and vacuolation of the spinous cell layer are seen.
- A cytology smear stained with PAP stain shows the pathognomonic perinuclear condensation of keratin microfilaments [2] (Fig. **5**).

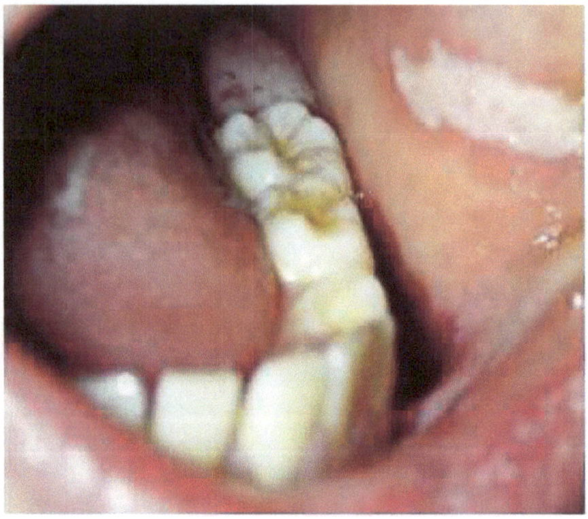

Fig. (5). White sponge nevus.

Treatment

• No specific treatment is required. Sometimes, maintenance of oral hygiene with chlorhexidine mouthwash is necessary.

Vesicular, Erythematous, and Ulcerated Lesions of Viral Etiology (Fig 6)

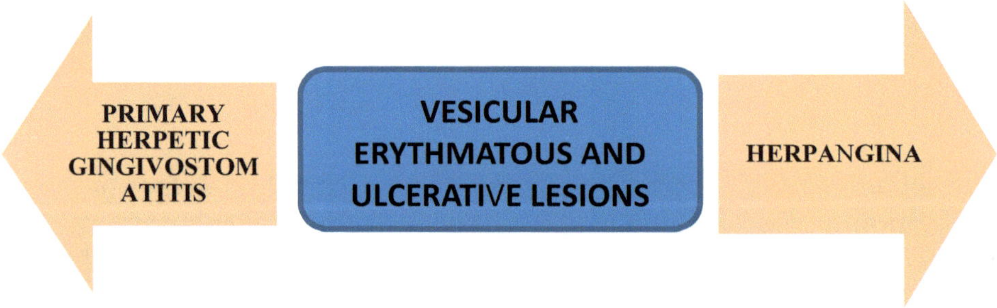

Fig. (6). Vesicular, erythematous, and ulcerated lesions of viral etiology.

Primary Herpetic Gingivostomatitis (Fig 7)

- Primary herpetic gingivostomatitis develops mostly in children and young adults. Painful vesicular eruptions develop on all mucosal surfaces and rupture to produce foul-smelling painful ulcers.
- The patient is febrile and has malaise and tender cervical lymphadenopathy.
- The lesions and acute illness last about 10 days and resolve with scar formation. Clusters of the ruptured vesicles may coalesce. It is caused by herpes simplex

virus type 1. This gains access to the patient via direct or airborne water droplet transmission from an infected individual.

- Laboratory evaluation through immunoblot testing to detect HSV1 circulating antibodies may be useful in children with acute herpetic gingivostomatitis. Murine monoclonal AB immunohistochemistry can identify the presence of intracellular HSV in formalin-fixed paraffin-embedded sections. DFA and PCR can be employed.
- Histopathologically, the characteristic feature is the presence of altered epithelial cells exhibiting ballooning degeneration, margination of chromatin and multinucleation [3].

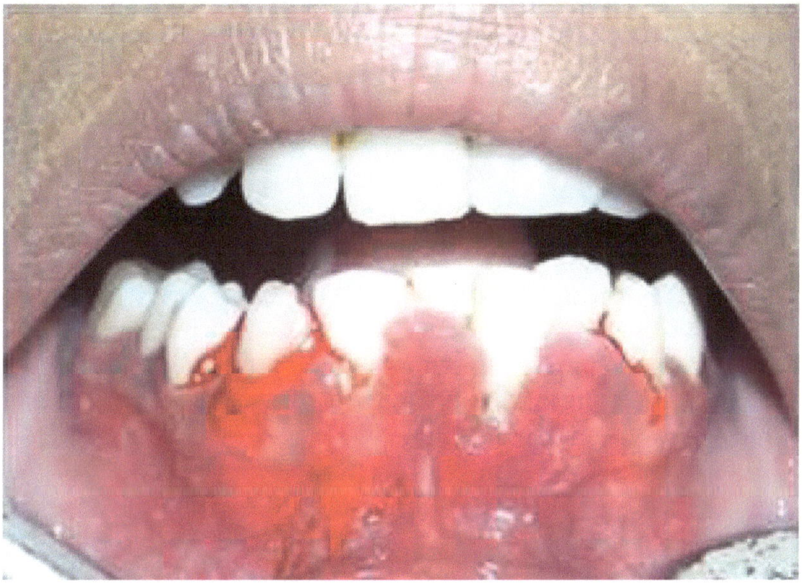

Fig. (7). Primary Herpetic Gingivostomatitis.

Treatment

- Antiviral agents like Acyclovir, penciclovir, docasonal, valacyclovir and famciclovir are advised.
- Supportive treatment with analgesics, popsicles, avoidance of citrus or spicy foods and glyoxide rinse for oral hygiene.
- Topical application of Diphenhydramine, Lidocaine, Benzocaine, Magnesium hydroxide, Aluminium hydroxide, Corticosteroids and Nystatin helps to relieve pain thereby easing the process of eating and drinking.
- Also, topical application of Idoxuridine on the tongue can be given as a part of palliative therapy.

Herpangina (Fig 8).

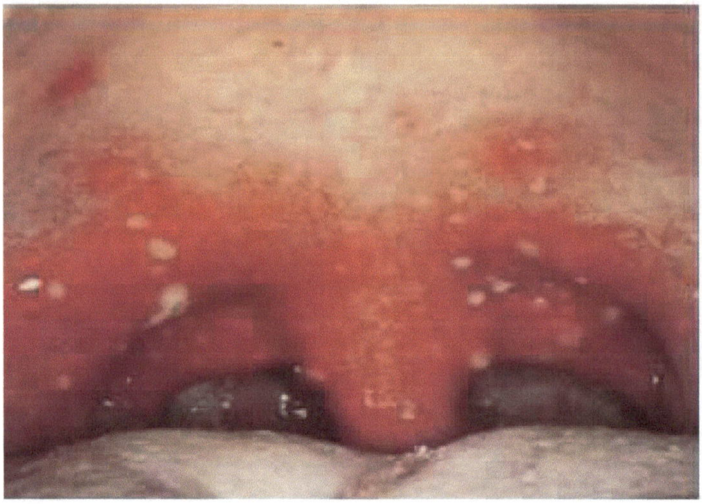

Fig. (8). Herpangina

- Principally caused by group A Coxsackie virus, but also by group B Coxsackie viruses and Echoviruses. Greatest incidence in the summer and early fall among the 3-10 years old age group.
- Prodrome of fever, sore throat, and dysphagia may precede by 1-2 days from the development of exanthem. Gray, pinhead size vesicles rupture to form large, fibrin-covered ulcers. Usually present on the anterior tonsillar pillars, posterior pharynx, and soft palate. Average of 5 lesions although some cases can have up to 16. In addition to fever and oral lesions, other symptoms like headache, vomiting, and abdominal pain may occur.
- The infection is self-limited, symptoms are mild, and lesions resolve within 3-5 days. Decreased Per so intake may lead to dehydration.
- In addition to all these, Hand foot and mouth disease is important.
- Hand Foot and Mouth Disease usually occur in the summer and fall and is caused by infections with 2 enteroviruses, Coxsackie A16 being the most common.
- Transmission is faecal-oral and less commonly oral-oral. Viruses may shed for months after infection.
- Common in toddlers and school-aged children.
- 1-2 days of fever and sore throat followed by an outbreak of vesicles on the buccal mucosa and tongue. The lesions are slightly painful. Vesicles are also found on the palms, soles, extremities, and buttocks area. Genital lesions are rare [4].

Treatment

- Symptomatic treatment is advised.
- Fever can be managed by Acetaminophen or Ibuprofen.
- Supportive therapy includes a regular intake of water.

Pigmented lesions (Fig 9)

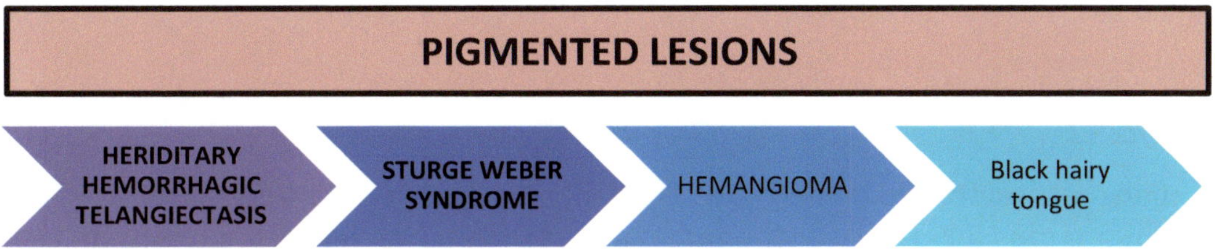

Fig. (9). Pigmented lesions.

Hereditary Hemorrhagic Telangiectasia (Rendu-Osler-Weber syndrome) (Fig 10)

- Hereditary hemorrhagic telangiectasia (HHT or Osler-Weber-Rendu syndrome) is an autosomal dominant inherited disorder characterized by malformations of various blood vessels (vascular dysplasia), potentially resulting in bleeding (haemorrhaging).
- Chronic nose bleeds are often the first sign, and malformation of various blood vessels may result in abnormalities affecting the lungs, brain, spinal cord, and liver. One gene that causes HHT (*ENG*), and the protein it produces (encodes), is called endoglin. Another gene that causes HHT is the activin receptor-like kinase 1 (*ACVRL1*) gene. Mutations in another gene that primarily causes familial pulmonary hypertension, *BMPR9*, are occasionally associated with the vascular features of HHT. Patients with HHT exhibit frequent epistaxis.
- The nasal and oropharyngeal mucosa exhibit numerous scattered red papules, which blanch when diascopy is used. The papules represent a superficial collection of dilated capillary spaces. The red macules are normally seen on the vermillion zone of the lips, tongue, and buccal mucosa.
- Moderate cases can be managed by selective electrosurgery or electrocautery. Mild cases might be managed by laser ablation.
- Investigational therapies include antifibrinolytic agents like tranexamic acid, bevacizumab, estrogen, and progesterone therapy [5].

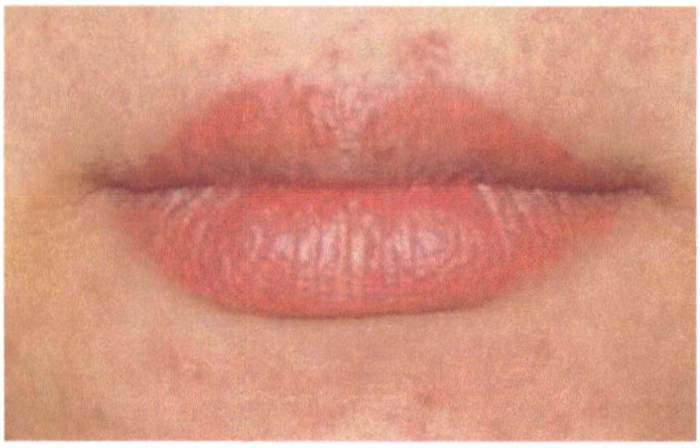

Fig. (10). Hereditary hemorrhagic telangiectasis.

Treatment

- Cutaneous lesions are treated with laser therapy such as Nd; YAG laser.
- Thalidomide due to its anti-angiogenic effects is nowadays advised for the management of these lesions.

Hemangioma (Fig 11)

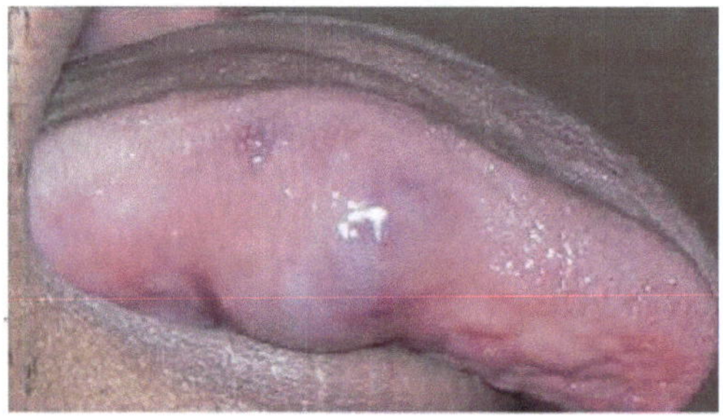

Fig. (11). Hemangioma on tongue.

- The term hemangioma has traditionally been used to describe a variety of vascular developmental anomalies. They are benign tumours of infancy that display a rapid growth phase with endothelial cell proliferation followed by gradual involution. Hemangiomas are the most common tumours of infancy, occurring in 5-10% of1-year-old children. Females are more commonly affected than males. The head and neck are the commonest locations.
- Fully developed hemangiomas are rarely present at birth, although a pale macule with threadlike telangiectasias' may be noted on the skin. The tumour will demonstrate a very rapid growth pattern during the first few weeks of life. Superficial tumours of the skin appear raised and bosselated with a bright red colour, which is firm and rubbery to palpation, and the blood cannot be evacuated by applying pressure. Deeper tumours may have a bluish hue. About half of all the hemangiomas show complete resolution by 5 years of age, with 90% resolving by age 9.

- Radiologically, there is a multilocular radiolucent defect with a honeycomb or soap bubble appearance, or large malformations can cause cortical expansion, and sometimes a sunburst radiographic appearance is noted. Angiography can help determine the vascular nature of the tumour.
- Microscopically, a highly cellular endothelial proliferation possessing plump, endothelial cells and forming occasionally indistinct vascular lumina might be noted in the initial stages. As the lesion matures, the endothelial cells get flattened and the small well-formed capillary-sized vascular spaces become more evident. GLUT1 is an IHC marker that is consistently positive in hemangioma in infancy [6].

Treatment

- Systemic corticosteroids are sometimes used for life-threatening conditions.
- Laser therapy such as Flashlamp pulsed dye lasers can be used.
- Larger and difficult lesions can be managed by sclerotherapy and surgical excision. Sclerotherapy agents like alcohol and sodium tetradecyl sulfate can be used. Propanolol can be used as a first-line drug as its effect is evident by an immediate colour change and reduction in tumour growth.

Sturge Weber Syndrome ('Encephalo- Trigeminal Angiomatosis') (Fig 12)

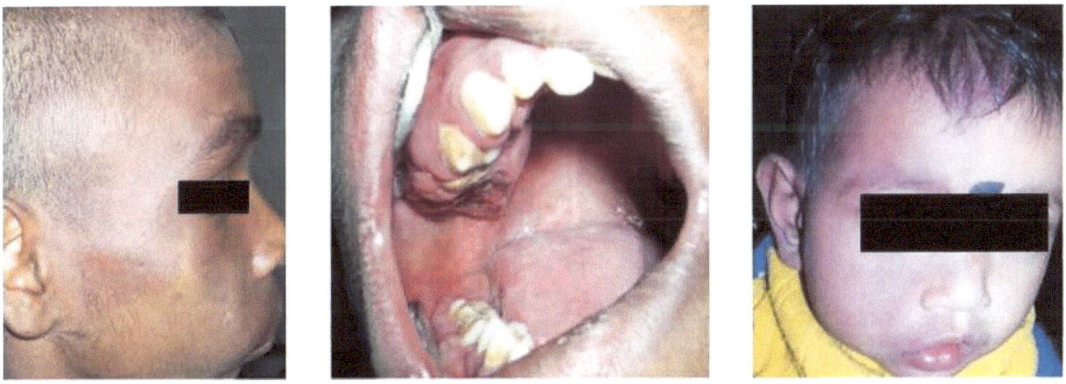

Fig. (12). Port wine stain.

- Sturge Weber angiomatosis is a nonhereditary developmental condition that may arise due to the persistence of vascular plexus around the cephalic portion of the neural tube.
- The patients are born with a dermal capillary vascular malformation of the face known as a port-wine stain because of the deep purple colour.
- It usually has a unilateral distribution along with one or more divisions of the trigeminal nerve.

- Imaging studies of the brain may reveal gyriform tramline calcifications. Convulsion, contralateral hemiplegia, and glaucoma may be there. Hypervascular changes in the ipsilateral mucosa may be there.
- The gingiva may exhibit slight vascular hyperplasia or massive hemangiomatous proliferation that resembles a pyogenic granuloma [7].

Treatment

- Symptomatic treatment is given for seizures, headaches, and glaucoma.
- Nd: YAG laser is used for hemostasis in cases of epistaxis.

Black Hairy Tongue (Fig. 13)

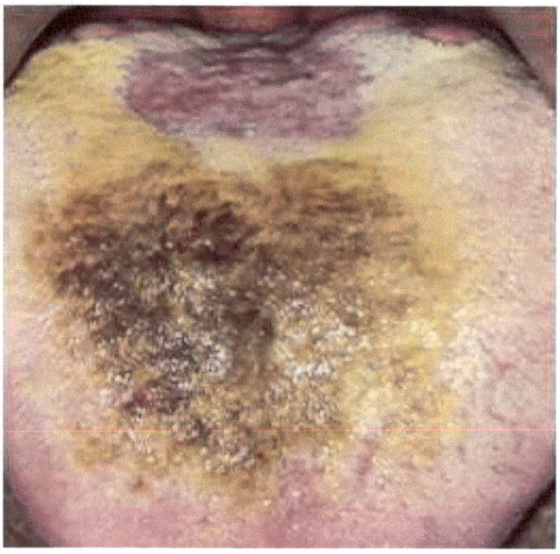

Fig. (13). Black hairy tongue.

- Hairy tongue is characterized by a marked accumulation of keratin on the filiform papilla of the dorsal surface of the tongue, resulting in a hair-like-like appearance.
- Condition represents an increase in keratin production or a decrease in the normal keratin desquamation.
- The elongated papillae are usually brown, yellow, or black because of the growth of pigment-producing bacteria or staining from tobacco or food [8].

Treatment

- This condition is usually self-limiting with a good prognosis. Normally, no treatment is advised. Maintaining good oral hygiene helps to prevent such conditions. Reassurance of the patient and the family members is important to alleviate the fear and anxiety.

- Recommendations- Avoidance of diet or medicines that have the potential to cause the lesion, maintenance of good oral hygiene, along with regular tongue cleaning (with a tongue cleaner or soft toothbrush).

Autoimmune Disorders (Fig 14)

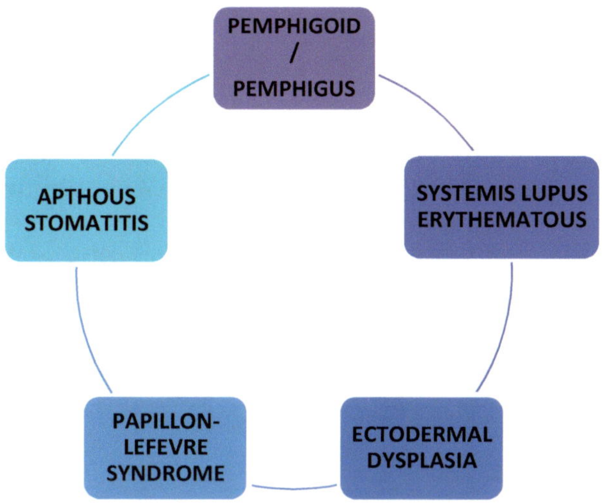

Fig. (14). Autoimmune Disorders.

Pemphigus/Pemphigoid (Fig 15)

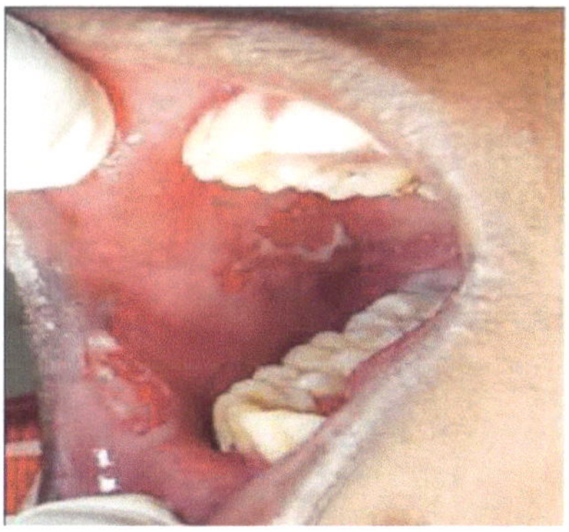

Fig. (15). Pemphigus.

- Pemphigus Vulgaris is a rare autoimmune vesiculobullous disease that is characterized by painful blisters and erosions on the skin and mucous membrane, most commonly inside the mouth. Pemphigus vulgaris accounts for 70% of all pemphigus cases worldwide.

- The pathogenesis is owing to autoantibodies directed against desmoglein1 and 3.
- Clinically, it is characterized by ragged and shallow painful erosion and ulcerations on the mucous membrane, along with sloughing out and blistering of the mucosa.
- Nikolsky sign is positive.
- Histopathologically, the entire epithelium above the basal layer is stripped, giving a characteristic 'Tombstone' appearance. Suprabasillar split present. Tzanck cells - intraepithelial acantholytic cells are evident in the spinous layer.
- Subbasillar split is seen in Pemphigoid.
- Clinically it is characterised by ocular, mucocutaneous and genital features.
- Pemphigus is confirmed by direct immunofluorescence staining of perilesional skin biopsy sections to reveal immunoglobulin (Ig)G antibodies or complements on the cell surfaces of keratinocytes.
- Other dermatologic conditions of note are Dermatitis-including Seborrheic, Atopic or Diaper dermatitis.
- Hair loss-Alopecia areata, Tinea capitis, Telogen effluvium, Trichotillomania.
- Eczema herpeticum, Annular lesion including Tinea corporis, Granuloma annulare [9, 10].

Treatment

- Medical management includes administration of systemic corticosteroids to control the disease usually moderate to high doses of oral prednisone or prednisolone, or as pulsed intravenous methylprednisolone.
- Rituximab is an FDA-approved drug for the same.
- The available treatment includes aggressive systemic corticosteroid therapy, pulsed intravenous corticosteroids, steroid-sparing drugs (such as Cyclophosphamide), immunosuppressants, intravenous immunoglobulins, Rituximab, and plasma exchange therapy.

Systemic Lupus Erythematosus (Fig 16a, 16b)

- SLE is a multiorgan disease with oral and dermatological manifestations. Inflammation caused by lupus can affect many different body systems — including joints, skin, kidneys, blood cells, brain, heart, and lungs.
- The characteristic feature is a Butterfly rash over the Malar and nose region.
- The most common signs and symptoms include:
- Fatigue
- Fever
- Joint pain, stiffness and swelling
- Butterfly-shaped rash on the face that covers the cheeks and bridge of the nose or rashes elsewhere on the body
- Skin lesions that appear or worsen with sun exposure (photosensitivity)

- Fingers and toes that turn white or blue when exposed to cold or during stressful periods (Reynaud's phenomenon)
- Shortness of breath
- Chest pain
- Dry eyes
- Headaches, confusion, and memory loss
- Oral manifestations of SLE are frequently encountered and may include oral ulceration, honeycomb plaque, raised keratotic plaque, nonspecific erythema, purpura, petechiae, and cheilitis.
- Antinuclear antibodies are found in the majority of SLE patients.
- Histopathology
- Fibrinoid necrosis at the dermo-epidermal junction with liquefactive degeneration and atrophy of epidermis.
- More mucin deposition in the reticular dermis than discoid lupus.
- Edema, small haemorrhages, and a mild infiltrate of inflammatory cells, principally lymphocytes, in the upper dermis
- Eosinophils in drug-induced cases and urticarial lesions [11].

Treatment

SLE treatment consists primarily of immunosuppressive drugs that inhibit the activity of the immune system. Hydroxychloroquine and corticosteroids (*e.g.*, prednisone) are often used to treat SLE. The FDA approved belimumab in 2011, the first new drug for SLE in more than 50 years.

- In 2007, the European league against Rheumatism issued recommendations for SLE treatment.
- In an individual without any major organ involvement, glucocorticosteroids and antimalarial drugs such as hydroxychloroquine can be prescribed.
- Immunosuppressive drugs such as Methotrexate, Azathioprine and Mycophenolate mofetil can also be prescribed in refractory cases or in cases where long-term steroids must be prescribed.
- Corticosteroid therapy is the treatment of choice.
- Biological therapies using Rituximab, Belimumab, Interferon antagonists, and Peptide-based therapies are newer modalities in targeting this condition.
- Wearing protective clothing is advocated for the affected patients while venturing in sunlight to avoid flaring of disease and to avoid a photosensitive rash.

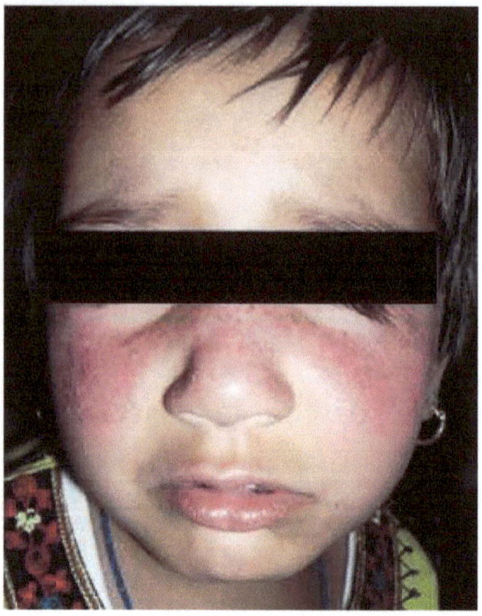

Fig. (16a). Extraoral picture showing the characteristic butterfly shaped malar rash.

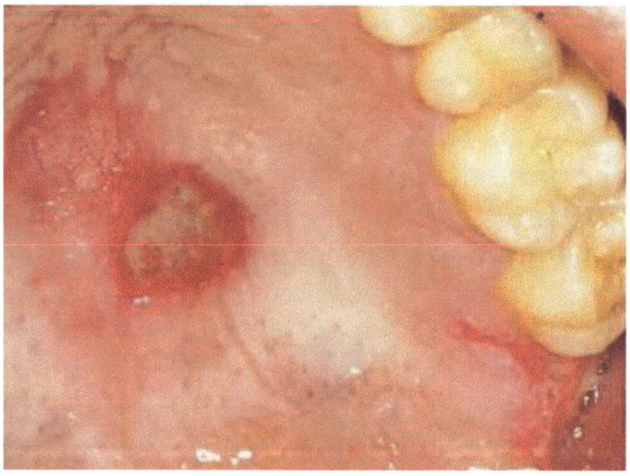

Fig. (16b). Intraorally presence of grayish yellow plaque like ulcer on hard palate surrounded by erythema.

Ectodermal Dysplasia (Fig. 17a, 17b, 17c)

- Ectodermal dysplasias (ED) are a group of inherited disorders that affect the outer layer of tissue of the embryo (ectoderm) that helps make up the skin, sweat glands, hair, teeth, and nails.
- Symptoms of ED can range from mild to severe and may include teeth abnormalities; abnormal, tapering, pointed or smaller crown, brittle, sparse or absent hair; abnormal fingernails; inability to perspire (hypohidrosis); various skin problems; and other symptoms.
- Two classic forms of this syndrome are anhidrotic/hypohidrotic and hidrotic [12 - 14].

Treatment

- Prosthetic replacement of missing teeth with over-dentures and dentures.
- Crown placement over misshaped & distorted teeth and restorative procedures as indicated.

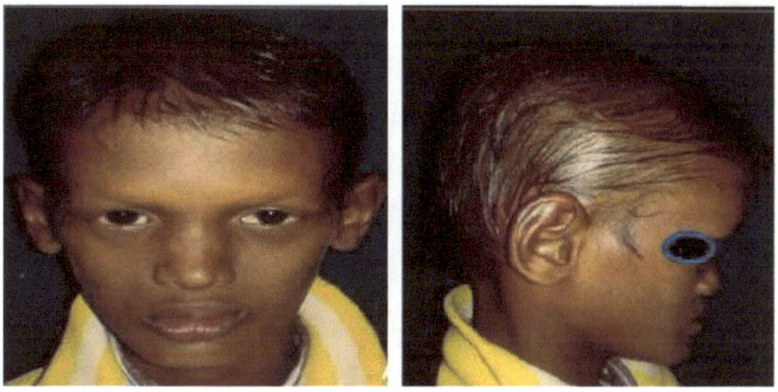

Fig. (17a). Frontal and Profile view showing frontal bossing, protuberant lips due to loss of vertical dimension and scarce hair.

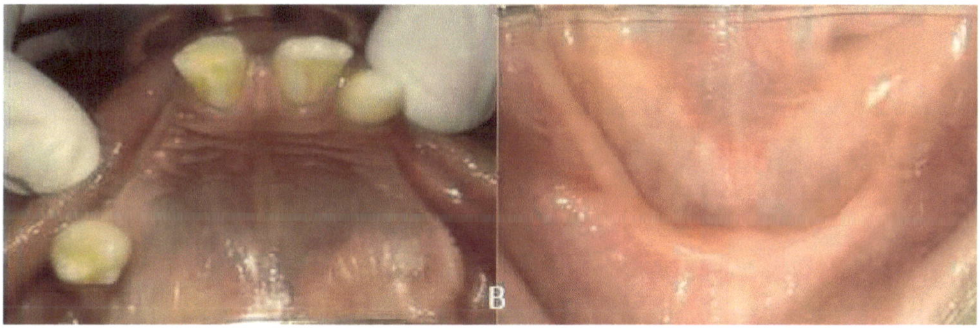

Fig. (17b). Intraoral view showing partial anodontia with misshapen teeth.

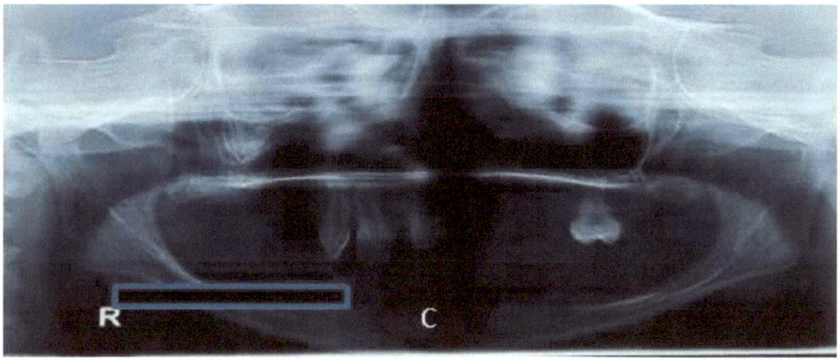

Fig. (17c). Panoramic orthpantomogram showing partial anodontia.

Papillon–Lefèvre Syndrome (PLS) (Fig 18a, 18b)

- It is a rare autosomal recessive disorder, characterized by diffuse palmoplantar keratoderma and precocious aggressive periodontitis, leading to premature loss of deciduous and permanent dentition at an early age. **PLS** was first described by two French physicians, Papillon and Lefevre.
- Mutation of the Cathepsin C gene is held responsible.
- Various etiopathogenic factors are associated with the syndrome, like immunologic alterations, genetic mutations, and the role of bacteria [15].

Treatment

- Oral retinoids such as Acitretin, Etretinate and Isotretinoin are prescribed.

However, Isotretinoin should be prescribed cautiously because of its adverse effects.

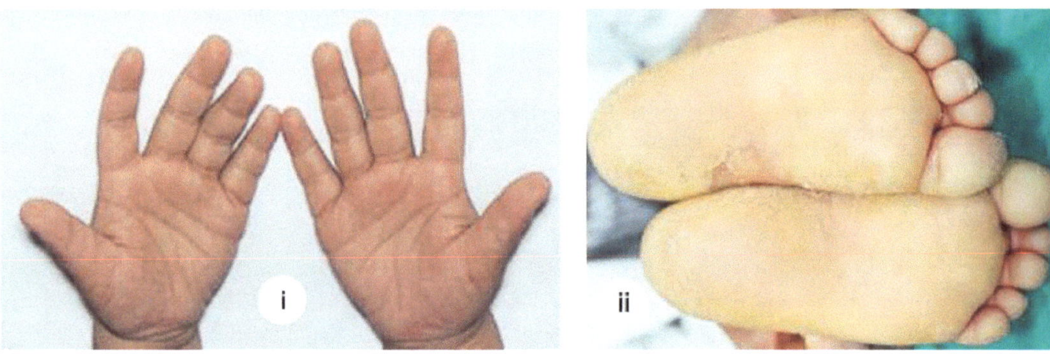

Fig. (18a). Panoramic orthpantomogram showing partial anodontia.

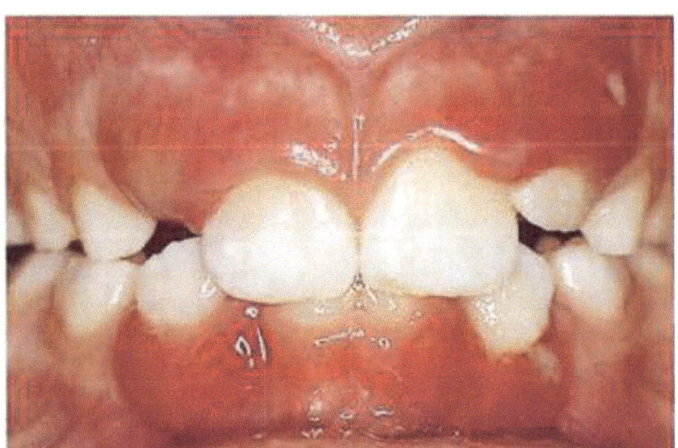

Fig. (18b). Panoramic orthpantomogram showing partial anodontia.

Aphthous Stomatitis

- Recurrent aphthous stomatitis is a common disease.
- Within the oral cavity, RAS is the most common condition affecting oral mucosal surfaces. The peak age of onset is within 10-19 years.
- These are also called Canker sores. RAS occurs in three major clinical forms- Aphthous major, aphthous minor, and herpetiform aphthae. Behcet syndrome is an important syndrome associated with an aphthous ulcer.
- The lesions exhibit as recurrent multiple, painful small, round, or ovoid ulcers, with circumscribed margins, having yellow or grey floors and being surrounded by an erythematous halo (Fig **19**).
- TNF alpha is a proinflammatory cytokine associated with the development of apthae.
- Several factors might be found to be associated with the development of aphthous ulcers- which include extremes of temperature, hormonal changes, stress, GI disturbances, smoking, genetic anomaly, immunological impairment *etc* [16].

Treatment

- Management includes dietary supplements of Vit B12, folic acid and iron.
- High-potency corticosteroids can be applied topically two to four times a day.
- Anti-inflammatory agents like Amlexanox paste (5%), and metalloproteinase inhibitors (such as Tetracycline, and Doxycycline) are used.
- Symptomatic treatment with topical anaesthetic agents like Xylocaine can be used.

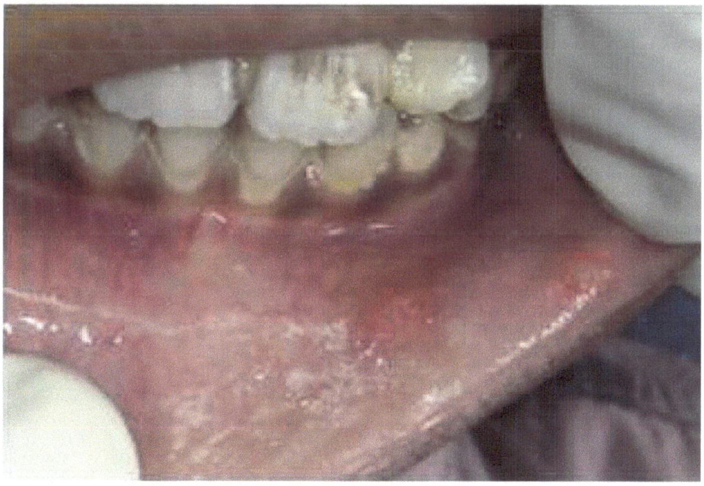

Fig. (19). Aphthous stomatitis.

Lesions of Idiopathic Etiology

Pterygoid Ulcer or Bednar's Ulcer (Fig. 20)

These are a type of oral ulceration which occurs in infants. The lesions are located medial to the greater palatine fossa and there is superficial ulceration. It is caused by trauma [17].

Treatment

- No treatment is required as most lesions heal spontaneously.
- Mother is advised to correct the position for nursing and to enlarge the size of the nipple pore.
- These ulcers heal spontaneously within a period of one to four weeks.

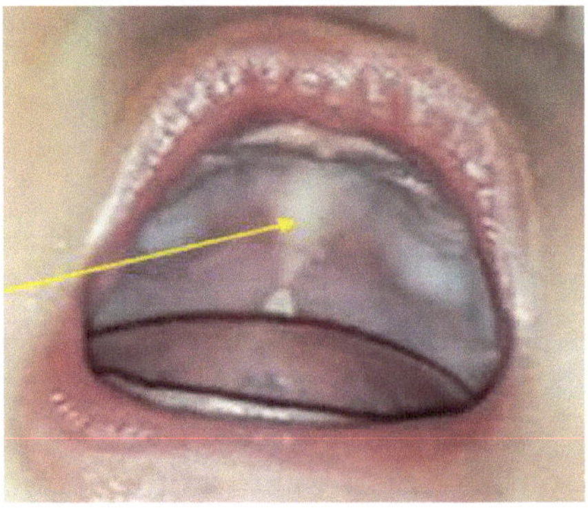

Fig. (20). Bednar's ulcer.

Lesions of Bacterial Origin (Fig. 21)

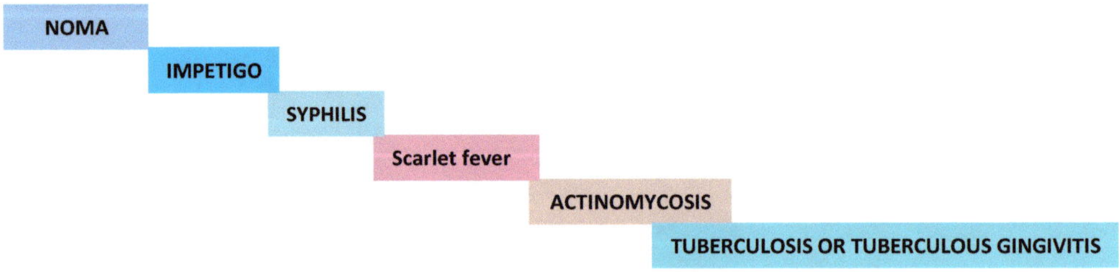

Fig. (21). Lesions of Bacterial Origin.

Impetigo (Fig. 22)

- It is an acute superficial purulent infection of the skin, which is initially vesicular but later becomes crusted. Two types of impetigo are described, which include Impetigo contagious or non-bullous impetigo and bullous impetigo.

- Non-bullousus impetigo is caused by group A *Streptococci* and bullous impetigo is caused by group II Streptococci.
- Non-bullousus impetigo occurs in the face and perioral region.
- Bullous impetigo occurs as scattered, thin-walled, bulla arising on normal skin and containing clear yellow or mildly turbid fluid with little or no surrounding erythema.
- The lesions are discrete and located on the trunk.
- They are normally associated with the deficiency of cell-mediated immunity [18].

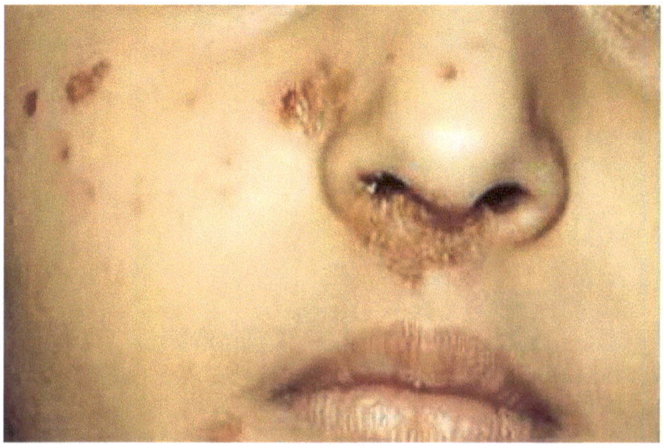

Fig. (22). Impetigo.

Staphylococcal Scalded Shock Syndrome

- This is a spectrum of bullous impetigo which is seen in neonates and infants.
- The disease begins abruptly with diffuse erythema and fever.
- It is caused by a Staphylococcal toxin called Exfoliating.

Treatment

- Topical and/or oral antibiotics are prescribed as anti-streptococcal therapy.

Scarlet Fever

- Children and young adults with scarlet fever develop a sudden onset of fever and sore throat. There may also be headaches, malaise, irritability, and nausea. The pharynx will appear red and swollen, and the cervical lymph nodes will be tender and swollen. The characteristic feature is the presence of a red, macular, skin rash on the chest, axilla, and groin. The face is usually red with circumoral pallor.
- The tongue develops a white coat within which reddened and swollen fungiform papillae stand out (Strawberry tongue). Later, the tongue becomes swollen, irregular, and beefy (Fig. **23**).

- Scarlet fever is caused by group A beta-hemolytic *Streptococci,* especially *Streptococcus scarlatina and S pyogenes.* Transmission is via infected aerosolized droplets. The skin rash is usually caused by an erythrogenic exotoxin.
- Leukocytosis is observed and Ant streptolysin O titer is elevated in 80% of cases [18].

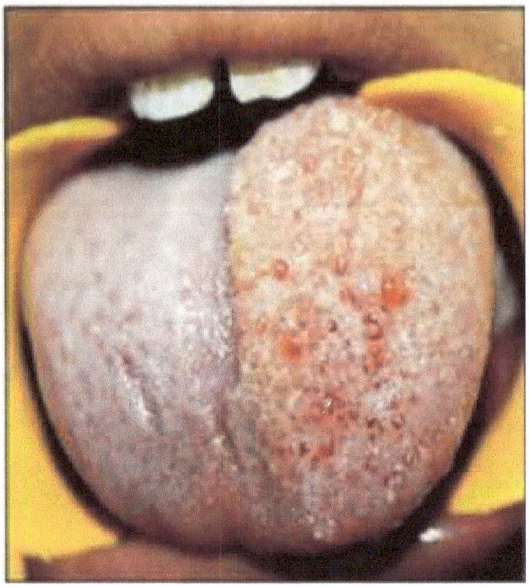

Fig. (23). Strawberry tongue.

Treatment

- No treatment modality is available for this condition.
- Antibiotic administration, such as Cephalexin, Dicloxacillin, *etc.,* can help in alleviating the symptoms and complications.
- Oral phenoxy methyl penicillin/Benzathine penicillin G (intra-muscular) is an effective treatment.

Syphilis

- It is a Spirochetal disease caused by *Treponema pallidum. Children typically are affected by congenital syphilis.* The classic Hutchinson triad of Congenital syphilis is characterized by – Hutchinson teeth, ocular interstitial keratitis, and eighth nerve deafness.
- The early findings within 2-3 weeks of birth encompass growth retardation, fever, jaundice, anaemia, hepatosplenomegaly, rhinitis, rhagades and desquamative maculo papular ulcerative or vesiculobullous skin eruptions.
- The screwdriver-shaped incisors with tapering towards the incisal edges and mulberry molars showing globular occlusal surface projections resembling

shrubs of a mulberry tree are the pathognomonic notable features. Saber shins, saddle nose, frontal bossing and rhagades can be found.

- The diagnosis of Syphilis can be confirmed by demonstrating the organism in dark field microscopy.
- Specific and sensitive serological assays for Syphilis include fluorescent treponemal antibody adsorption (FTA-ABS), and *T. Pallidum* haemagglutination assay (TPHA). Other bacterial infections of significance in children are acute otitis media, sinusitis, pharyngitis, conjunctivitis, pneumonia, UTI, and gastroenteritis [18].

Treatment

- Penicillin is the drug of choice.
- Tetracycline is given to patients who are allergic to penicillin.
- Surgical correction of facial defects is advised in some cases.

Oral Tuberculosis (Fig 24)

- Tuberculosis is a systemic infectious disease of worldwide prevalence and varying clinical manifestations.
- It is a granulomatous disease caused by acid-fast bacillus *Mycobacterium tuberculosis.*
- Transmission occurs via aerosolized droplets, which seed organisms to the lungs that persist viably within macrophages after ingestion.
- Lungs, pharynx, intestine, cervical lymph node and oral mucosa are commonly affected sites.
- Primary intestinal TB can occur from ingestion of unpasteurized milk containing Bovine tubercle bacilli.
- These organisms and macrophages become contained or walled off within a granuloma. Often called the primary infection, the site is asymptomatic.
- Active TB develops because of the reactivation of the primary disease process. Lung destruction and lymphatic or hematogenous spread can occur. Low-grade fever or lassitude may occur.
- Anorexia, weight loss, fever, and night sweats can also take place. Persistent dry cough, hemoptysis, abundant sputum, and pleuritic pain are usual features of TB.
- The most usual form of Oral TB is an irregular ragged, ulcerative lesion of the mucosa that has undermined edges, yellowish granular base, and minimal induration.
- The posterior ventrolateral aspect of the tongue is commonly affected. Palate, gingiva, lips, buccal mucosa, salivary glands, and alveolar mucosa might be affected.

- Preexisting epithelial trauma, impaired immune response, other medical compromising conditions, poor oral hygiene, cysts, or tumours can facilitate the occurrence.
- Radiographically, patchy irregular infiltrations and cavitations in the upper apical lobe of the lungs may be seen. Multiple small calcific nodules and/or pneumonic/fibrous areas may be seen. Tubercular involvement of cervical lymph nodes is known as Scrofula.
- Histopathologically, a granulomatous pattern with epithelioid cells, Langhans type giant cells, lymphocytes, and central caseation necrosis are the typical features. Ziehl Nielsen stain shows fuschia colored bacilli. Nonacid fast bacilli appear blue or green [18].

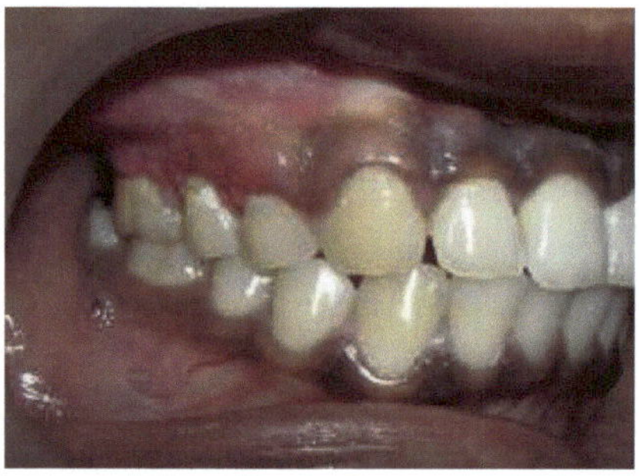

Fig. (24). Tubercular gingivitis.

Treatment

- Anti-tubercular regimen helps to control the oral lesions.
- All patients (including TB-HIV co-infected) who have not been treated previously should receive 2 months of Isoniazid (H), Rifampicin (R), Pyrazinamide (Z) and Ethambutol (E), during the intensive phase (IP). The continuation phase (CP) consists of Isoniazid and Rifampicin given for 4 months.

Actinomycosis (Fig. 25)

- It is a chronic infectious granulomatous and fibrosing disease caused by anaerobic, gram-positive, non-acid fast branched filamentous bacteria. Actimycoses can be cervicofacial, abdominal, thoracic, and cutaneous in nature, among which the Cervicofacial form is the commonest. *A Israeli, A viscosus, A naeslundi, A odontolyticus* are the causative organisms.
- The disruption of the mucosal barrier along with trauma can play a role in the entry of the microbes. The acute form of the disease is rapidly progressive and characterized by suppuration with multiple draining sinuses and the presence of pus containing yellow sulfur granules. The skin overlying the abscess is purplish

red, indurated, and has a wooden, fluctuant feel. The chronic form is slowly progressive and indurated in which fibrosis predominates and little pus is present.

- The oral mucous membrane, tongue, perimandibular area, maxilla, paranasal sinuses, eye, ear, face, neck, salivary glands are commonly affected.
- The microscopic picture is one of granulation tissue accompanied by tissue necrosis, abscess formation, and the presence of microcolonies of so-called sulfur granules consisting of branching organisms within the abscesses. The colonies are floating in a sea of polymorphonuclear leukocytes, macrophages, and giant cells in the periphery. This gives the appearance of so-called 'Ray fungus'.
- Methenamine silver stain can demonstrate the organisms better [19].

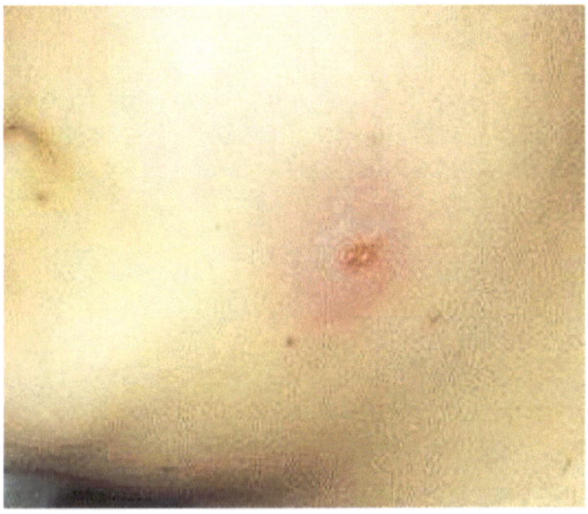

Fig. (25). Draining sinus tract in a child with actinomycosis.

Treatment

- Surgical resection of infected tissue along with the long course of penicillin and erythromycin is the standard line of treatment.

Noma (Cancrum Oris, Gangrenous stomatitis)

- The term Noma is derived from the Greek word nomein, meaning to devour. Noma is a rapidly progressive, polymicrobial opportunistic gangrenous mucositis and stomatitis infection, caused by pathogenic oral flora. *Prevotella intermedia, Borellia vincenti and Fusobacterium nucleatum* are key players.
- Noma usually affects children in the age group of 1-10 years, especially in malnourished and immunocompromised cases, and in areas of poor sanitation and hygiene.
- Noma usually begins as a small ulcer of the gingival mucosa that rapidly spreads and involves the surrounding tissues of the jaws, lips, and cheeks by gangrenous necrosis. The overlying skin becomes inflamed, edematous, and necrotic, which

sloughs out. The gangrenous tissues give off an extremely fetid odour. Significant pain, fever, malaise, tachycardia, tachypnoea, anaemia, leukocytosis, and regional lymphadenopathy are typical (Fig. **26**).

- The microscopic picture of Noma is one of central necrosis and a peripheral zone consisting of thrombovasculitis, haemorrhage, dense inflammatory cell infiltrate and the presence of microorganisms [20].

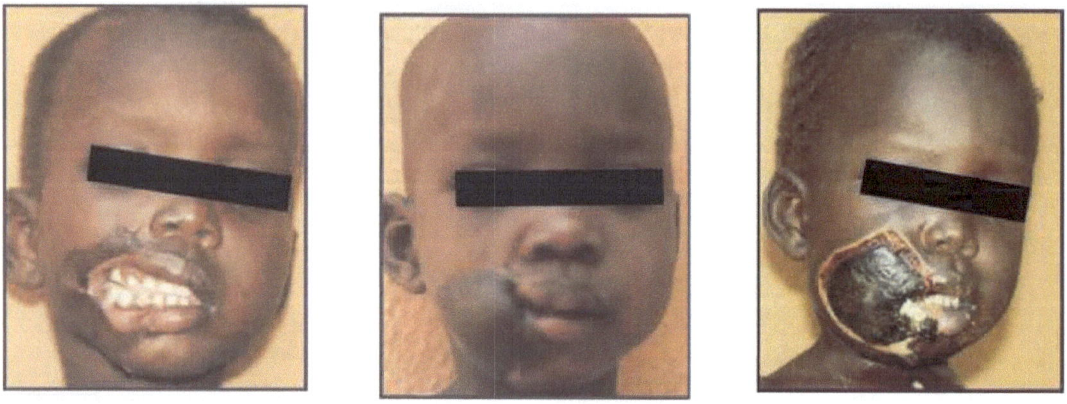

Fig. (26). Different cases of Noma. (Courtesy: http://www.fdiworldental.org/publications/oral-health-atlas/oral-health-atlas-(2015).aspx).

Treatment

- Parenteral administration of antibiotics along with nutritional supplements and rehydration helps to stop the disease progression.

SOFT TISSUE ENLARGEMENTS

Reactive

Mucocele (Fig 27)

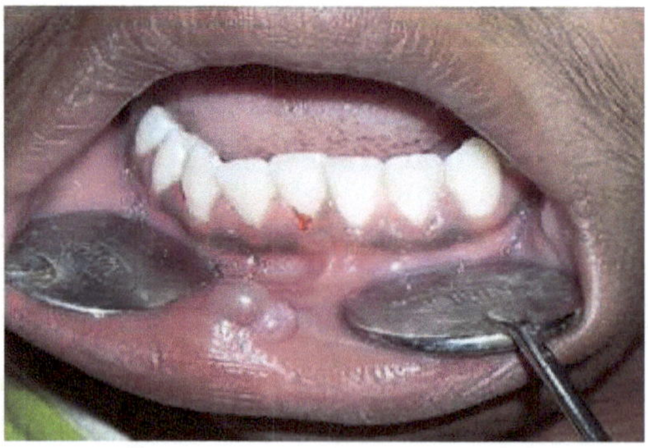

Fig. (27). Mucocele.

- Mucocele is a common lesion of the oral mucosa that results from rupture of the salivary gland duct and spillage of mucin to surrounding soft tissues. This spillage is owing to local trauma or obstruction of salivary gland ducts.
- The mucoceles are not true cysts because of the lack of an epithelial lining. Mucoceles typically appear as dome-shaped mucosal swellings that can range from 1-2 mm to scvcral cm in sizc.
- They are most common in children and young adults. The spilled mucin below the mucosal surface imparts a bluish translucent hue to the swelling, but deeper mucoceles may be normal in colour.
- The lesion is characteristically fluctuant, but some mucoceles feel firmer on palpation. Many patients relate a history of recurrent swelling that periodically may rupture and release its contents.
- The lower lip is the commonest site for the mucocele, followed by the floor of the mouth, anterior ventral tongue, buccal mucosa, palate, and retromolar pad.
- On microscopic examination, the mucocele shows an area of spilt mucin surrounded by granulation tissue response. The inflammation usually includes numerous foamy histiocytes(macrophages).
- Minor salivary gland duct residues along with a chronic inflammatory cell infiltrate may be found. Some mucoceles rupture and heal by themselves. Many chronic lesions require surgical intervention along with the adjacent surrounding minor salivary glands into the depths [21].

Treatment

• It involves local excision of lesion along with the removal of involved minor salivary gland acini.

Ranula (Fig 28)

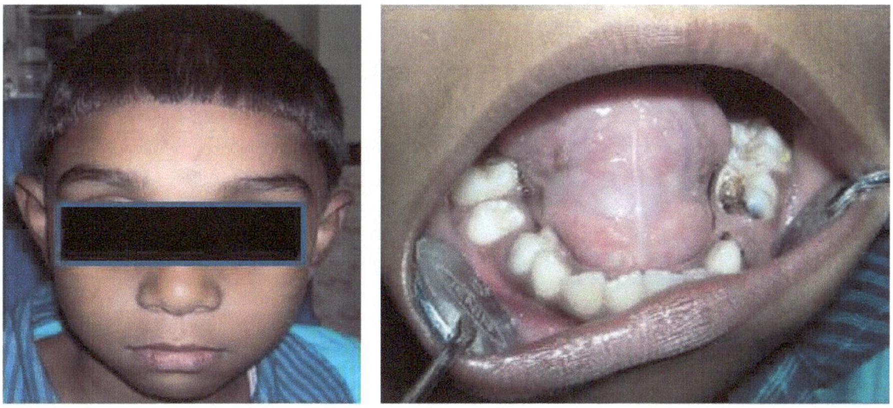

Fig. (28). Case of Ranula.

- Large, soft mucous possessing swelling on the floor of the mouth.
- It is produced by a defect in Wharton's duct or sublingual duct.

Treatment

- Marsupialization is carried out. It involves the Partsch procedure to form a surface connection of a severed duct [21].

B). Tumors or Neoplasms

(I). Benign Tumours of Epithelial Origin

Oral Papilloma (HPV)

- It is a benign, exophytic papillary growth of the stratified squamous epithelium.
- It may be sessile or pedunculated and white (keratinized) or pink (nonkeratinized), having verruciform or pebbly surface projections.
- HPV types 6 and 11 are mostly held responsible.
- Most lesions are solitary and commonly occur on the soft palate, uvula, ventral and dorsal surfaces of the tongue gingival and buccal mucosa.
- Papillary proliferation of stratified squamous epithelium with variable hyperkeratosis or parakeratosis.
- Hyperplasia and mitotic activity restricted to basal/parabasal layers
  Retention of cellular polarity and normal maturation in suprabasal layers
  Papillary (finger-like) projections exhibit prominent fibrovascular cores
  Koilocytes-Virally altered epithelial clear cells present (Fig **29**).
  Hyalinization at the tips of cores may be seen occasionally.
- Recurrence rate minimal and related to incomplete excision
- Since mucosal HPV infections may persist for 1 - 2 years, the patient may be at mildly elevated risk for additional squamous papillomas.
- Dysplasia is infrequently encountered in squamous papillomas; not considered a premalignant condition.
- No known association with oral or oropharyngeal squamous cell carcinoma [22, 23].
- However, in some of the cases of p16+ and especially HIV+ individuals, a close association between HPV and oropharyngeal SCC has been reported.

Treatment

- Simple surgical excision is the treatment of choice for the base of the lesion and a small area of surrounding normal tissue.
- The patient should be kept on follow-up as these lesions tend to recur.

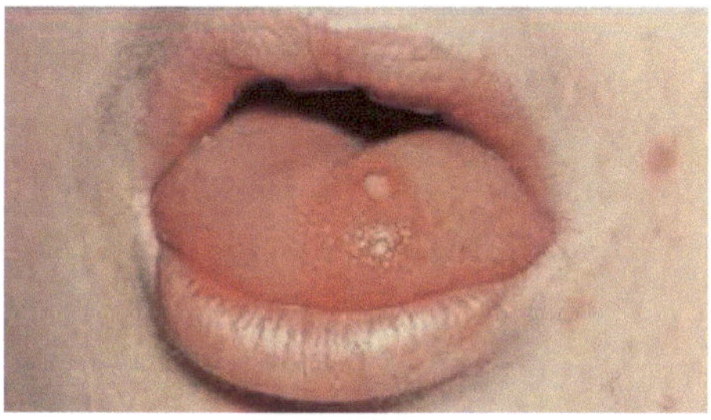

Fig. (29). Oral lesion of tongue due to oral papilloma.

II). Benign Tumours of Mesenchymal Origin

Pyogenic Granuloma: (Fig 30)

- Pyogenic granuloma is a common tumour-like growth of the oral cavity, which is mostly observed in children and young adults.
- It is a smooth or lobulated mass usually pedunculated, although some lesions are sessile.
- The surface is characteristically ulcerated and ranges from pink to purplish. Typically, it is a painless mass but tends to bleed easily owing to a large amount of vascularity.
- Gingiva is the most affected site, followed by the lips, tongue, buccal mucosa and palate.
- Pyogenic granuloma can develop in pregnancy associated with increased levels of estrogen and progesterone. Histopathology shows variably shaped and sized endothelial lined blood vessels and scattered inflammation [24].

Treatment

- Surgical excision is the treatment of choice.

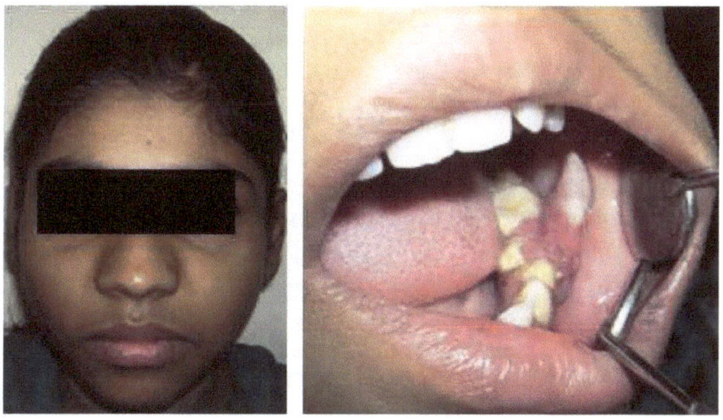

Fig. (30). Pyogenic granuloma.

CONCLUSION

In pediatric patients various intraoral lesions are present that require accurate diagnosis, treatment, and counselling. A pediatric dentist plays a key role in early diagnosis and referral for further dental evaluation. Sometimes the oral lesions may be associated with underlying systemic conditions, therefore, thorough medical history and general examination play a vital role. New insights into the cause and treatment of various oral lesions in children have made the prevention and treatment of various untreatable conditions possible. Thus, regular review of oral tissues and early detection of these oral conditions may be life-saving for pediatric patients.

CONSENT FOR PUBLICATION

Not applicable.

CONFLICT OF INTEREST

The author(s) declare no conflict of interest, financial or otherwise.

ACKNOWLEDGEMENT

Declared none.

REFERENCES

[1] Majorana A, Bardellini E, Flocchini P, Amadori F, Conti G, Campus G. Oral mucosal lesions in children from 0 to 12 years old: ten years' experience. Oral Surg Oral Med Oral Pathol Oral Radiol Endod 2010; 110(1): e13-8.
[http://dx.doi.org/10.1016/j.tripleo.2010.02.025] [PMID: 20452255]

[2] Marcushamer M, King DL, McGuff S. White sponge nevus: case report. Pediatr Dent 1995; 17(7): 458-9.
[PMID: 8786915]

[3] Nevet A, Yarden-Bilavsky H, Ashkenazi S, Livni G. C-Reactive protein levels in children with primary herpetic gingivostomatitis. Isr Med Assoc J 2014; 16(11): 700-2.
[PMID: 25558699]

[4] Cherry JD, *et al.* 4. Cherry JD, et al. Herpangina. Textbook of Pediatric Infectious Diseases. 6th ed. 2009; 1.

[5] Velegrakis GA, Prokopakis EP, Papadakis CE, Helidonis ES. Nd:YAG laser treatment of recurrent epistaxis in heredity hemorrhagic telangiectasia. J Otolaryngol 1997; 26(6): 384-6.
[PMID: 9438937]

[6] Corrêa PH, Nunes LCC, Johann ACBR, Aguiar MCF, Gomez RS, Mesquita RA. Prevalence of oral hemangioma, vascular malformation and varix in a Brazilian population. Braz Oral Res 2007; 21(1): 40-5.
[http://dx.doi.org/10.1590/S1806-83242007000100007] [PMID: 17384854]

[7] Godge P, Sharma S, Yadav M, Patil P, Kulkarni S. Sturge Weber syndrome: a case report. Rev Odonto Ciênc 2011; 26(4): 366-9.

[http://dx.doi.org/10.1590/S1980-65232011000400016]

[8] Gurvits GE, Tan A. Black hairy tongue syndrome. World J Gastroenterol 2014; 20(31): 10845-50. [http://dx.doi.org/10.3748/wjg.v20.i31.10845] [PMID: 25152586]

[9] Harman KE, Albert S, Black MM. Guidelines. Br J Dermatol 2003; 149(5): 926-37. [http://dx.doi.org/10.1111/j.1365-2133.2003.05665.x] [PMID: 14632796]

[10] Beissert S, Mimouni D, Kanwar AJ, Solomons N, Kalia V, Anhalt GJ. Treating pemphigus vulgaris with prednisone and mycophenolate mofetil: a multicenter, randomized, placebo-controlled trial. J Invest Dermatol 2010; 130(8): 2041-8. [http://dx.doi.org/10.1038/jid.2010.91] [PMID: 20410913]

[11] Mok CC, Lau CS. Pathogenesis of systemic lupus erythematosus. J Clin Pathol 2003; 56(7): 481-90. [http://dx.doi.org/10.1136/jcp.56.7.481] [PMID: 12835292]

[12] Hekmatfar S, Jafari K, Meshki R, Badakhsh S. Dental management of ectodermal dysplasia: two clinical case reports. J Dent Res Dent Clin Dent Prospect 2012; 6(3): 108-12. [PMID: 22991648]

[13] Pavarina AC, Machado AL, Vergani CE, Giampaolo ET. Overlay removable partial dentures for a patient with ectodermal dysplasia: A clinical report. J Prosthet Dent 2001; 86(6): 574-7. [http://dx.doi.org/10.1067/mpr.2001.119981] [PMID: 11753305]

[14] Richter MK. Ectodermal dysplasia, twenty years later and little has changed. Pediatr Dent 2001; 23(5): 394. [PMID: 11699160]

[15] Muppa R, Duddu M, Prameela B, Dandempally A. Papillon-lefevre syndrome: A combined approach from the dermatologist and dentist - A clinical presentation. Indian J Dermatol 2011; 56(6): 740-3. [http://dx.doi.org/10.4103/0019-5154.91843] [PMID: 22345785]

[16] Amadori F, Bardellini E, Conti G, Majorana A. Oral mucosal lesions in teenagers: a cross-sectional study. Ital J Pediatr 2017; 43(1): 50. [http://dx.doi.org/10.1186/s13052-017-0367-7] [PMID: 28569171]

[17] Pedra C, Terra CM, Ejzenberg B, Baldacci ER, Okay Y. Oral palatine ulcers of a traumatic nature in infants: Bednar's aphthae. Int J Pediatr Otorhinolaryngol 1996; 35(1): 39-49. [http://dx.doi.org/10.1016/0165-5876(95)01282-6] [PMID: 8882108]

[18] Irani S. Orofacial bacterial infectious diseases: An update. J Int Soc Prev Community Dent 2017; 7(8) (Suppl. 2): 61. [http://dx.doi.org/10.4103/jispcd.JISPCD_290_17] [PMID: 29184830]

[19] Valour F, Sénéchal A, Dupieux C, *et al.* Actinomycosis: etiology, clinical features, diagnosis, treatment, and management. Infect Drug Resist 2014; 7: 183-97. [PMID: 25045274]

[20] McGurk M, Marck R. Treatment of Noma: medical missions in Ethiopia. Br Dent J 2010; 208(4): 179-82. [http://dx.doi.org/10.1038/sj.bdj.2010.159] [PMID: 20186205]

[21] Huzaifa M, Soni A. Mucocele and Ranula.StatPearls. Treasure Island, FL: StatPearls Publishing 2021. Updated 2021 Feb 13 Internet

[22] Abbey LM, Page DG, Sawyer DR. The clinical and histopathologic features of a series of 464 oral squamous cell papillomas. Oral Surg Oral Med Oral Pathol 1980; 49(5): 419-28. [http://dx.doi.org/10.1016/0030-4220(80)90286-8] [PMID: 6154913]

[23] Kreimer AR, Pierce Campbell CM, Lin HY, *et al.* Incidence and clearance of oral human papillomavirus infection in men: the HIM cohort study. Lancet 2013; 382(9895): 877-87. [http://dx.doi.org/10.1016/S0140-6736(13)60809-0] [PMID: 23827089]

[24] Pagliai KA, Cohen BA. Pyogenic granuloma in children. Pediatr Dermatol 2004; 21(1): 10-3. [http://dx.doi.org/10.1111/j.0736-8046.2004.21102.x] [PMID: 14871318]

SUBJECT INDEX

A

B

C

D

E

F

G

H

I

N

O

P

R

S

T

www.ingramcontent.com/pod-product-compliance
Lightning Source LLC
LaVergne TN
LVHW070944210926
848482LV00002B/93
* 9 7 8 9 8 1 5 0 5 1 5 0 6 *